HIGH-RISK ATHEROSCLEROTIC PLAQUES

Mechanisms, Imaging, Models, and Therapy

HIGH-RISK ATHEROSCLEROTIC PLAQUES
Mechanisms, Imaging, Models, and Therapy

EDITED BY

Levon Michael Khachigian

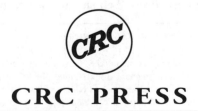

CRC PRESS

Boca Raton   London   New York   Washington, D.C.

Library of Congress Cataloging-in-Publication Data

High-risk atherosclerotic plaques: mechanisms, imaging, models, and therapy / edited by
  Levon Khachigian.
    p. ; cm.
  Includes bibliographical references and index.
  ISBN 0-8493-3028-9 (alk. paper)
    1. Atherosclerotic plaque. I. Khachigian, Levon.
  [DNLM: 1. Arteriosclerosis—diagnosis. 2. Arteriosclerosis—therapy. 3. Diagnostic
  Imaging. 4. Heart Diseases—etiology. WG 550 H638 2004]
  RC692.H535 2004
  616.1'36—dc22

                                                                    2004054450

Visit the CRC Press Web site at www.crcpress.com

© 2005 by CRC Press

No claim to original U.S. Government works
International Standard Book Number 0-8493-3028-9
Library of Congress Card Number 2004054450
Printed in the United States of America 1 2 3 4 5 6 7 8 9 0
Printed on acid-free paper

Preface

Instability of atherosclerotic plaques is the primary cause of acute coronary syndromes comprising unstable angina, myocardial infarction, and sudden death. "Vulnerable" or "high-risk" plaques are associated with inflammation, apoptosis, rupture, and thrombosis. Greater understanding of the cellular and molecular pathogenesis of high risk plaques, together with our ability to visualize and diagnose these lesions, will lead to the more effective management of acute coronary syndromes.

This book brings together timely, authoritative, in-depth reviews by renowned international cardiologists and scientists covering the definition, structure, cellular and molecular mechanisms of high-risk plaque development, animal models of vulnerable plaque, plaque imaging, and current and future therapies.

Prediman Shah (Chapter 1) and Martin Bennett (Chapter 2) describe the cellular and molecular mechanisms of plaque vulnerability, with emphasis on plaque size, cellular composition, thrombosis, and the critical role of apoptosis. Harry Lowe et al. (Chapter 3) discuss the advantages and limitations of large and small animal models of vulnerable plaques. Johannes Schaar et al. (Chapter 4) provide an overview of current and future imaging and diagnostic approaches including angiograms, angioscopy, optical coherence tomography, intravascular ultrasound, palpography, thermography, Raman spectroscopy, near-infrared spectroscopy, and magnetic resonance imaging.

Paul Schoenhagen et al. (Chapter 5) focus on intravascular ultrasound. Fabian Moselewski et al. (Chapter 6) discuss optimal coherence tomography. Stephen Worthley and Juan Badimon (Chapter 7) describe magnetic resonance imaging. John Davies et al. (Chapter 8) devote their work to single photon emission computed tomography and positron emission tomography. Konstantinos Toutouzas et al. (Chapter 9) discuss catheter-based techniques of coronary thermography. Finally, Len Kritharides et al. (Chapter 10) review current and future local and systemic strategies for the therapeutic management of vulnerable plaques.

I am confident this book will serve as a valuable practical and informative resource for vascular biologists, interventionalists, cardiologists, and radiologists alike.

Levon Khachigian
Sydney, Australia

About the Editor

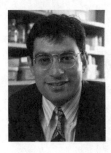 **Professor Levon Michael Khachigian (BSc(Hons), PhD, DSc)** is a Principal Research Fellow of the National Health and Medical Research Council of Australia and Head of the Transcription and Gene Targeting Laboratory at The Centre for Vascular Research, University of New South Wales and Prince of Wales Hospital, Sydney.

His research, encompassed in over 100 journal articles and book chapters, has greatly increased our understanding of the fundamental transcriptional mechanisms that led to the inappropriate expression of harmful genes in cells of the artery wall. It has also led to his generation of novel DNA-based drugs that block arterial renarrowing after balloon angioplasty in a variety of experimental models. More recently, he has been unravelling the mechanisms behind tumor growth control and other neovascular pathologies by inhibiting angiogenesis.

Professor Khachigian has been a major contributor to the broader workings of science on matters of policy, advocacy, consultancy, peer-review, mentorship, and societal service. For example, he is National Executive Director and President-Elect of the Australian Society for Medical Research, and Immediate-Past President of the Australian Vascular Biology Society. He has served on numerous grant review, fellowship, and policy formulation panels for the National Health and Medical Research Council of Australia and the National Heart Foundation of Australia. He sits on the editorial boards of five international journals.

Professor Khachigian has won many highly competitive awards for innovative research including the Commonwealth Health Minister's Award for Excellence in Health and Medical Research, the Gottschalk Award from the Australian Academy of Science, Eureka Prize for Scientific Research from the Australian Museum, RT Hall Prize from the Cardiac Society of Australia and New Zealand, AMGEN Medical Researcher Award, Eppendorf Award for the Young Australian Researcher, Quantum Scientific Research Award, Young Tall Poppy Award, and numerous named research awards for research excellence from the Heart Foundation of Australia.

Professor Khachigian received his BSc with first-class honors in biochemistry, and PhD in cell and molecular biology from the University of New South Wales, then studied transcriptional control in the Department of Pathology, Brigham and Women's Hospital, Harvard Medical School. In 2004, he was awarded a DSc in vascular pathobiology and translational research from the University of New South Wales.

Contributors

Stephan Achenbach, MD
Massachusetts General Hospital and
Harvard Medical School
Boston, Massachusetts

Chourmouzios A. Arampatzis, MD, PhD
Erasmus Medical Center
Rotterdam, The Netherlands

Juan J. Badimon, PhD, FACC
Mount Sinai School of Medicine
New York, New York

Martin R. Bennett, BCh, PhD, FRCP
Addenbrooke's Hospital
Cambridge University
Cambridge, United Kingdon

David Brieger, PhD, FRACP
Concord Hospital
University of Sydney
Sydney, Australia

John Davies, MBBS, MRCP
Addenbrooke's Hospital
Cambridge University
Cambridge, United Kingdom

Pim J. de Feyter, MD, PhD
Erasmus Medical Center
Rotterdam, The Netherlands

S. Benedict Freedman, PhD, FRACP, FACC
Concord Hospital
University of Sydney
Sydney, Australia

Tim Fryer, PhD
Addenbrooke's Hospital
Cambridge University
Cambridge, United Kingdom

Frank J. Gijsen, PhD
Erasmus Medical Center
Rotterdam, The Netherlands

Jonathan Gillard, MD, FRCP
Addenbrooke's Hospital
Cambridge University
Cambridge, United Kingdom

Ik-Kyung Jang, MD, PhD
Massachusetts General Hospital and
Harvard Medical School
Boston, Massachusetts

Jason L. Johnson, MSc
Bristol Heart Institute
University of Bristol
Bristol, United Kingdom

Levon M. Khachigian, PhD, DSc
Centre for Vascular Research
University of New South Wales
Sydney, Australia

Leonard Kritharides, PhD, FRACP, FAHA
Concord Hospital
University of Sydney and
Centre for Vascular Research
University of New South Wales
Sydney, Australia

Harry C. Lowe, FRACP, PhD, FACC
Centre for Vascular Research
University of New South Wales
Sydney, Australia

Fabian Moselewski, MD
Massachusetts General Hospital and
Harvard Medical School
Boston, Massachusetts

Steven E. Nissen, MD, FACC
The Cleveland Clinic Foundation
Cleveland, Ohio

Evelyn Regar, MD, PhD
Erasmus Medical Center
Rotterdam, The Netherlands

James Rudd, PhD, MRCP
Addenbrooke's Hospital
Cambridge University
Cambridge, United Kingdom

Johannes A. Schaar, MD, PhD
Erasmus Medical Center
Rotterdam, The Netherlands

Paul Schoenhagen, MD, FAHA
The Cleveland Clinic Foundation
Cleveland, Ohio

Patrick W. Serruys, MD, PhD
Erasmus Medical Center
Rotterdam, The Netherlands

Prediman K. Shah, MD
Cedars Sinai Medical Center and
UCLA School of Medicine
Los Angeles, California

Cornelis J. Slager, PhD
Erasmus Medical Center
Rotterdam, The Netherlands

Christodoulos Stefanadis, MD, PhD
Hippokration Hospital and
Athens Medical School
Athens, Greece

Konstantinos Toutouzas, MD
Hippokration Hospital and
Athens Medical School
Athens, Greece

Sophia Vaina, MD
Hippokration Hospital and
Athens Medical School
Athens, Greece

A.F.W. van der Steen, PhD
Erasmus Medical Center
Rotterdam, The Netherlands

Arjen R.A. van der Ven, MD
Erasmus Medical Center
Rotterdam, The Netherlands

Peter Weissberg, MD, FRCP, FMedSci
Addenbrooke's Hospital
Cambridge University
Cambridge, United Kingdom

Jolanda J. Wentzel, PhD
Erasmus Medical Center
Rotterdam, The Netherlands

Richard D. White, MD, FACC, FAHA
The Cleveland Clinic Foundation
Cleveland, Ohio

Stephen G. Worthley, MBBS, PhD, FRACP
Wakefield Hospital
Adelaide, South Australia

About the Senior Authors

Juan J. Badimon is a professor of medicine and director of the Cardiovascular Biology Research Laboratory at the Cardiovascular Institute of the Mount Sinai School of Medicine in New York City. He earned a specialty degree in pharmacology from the School of Medicine of the University of Barcelona and the High Council for Scientific Research of Spain and a Ph.D. also from the University of Barcelona. He completed a postdoctoral research fellowship at the Atherosclerosis Research Unit of the Mayo Clinic and Foundation in Rochester, Minnesota. In 1983, he moved to Mount Sinai. From 1991 through 1995, he worked at the Cardiac Unit of Massachusetts General Hospital in Boston, after which he returned to Mount Sinai. Dr. Badimon's research focuses on atherothrombotic disease, cardiovascular diseases, restenosis, the use of MRI for plaque characterization, and assessing the effectiveness of hypolipidemic regimens. A more recent interest is the role of tissue factor in atherothrombosis and its potential role as new therapeutic target in antithrombotic therapy. Dr. Badimon was designated Professor Honoris Causa by the Catholic University of Buenos Aires, Argentina in 2001. He is a fellow of the American College of Cardiology and the American Heart Association and an associate editor of *Vessels and Thrombosis* and *Haemostasis*. He sits on the editorial board of the *Journal of the American College of Cardiology* and the scientific board of the Spanish Familial Hypercholesterolemia Foundation. Dr. Badimon is an *ad hoc* reviewer for several major publications.

   Martin R. Bennett trained in cardiology in Birmingham and Cambridge in the United Kingdom. His research training included working with Gerard Evan and earning a Ph.D. at the Imperial Cancer Research Fund Laboratories, London, followed by a postdoctoral position in Seattle, Washington, working with Steve Schwartz. He currently holds the British Heart Foundation Chair of Cardiovascular Sciences at the University of Cambridge, and is a consultant cardiologist. His major research interests are the vascular biology of atherosclerosis, with focus on the regulation of vascular smooth muscle cell apoptosis and cell proliferation. Dr. Bennett is currently on the editorial boards of *Circulation Research*, *Heart*, and *Arteriosclerosis, Thrombosis, and Vascular Biology*.

   John Davies graduated in Medicine in 1997 from Guy's Hospital, London. He completed his general medical training in hospitals around London, including Guy's and St George's. He then pursued training in cardiology as a specialist registrar at Middlesex Hospital. After 2 years of clinical cardiology training, Dr. Davies moved to Cambridge University to undertake a Ph.D. program as a British Heart Foundation Research Fellow. Dr Davies' research interest focuses on the biology of atherosclerosis, in particular the imaging and quantification of inflammation within atherosclerotic plaques using positron emission tomography.

Ik-Kyung Jang is an interventional cardiologist at Massachusetts General Hospital and associate professor of medicine at Harvard Medical School. He currently serves as a director of the Center for Cardiovascular Clinical Research and co-director of Cardiology Laboratory of Integrative Physiology and Imaging at the Massachusetts General Hospital.

Leonard Kritharides is a consultant cardiologist at Concord Hospital, an associate professor of medicine at the University of Sydney, and co-leader of the Macrophage Biology Group at the Centre for Vascular Research, University of New South Wales, Australia. He graduated from the University of Melbourne in 1984, completed physician training at the Royal Melbourne Hospital in 1990, and completed a Ph.D. program and postdoctoral studies on macrophage cholesterol metabolism and lipoprotein oxidation at the Heart Research Institute in Sydney. His major research interests are in clinical cardiology and in the cell biology and biochemistry of atherosclerosis.

Harry C. Lowe is a cardiologist at Concord Hospital, a senior lecturer in medicine at the University of Sydney. He is also a National Health and Medical Research Council of Australia (NHMRC) C.J. Martin Research Fellow at the Centre for Vascular Research (CVR) of the University of New South Wales, Australia. Following cardiology training in New Zealand and at St Vincent's Hospital in Sydney, Dr. Lowe completed a Ph.D. program at the CVR, investigating gene modification of the response to vascular injury. He then pursued postdoctoral studies and interventional cardiology training at Massachusetts General Hospital and Harvard Medical School. His major research interests include the investigation of animal models of cardiovascular disease and clinical cardiology.

Fabian Moselewski is a research fellow at the Division of Cardiology of Massachusetts General Hospital and at CIMIT — the vulnerable plaque program of the Department of Radiology at Massachusetts General Hospital. His research focuses on noninvasive cardiac imaging by multidetector CT and coronary calcium screening, as well as invasive modalities such as IVUS and optical coherence tomography with a special emphasis on the detection of vulnerable plaques.

Steven E. Nissen is medical director of The Cleveland Clinic's Cardiovascular Coordinating Center. Professor Nissen has authored more than 200 journal articles, book chapters, and CD-ROMs, mostly in the field of cardiovascular imaging. He was one of the pioneers in the development of intravascular ultrasound (IVUS), and his research during the past decade has focused on this imaging technique. In particular, he has examined the discrepancies between angiography and IVUS in the assessment of coronary atherosclerosis, pointing out the limitations of radiographic methods. Dr Nissen currently serves as the principal investigator for several large IVUS studies of atherosclerosis regression and progression. He is also a member of the Cardiorenal Advisory Panel of the U.S. Food and Drug Administration.

Johannes A. Schaar earned a Ph.D. (cum laude) in Wuerzburg and also studied in St. Louis and New York. He worked at the University in Essen under the mentorship of Professor Raimund Erbel. He currently conducts research at the Erasmus Medical Center in Rotterdam with Professor Anton van der Steen and Professor Patrick Serruys. His research focuses on the detection of vulnerable plaques. Dr. Schaar has been awarded several research grants from organizations such as the

German Heart Foundation and the Dutch Heart Foundation. He has written several book chapters about valve disease and vulnerable plaque detection and published in peer review journals on the subjects of pulmonary hypertension, aortic dissection, and vulnerable plaque detection.

Paul Schoenhagen is on staff at the Departments of Diagnostic Radiology and Cardiovascular Medicine of The Cleveland Clinic Foundation. He earned his M.D. from the Universitaet Tuebingen, Germany in 1992 and wrote his doctoral thesis in medicine at the Philipps Universitaet, Marburg, Germany, in 1991. He was elected a Fellow of the Council of Atherosclerosis, Thrombosis, and Vascular Biology of the American Heart Association in 2001. He received the second James E. Muller Vulnerable Plaque New Investigator Prize for clinical research in 2002. Since he arrived at The Cleveland Clinic in 1996, his work has focused on atherosclerosis imaging.

Patrick W. Serruys is professor of medicine and interventional cardiology and directs the Interventional Heart Center at Erasmus Medical Center in Rotterdam. His primary research interests are coronary artery disease and interventional cardiology, for which he has received numerous awards. In the late 1980s he was among the first researchers to apply the so-called stent — now the most commonly used intervention procedure in cardiology. Professor Serruys is a Fellow of the European Society of Cardiology and the American College of Cardiology. He is associate editor of *Circulation*, the leading journal in the field of cardiac and cardiovascular systems, and his scientific output exceeds 1200 papers.

Prediman K. Shah is a graduate of the University of Kashmir (India) and received post-graduate training at Albert Einstein College of Medicine and Montefiore Hospital in New York. Dr. Shah's main research interests are in the area of atherosclerosis, coronary artery disease and acute coronary syndromes. His current major focus of research includes understanding the molecular mechanisms of atherosclerosis, plaque rupture, thrombosis and restenosis, and development and testing of novel antiatherogenic and antirestenotic strategies. Dr. Shah and his colleagues introduced recombinant apoA-I Milano, the product of a naturally occurring apoA-I mutant gene, as a novel antiatherogenic therapy that is currently in human trials. They have also developed a new vaccine against atherosclerosis and demonstrated its atheroprotective effectiveness in animal models. Dr Shah's many other important scientific contributions have improved the understanding of the pathophysiology and treatment of coronary syndromes. Dr. Shah has published over 250 scientific papers and abstracts and has lectured all over the world as a visiting professor. He is a fellow of the American College of Cardiology, member of the European Academy of Sciences, and a member of the Editorial Boards of *Circulation, American Journal of Cardiology, International Journal of Heart Failure, Indian Heart Journal, Journal of Preventive Cardiology, Reviews in Cardiovascular Medicine, Current Cardiology Reports,* and *Journal of Cardiovascular Pharmacology and Therapeutics*. Dr. Shah has been the recipient of numerous awards including the Award of Excellence in Teaching from the Dean of UCLA School of Medicine, the Golden Apple Award from UCLA medical students, the Lifetime Achievement Award from the Los Angeles Chapter of the American Heart Association, the Gifted Teacher Award from the

American College of Cardiology, and the Lifetime Achievement Award from the Association for Eradication of Heart Attacks and Vulnerable Plaque.

Christodoulos Stefanadis is professor and chairman of the Department of Cardiology, Hippokration Hospital, Athens Medical School, Greece. After earning an M.D. at Athens Medical School and completing his postgraduate education at Ohio State University in the U.S., he became the chief of the Catheterization Laboratory at Hippokration Hospital. His research activities focus on the design of diagnostic and guiding catheters, covered stents, balloon valvuloplasty, elastic properties of the aorta, left atrium function, and vulnerable plaque.

Peter Weissberg graduated in medicine from the University of Birmingham, United Kingdom. He trained as a clinical cardiologist in and around Birmingham and was appointed lecturer in cardiovascular medicine at the University of Birmingham. Following a 2-year appointment as a Medical Research Council travelling fellow at the Baker Institute and Alfred Hospital in Melbourne, Australia, he was appointed to a British Heart Foundation Senior Research Fellowship at the University of Cambridge. In 1994, Dr. Weissberg was named the first British Heart Foundation Professor of Cardiovascular Medicine at the University of Cambridge. Professor Weissberg's research interests focus on the cell biology of atherosclerosis and, in particular, the cell and molecular biology of vascular smooth muscle cells. He has published numerous original research articles on the role of smooth muscle cells in the development and progression of vascular disease. He currently heads the Division of Cardiovascular Medicine in the Addenbrooke's Centre for Clinical Investigation in Cambridge and serves as an honorary consultant cardiologist at Addenbrooke's and Papworth NHS.

Richard D. White is clinical director of the recently established Center for Integrated Noninvasive Cardiovascular Imaging at The Cleveland Clinic. He was one of the pioneers in the development of cardiovascular magnetic resonance imaging (MRI). More recently, his clinical and academic work has significantly contributed to the development of cardiovascular multidetector computed tomography (MDCT).

Stephen G. Worthley graduated from Adelaide University, South Australia and completed his cardiology training at the Royal Adelaide Hospital. He completed a Ph.D. program (magnetic resonance imaging of atherosclerosis) at Mount Sinai Medical Center in New York under Professors Juan Badimon and Valentin Fuster in the late 1990s. He also won young investigator awards for his work with the North American Society of Cardiac Imaging. At the Monash Medical Centre in Melbourne, Victoria, he completed his interventional training and earned a medical degree with a focus on novel intravascular imaging of atherosclerosis in 2000. He is now the director of cardiovascular imaging at Wakefield and the Royal Adelaide Hospitals in Adelaide, and continues his academic work in the field of cardiac imaging.

Contents

1 Cellular and Molecular Mechanisms of Plaque Rupture

Prediman K. Shah

CONTENTS

1.1 INTRODUCTION

Cardiovascular disease is the leading cause of death for both men and women in the United States and much of the western world and is predicted to be the leading global killer by 2020.[1] Atherosclerosis is responsible for coronary heart disease, most strokes, and limb ischemia. Although some of the clinical manifestations associated with atherosclerosis result from progressive luminal narrowing by atherosclerotic plaques and exaggerated or paradoxical vasoconstriction, the superimposition of thrombus over an underlying disrupted plaque causes the most acute and serious clinical manifestations of this disease. Coronary thrombosis, therefore, is responsible for the vast majority of cases of unstable angina, acute myocardial infarction, and sudden death.[2-6]

1.2 RUPTURE OF ATHEROSCLEROTIC PLAQUE FOLLOWED BY THROMBOSIS

A large number of studies involving angiography, surgical exploration, angioscopy, biochemical markers, and autopsy evaluation have shown that coronary thrombosis is the proximate cause for abrupt coronary occlusion leading to acute myocardial infarction, unstable angina, and many cases of sudden cardiac death.[7-18]

Fissure or rupture of the fibrous cap is the underlying basis for 70 to 80% of coronary thrombi with extension of the thrombus into the plaque as well as into the lumen, and with propagation of the thrombus upstream from the site of cap rupture.[14,18-20] Coronary stenoses that contain plaques with ruptured fibrous caps and superimposed thromboses often produce distinctive patterns on contrast angiography characterized as complex lesions. These lesions have eccentric stenoses bearing irregular or overhanging margins and lucencies or filling defects.[9,21]

1.2.1 PLAQUE RUPTURE: RELATIONSHIP TO PLAQUE SIZE AND STENOSIS SEVERITY

Retrospective analyses of serial angiograms and prospective serial angiographic observations have suggested that in nearly 60 to 70% of patients with acute coronary syndromes, coronary angiograms performed weeks or months before the acute events had shown the culprit lesion sites to have <70% (often <50%) diameter narrowing.[2,15,16,21-27] Thus, plaques producing non-flow-limiting, less-than-severe stenoses account for more cases of plaque rupture and thrombosis than plaques producing more severe luminal stenoses. Paralleling the angiographic data, stress testing in stable coronary disease patients has shown that the site of ischemia on stress myocardial perfusion scintigraphy does not accurately predict the future sites of acute myocardial infarctions.[28] This seeming clinical and angiographic paradox may be attributed to several factors[29]:

1. Less stenotic plaques outnumber the more severely stenotic plaques.
2. More stenotic plaques are likely to promote collaterals that protect from clinically overt manifestations of coronary occlusion.
3. Angiography underestimates stenosis severity.
4. Less stenotic plaques may be more vulnerable to plaque rupture.

Recent studies have shown that in addition to plaque size, positive remodeling (outward expansion) versus negative remodeling (vessel shrinkage or contraction) can play an important role in determining the net effect of a plaque on lumen size. Outward remodeling of unstable or vulnerable plaques may minimize luminal encroachment despite large plaque size. Human studies using intravascular ultrasound have, in fact, shown that outward arterial expansion due to positive remodeling

TABLE 1.1
Features of Unstable or Vulnerable Plaque

Large lipid core ($\geq$40% plaque volume) composed of free cholesterol crystals, cholesterol esters, and oxidized lipids impregnated with tissue factor
Thin fibrous cap depleted of smooth muscle cells and collagen
Outward (positive) remodeling
Inflammatory cell infiltration of fibrous cap and adventitia (mostly monocyte–macrophages, some activated T cells and mast cells)
Increased neovascularity

is more common at culprit lesion sites in unstable angina, whereas inward or negative remodeling is more common in stable angina.[30–32] Similarly, computer models using the Laplace law show that larger lumens create greater circumferential stress on the fibrous caps, thereby increasing their likelihood of rupture.[33]

Finally, recent histomorphometric data have shown that plaques with prominent outward remodeling on average contain larger lipid cores and more inflammatory cells than plaques without outward remodeling.[34] These histological features are known to be more prevalent in ruptured plaques and by inference in plaques at risk for rupture (vulnerable plaques).

1.2.2 PLAQUE RUPTURE: RELATIONSHIP TO PLAQUE COMPOSITION

Detailed histological assessment of ruptured plaques has shown several distinctive features which, when present before plaque ruptures, are also believed to indicate vulnerability to plaque rupture (Table 1.1). This hypothesis is the basis for the concept of plaque vulnerability. Plaques that rupture tend to be large; demonstrate outward or positive remodeling; have large lipid cores often occupying $\geq$40% plaque volume; show inflammatory cell infiltration of the fibrous caps and adventitia; possess thin caps depleted of collagen, glycosaminoglycans, and smooth muscle cells; and have increased adventitial and plaque neovascularity.[2,4,30,35–44]

1.2.2.1 Lipid Core

The extracellular lipid core is composed of free cholesterol, cholesterol crystals, and cholesterol esters derived from lipids that have infiltrated the arterial wall and also lipids derived from the deaths of foam cells, mostly macrophages. Accumulation of large quantities of free cholesterol has been shown to induce macrophage apoptosis through the activation of an endoplasmic reticulum-mediated gene program that can be abrogated by partial deficiency of the Niemann–Pick gene. This enhanced apoptosis of macrophage-foam cells may thus contribute to expansion of the acellular lipid core.[35,45]

It has also been suggested that red cell membranes may contribute to expansion of the lipid core when intraplaque hemorrhage occurs.[46] Such hemorrhage may occur from rupture of neovessels that are abundant in atherosclerotic plaques. A large eccentric lipid core may confer a mechanical disadvantage to the plaque by redistributing circumferential stress to the shoulder regions of the plaque which are the sites of fibrous cap rupture in nearly 60% of cases of plaque rupture.[33,36,47–49]

Transcriptional profiling has recently shown selective expression of a novel gene, perilipin, in ruptured human plaques. This is of considerable interest because perilipin inhibits lipid hydrolysis and may contribute to an accumulation of lipids in the core, thereby contributing to plaque vulnerability.[50] In addition, the lipid core contains prothrombotic oxidized lipids and is impregnated with procoagulant tissue factor derived from apoptotic macrophages. Tissue factor makes the lipid core highly thrombogenic when exposed to circulating blood.[51–55]

1.2.2.2 Plaque Inflammation

A number of histopathological studies have shown that ruptured plaques contain more inflammatory cells than intact plaques. These cells are mostly monocyte–macrophages, but also include activated T cells and degranulating mast cells. Inflammation is often found adjacent to the sites of fibrous cap ruptures, around the lipid cores, and in the adventitia around areas of neovascularization.[38,50–60] Inflammatory cells are probably recruited into the atherosclerotic plaques by adhesion molecules such as vascular cell adhesion molecules (VCAM)-1 and chemokines such as monocyte chemoattractant protein (MCP)-1.[61] They are then activated in the vessel walls. Another potential avenue for the entry and recruitment of inflammatory cells inside the atherosclerotic lesion may be through the adventitial neovasculature, which is enhanced in atherosclerosis.[62–67]

Factors that contribute to recruitment and activation of inflammatory cells and the inflammatory response in atherosclerosis include oxidized lipids, cytokines such as macrophage colony-stimulating factor (M-CSF), increased angiotensin II activity, elevated arterial pressure, diabetes, obesity, insulin resistance, smoking, chronic infections remote from the arterial wall, possible infectious organisms in the vessel wall (*Chlamydia pneumoniae*, cytomegalovirus, etc.), and activation of the immune system with release of pro-inflammatory mediators such as interferon gamma, CD40 ligands and others in response to antigens such as oxidized LDL, heat-shock proteins, beta microglobulin, and possibly others.[4,61] In addition, a deficiency of natural anti-inflammatory molecules such as IL-10 and transforming growth factor beta may also promote plaque inflammation.[68–70]

1.2.3 PATHOPHYSIOLOGIC LINK BETWEEN PLAQUE INFLAMMATION AND PLAQUE RUPTURE

The structural components of the fibrous cap include matrix molecules such as collagen, elastin, and proteoglycans derived from smooth muscle cells. The cap protects the deeper components of the plaque from contact with circulating blood, but thins out in the vicinity of rupture. Thinning of the fibrous cap is generally considered a prelude to rupture and a sign of vulnerability. Fibrous caps from ruptured plaques contain less extracellular matrix (collagen and proteoglycans) and fewer smooth muscle cells than caps from intact plaques.[39]

A number of investigators have hypothesized that depletion of matrix components, specifically fibrillar collagens, from the fibrous cap due to an imbalance

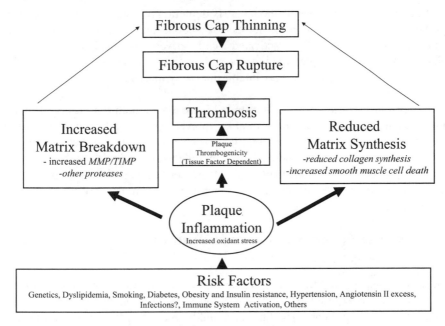

FIGURE 1.1 Central role of inflammation in plaque rupture and thrombosis.

between synthesis and breakdown leads to cap thinning. This predisposes the fibrous cap to rupture, either spontaneously or in response to hemodynamic or other triggers (Figure 1.1)[2,4] Enhanced matrix breakdown has been attributed primarily to a host of matrix-degrading metalloproteinases (MMPs) expressed in atherosclerotic plaques by inflammatory cells (macrophages, foam cells) and to a lesser extent by smooth muscle cells and endothelial cells.[71–80] This family of enzymes can degrade all components of the extracellular matrix and has been shown to be catalytically active *in vitro* and *in vivo*.[72,81–83] The activities of MMPs are tightly regulated at the level of gene transcription and also by their secretion in an inactive zymogen form that requires extracellular activation and co-secretion of the tissue inhibitors of metalloproteinases (TIMPs).[82] Thus, increased gene transcription, enhanced activation, and reduced activity of TIMPs can individually or together create an environment for increased matrix degradation.

All the components necessary for the activation of the MMP pathway exist in atherosclerotic plaques. Latent forms of MMPs can be activated by plasmin (produced by the plasminogen activator [uPA] from plasminogen by macrophages), trypsin, and chymase derived from degranulating mast cells. Increased MMP production can be induced by oxidized lipids, reactive oxygen species, chlamydial heat shock protein (HSP), CD-40 ligation, inflammatory cytokines, tenascin-C derived from macrophages, and hemodynamic stress.[59,77,78,84–90] In addition to MMPs, increased expression of cysteine and aspartate proteases of the cathepsin family and reduced expression of their cystatin-c inhibitor in human atherosclerotic lesions may also contribute to increased matrix breakdown in atherosclerosis.[91,92]

In addition to matrix degradation, matrix depletion may also result from reduced synthesis due to a decrease in the number of smooth muscle cells or a reduction in their synthetic function.[38,39] The activated T cell-derived cytokine, interferon gamma, inhibits collagen gene expression in smooth muscle cells *in vitro*. This suggests that activated T cells in the plaque may inhibit matrix synthesis by producing interferon gamma.

Several investigators have demonstrated increased smooth muscle cell death by apoptosis in human plaques, and several key players of the death-signaling pathway have been identified in atherosclerotic lesions.[93–104] Other stimuli that may induce smooth muscle cell death in atherosclerosis include oxidized lipids and the epidermal growth factor (EGF)-like domain of macrophage-derived tenascin-C (normally cryptic, but exposed when MMPs cleave the intact tenascin-C molecule)[104a] and apo C1-enriched HDL.[105]

1.2.4 ROLE OF PLAQUE INFLAMMATION IN THROMBOSIS FOLLOWING PLAQUE RUPTURE

Thrombosis is triggered following plaque rupture when thrombogenic components of the plaque are exposed to circulating blood. Thrombogenic components include collagen and the lipid core. The lipid core tends to be the most thrombogenic part of the plaque in part due to direct platelet activating effects of oxidized lipids but in large measure due to impregnation of the lipid core with a catalytically active tissue factor that activates the extrinsic clotting cascade leading to thrombin generation and thrombus formation at sites of plaque rupture.[52,54,55]

The major source of tissue factor in the lipid core appears to be the apoptotic macrophage.[104] Thus, inflammatory cells contribute mainly to plaque thrombogenicity by providing sources of tissue factor. Lipid ingestion, exposure to oxidized lipids, cytokines such as CD40 ligand, and other pro-inflammatory stimuli activate macrophages to produce tissue factor.[4]

1.2.5 INSIGHTS FROM EXPERIMENTAL MODELS OF PLAQUE RUPTURE

Despite numerous attempts, no convincing and consistently reproducible animal model of spontaneous atherosclerotic plaque rupture and thrombosis is currently available. In the past, investigators injected catecholamine, lipopolysaccharide (LPS), and Russell's viper venom to trigger thrombosis in rabbits with atherosclerosis, but such models bear little resemblance to human plaque rupture or thrombosis.[106] In another rabbit model, Rekhter and colleagues used a balloon incorporated in the arterial wall to study the role of lipid accumulation and macrophage infiltration on vulnerability to rupture. However, this model also bears little resemblance to human disease.[107] Similarly, endothelin injections in apo E-null mice have been shown to trigger acute myocardial necrosis, but coronary plaque rupture and thrombosis were not the underlying mechanisms.[108]

Recent research with apo E-null mice revealed frequent atherosclerotic lesions resembling vulnerable plaques in the innominate arteries. Although intraplaque hemorrhages were observed, frank ruptures and thromboses were not demonstrated.[109]

Other investigators described findings suggestive of plaque rupture and thrombosis in the innominate arteries of genetic variations of apo E-null mice fed a lard-based high-fat diet.[110] Rekhter reported evidence of plaque rupture in the aortic plaques of apo E-null mice after corticotropin-releasing factor was injected intracranially to simulate a stress response and presented the data at the annual Vascular Biology meeting held in Geneva in 2000.

Over-expression of MMP-1 failed to produce plaque rupture in mice. A paradoxical reduction in atherosclerosis was actually observed with MMP-1 over-expression, raising some questions about the role of MMPs as critical mediators of plaque rupture.[111] Calara et al. reported findings suggestive of plaque rupture and thrombosis in apo E- and low density lipoprotein (LDL) receptor-null mice, but the overall frequency was quite low.[112] Von der Thüsen and colleagues reported evidence of plaque rupture in murine models of atherosclerosis in response to vasopressor infusion when the pro-apoptotic gene p53 was over-expressed locally in carotid plaques.[113] However, this model again suffers from the drawback that both p53 over-expression and pressor stimuli were required, making it less of a model of spontaneous plaque rupture and thrombosis. Despite these limitations, the search for a model of spontaneous plaque rupture and thrombosis continues.

1.2.6 PLAQUE RUPTURE: POTENTIAL ROLE OF EXTRINSIC TRIGGERS

Sudden rupture of a vulnerable plaque may occur spontaneously without obvious triggers. In contrast, a rupture may follow a particular event, such as extreme physical activity (especially in someone unaccustomed to regular exercise), severe emotional trauma, sexual activity, exposure to illicit drugs (cocaine, marijuana, amphetamines), exposure to cold, or acute infection.[114–122]

While plaque rupture often leads to thrombosis with the clinical manifestations of an acute coronary syndrome, it may also occur without clinical consequences (silent plaque rupture). In approximately 40 to 80% of cases of acute coronary syndrome, multiple plaque ruptures have been demonstrated in arteries remote from the acute culprit site.[123] The thrombotic response to a plaque rupture is probably regulated by the thrombogenicity of the exposed plaque constituents, the local hemorrheology (determined by the severity of underlying stenosis), shear-induced platelet activation, and also by systemic thrombogenicity and fibrinolytic activity.[2,4] Lipid-rich plaques may be more thrombogenic than fibrous plaques, probably because of the high content of tissue factor in the lipid core.[55] The major source of tissue factor appears to be the macrophage. Apoptosis of macrophages may impregnate the lipid cores with tissue factor-laden microparticles, making the lipid cores highly thrombogenic.[53] Inflammatory cells, therefore, may be critical in influencing plaque thrombogenicity.

Recent studies in our laboratory have shown that plaques of smokers contain more tissue factor and inflammatory cells (macrophages) compared to non-smokers, perhaps contributing to the high thrombotic risk in smokers.[124] Furthermore, coronary collaterals may also influence the clinical consequences of acute coronary occlusion. Several investigators have suggested that organization and healing at the site of plaque rupture and thrombosis may eventually lead to rapid progression of plaque and worsening of stenosis, thereby providing a mechanism for atherosclerosis progression.[125]

1.2.7 THROMBOSIS WITHOUT PLAQUE RUPTURE: PLAQUE EROSION AND CALCIFIED NODULES

Coronary thrombi have been observed overlying atherosclerotic plaques in 20 to 40% of cases, without rupture of the fibrous cap.[2,4,13,126,127] Such thrombi occur over plaques with superficial endothelial erosions. These erosions are particularly common in young victims of sudden death, in smokers, and in women. Plaques under such thrombi do not have large lipid cores, but rather proteoglycan-rich matrices. The prevalence of inflammation is also lower than that in plaque rupture. The precise mechanisms of thrombosis in this scenario are unknown. It is conceivable that thrombosis in such cases is triggered by an enhanced systemic thrombogenic state (enhanced platelet aggregability, increased circulating tissue factor levels, depressed fibrinolytic state).[2,4]

Activated circulating leucocytes may transfer active tissue factor by shedding microparticles and transferring them onto adherent platelets.[128,129] It is possible that these circulating sources of tissue factor (rather than plaque-derived tissue factor) contribute to thromboses at sites of superficial endothelial denudation such as in plaque erosion. In addition, endothelial cell apoptosis may also increase local thrombogenicity, accounting for both endothelial denudation and thrombosis in plaque erosion. Furthermore, severe deficiencies of antithrombotic molecules, thrombomodulin, and protein-c receptor, on advanced atherosclerotic lesions may also contribute to thrombosis.[130] Erosion of a calcified nodule within an atherosclerotic plaque has also been reported as an uncommon basis for thrombosis.

1.2.8 DETERMINANTS OF PLAQUE VULNERABILITY AND RUPTURE: IMPLICATIONS FOR PLAQUE STABILIZATION THROUGH CHANGE IN PLAQUE PHENOTYPE

Several angiographic studies have shown that risk factor modification leads to reduced new lesion formation, less lesion progression and, in some cases, actual regression. However, these studies have also shown that the magnitude of vaso-occlusive clinical event reduction is far greater than that accounted for by the relatively small changes in stenosis severity. This apparent discrepancy led to the following hypotheses:

1. Risk factor modification may induce plaque regression and reverse remodeling with little net change in stenosis severity.
2. Risk factor modification may not change plaque mass or stenosis severity and might reduce the propensity for plaque rupture and thrombosis by changing the composition of the plaque.

The latter possibility is referred to as plaque stabilization.[2,4,131–136]

Studies in animals have in fact shown that lowering lipids through diet, statin therapy, or direct administration of apo A-I and high density lipoprotein (HDL)-like particles can deplete lipids, reduce inflammation, sometimes reduce MMP and tissue factor levels, and increase the collagen content of atherosclerotic lesions.[137–143] Thus, plaque composition change can be achieved in animal models.

Our laboratory demonstrated that 3 months of therapy with pravastatin also favorably modifies human carotid plaque composition to a more stable phenotype, providing the first human data paralleling the results from animal models.[144] It can be postulated, therefore, that reducing lipids and inflammation in atherosclerotic plaques may help lower the risk of plaque rupture and subsequent thrombosis. Also, such a plaque-stabilizing effect may account for the clinical benefits of risk factor modification by lifestyle changes and drug therapy (lipid-modifying drugs, angiotensin converting enzyme, and angiotensin-II receptor blockers).[2,4] Future additional approaches may include direct administration of HDL and its apolipoproteins and novel HDL-boosting compounds such as the rexinoids.[145–147]

1.3 CONCLUDING REMARKS

Atherosclerosis is a chronic disease characterized by lipid deposition, matrix deposition, neoangiogenesis and inflammation, vessel wall remodeling, and abnormal vasomotor regulation. Inflammatory gene activation appears to be a common pathophysiologic underpinning in the evolution and progression of atherosclerosis. The natural history of atherosclerotic vascular disease is characterized by episodes of plaque rupture and superficial endothelial erosion leading to thrombus formation, which is the proximate event responsible for acute ischemic syndromes. A body of evidence assigns a central role for inflammation in the process of plaque rupture and subsequent thrombosis with multiple risk factors serving as potential pro-inflammatory triggers. Risk factor modification appears to reduce acute vaso-occlusive events primarily by changing the plaque phenotype from one that is vulnerable to rupture into the one that is less prone to rupture. This process of plaque stabilization represents a novel paradigm in atherosclerosis management.

ACKNOWLEDGMENTS

Generous support from Sam Spaulding, United Hostesses Charities and the Ornest Family Foundation is acknowledged. Contributions of many colleagues and collaborators at the Atherosclerosis Research Center of Cedars Sinai Medical Center are also gratefully acknowledged.

REFERENCES

1. Murray CJ and Lopez AD. Global mortality, disability and contribution of risk factors: Global Bureau of Disease Study. *Lancet* 1997; 349: 1436–1442.
2. Falk E, Shah PK, and Fuster V. Coronary plaque disruption. *Circulation* 1995; 92: 657–671.

3. Virmani R, Burke AP, and Farb A. Plaque rupture and plaque erosion. *Thromb Haemost* 1999; 82 Suppl 1: 1–3.
4. Shah PK. Pathophysiology of coronary thrombosis: role of plaque rupture and plaque erosion. *Progr Cardiovasc Dis* 2002; 44: 357–368.
5. Libby P. Current concepts of the pathogenesis of the acute coronary syndromes. *Circulation* 2001; 104: 365–372.
6. DeWood MA, Spores J, Notske R, et al. Prevalence of total coronary occlusion during the early hours of transmural myocardial infarction. *New Engl J Med* 1980; 303: 897–902.
7. DeWood MA, Spores J, Hensley GR, et al. Coronary arteriographic findings in acute transmural myocardial infarction. *Circulation* 1983; 68: 39–49.
8. DeWood MA, Stifter WF, Simpson CS, et al. Coronary arteriographic findings soon after non-Q-wave myocardial infarction. *New Engl J Med* 1986; 315: 417–423.
9. Levin DC and Fallon JT. Significance of the angiographic morphology of localized coronary stenoses: histopathologic correlations. *Circulation* 1982; 66: 316–320.
10. Sherman CT, Litvack F, Grundfest W, et al. Coronary angioscopy in patients with unstable angina pectoris. *New Engl J Med* 1986; 315: 913–919.
11. Kruskal JB, Commerford PJ, Franks JJ, and Kirsch RE. Fibrin and fibrinogen-related antigens in patients with stable and unstable coronary artery disease. *New Engl J Med* 1987; 317: 1361–1365.
12. Folts JD. Platelet aggregation in stenosed coronary or cerebral arteries: a mechanism for sudden death? *Wis Med J* 1980; 79: 24–26.
13. Davies MJ and Thomas A. Thrombosis and acute coronary artery lesions in sudden cardiac ischemic death. *New Engl J Med* 1984; 310: 1137–1140.
14. Falk E. Plaque rupture with severe pre-existing stenosis precipitating coronary thrombosis: characteristics of coronary atherosclerotic plaques underlying fatal occlusive thrombi. *Br Heart J* 1983; 50: 127–134.
15. Ambrose JA, Winters SL, Stern A, et al. Angiographic morphology and the pathogenesis of unstable angina pectoris. *J Am Coll Cardiol* 1985; 5: 609–616.
16. Ambrose JA, Winters SL, Arora RR, et al. Coronary angiographic morphology in myocardial infarction: a link between the pathogenesis of unstable angina and myocardial infarction. *J Am Coll Cardiol* 1985; 6: 1233–1238.
17. Gorlin R, Fuster V, and Ambrose JA. Anatomic–physiologic links between acute coronary syndromes. *Circulation* 1986; 74: 6–9.
18. Friedman M. Pathogenesis of coronary thrombosis, intramural and intraluminal hemorrhage. *Adv Cardiol* 1970; 4: 20–46.
19. Friedman M. The pathogenesis of coronary plaques, thromboses, and hemorrhages: an evaluative review. *Circulation* 1975; 52: 34–40.
20. Constantinides P. Atherosclerosis — a general survey and synthesis. *Surv Synth Pathol Res* 1984; 3: 477–498.
21. Ambrose JA, Hjemdahl-Monsen C, Borrico S, et al. Quantitative and qualitative effects of intracoronary streptokinase in unstable angina and non-Q wave infarction. *J Am Coll Cardiol* 1987; 9: 1156–1165.
22. Ambrose JA, Winters SL, Arora RR, et al. Angiographic evolution of coronary artery morphology in unstable angina. *J Am Coll Cardiol* 1986; 7: 472–478.
23. Ambrose JA and Monsen C. Significance of intraluminal filling defects in unstable angina. *Am J Cardiol* 1986; 57: 1003–1004.
24. Little WC, Constantinescu M, Applegate RJ, et al. Can coronary angiography predict the site of a subsequent myocardial infarction in patients with mild-to-moderate coronary artery disease? *Circulation* 1988; 78: 1157–1166.

25. Hackett D, Davies G, and Maseri A. Pre-existing coronary stenoses in patients with first myocardial infarction are not necessarily severe. *Eur Heart J* 1988; 9: 1317–1323.

26. Giroud D, Li JM, Urban P, Meier B, and Rutishauer W. Relation of the site of acute myocardial infarction to the most severe coronary arterial stenosis at prior angiography. *Am J Cardiol* 1992; 69: 729–732.

27. Brown G, Albers JJ, Fisher LD, et al. Regression of coronary artery disease as a result of intensive lipid- lowering therapy in men with high levels of apolipoprotein B. *New Engl J Med* 1990; 323: 1289–1298.

28. Naqvi TZ, Hachamovitch R, Berman D, Buchbinder N, Kiat H, and Shah PK. Does the presence and site of myocardial ischemia on perfusion scintigraphy predict the occurrence and site of future myocardial infarction in patients with stable coronary artery disease? *Am J Cardiol* 1997; 79: 1521–1524.

29. Shah PK. Plaque size, vessel size and plaque vulnerability: bigger may not be better. *J Am Coll Cardiol* 1998; 32: 663–664.

30. Schoenhagen P, Ziada KM, Kapadia SR, Crowe TD, Nissen SE, and Tuzcu EM. Extent and direction of arterial remodeling in stable versus unstable coronary syndromes: an intravascular ultrasound study. *Circulation* 2000; 101: 598–603.

31. von Birgelen C, Klinkhart W, Mintz GS, et al. Plaque distribution and vascular remodeling of ruptured and nonruptured coronary plaques in the same vessel: an intravascular ultrasound study *in vivo*. *J Am Coll Cardiol* 2001; 37: 1864–1870.

32. Takano M, Mizuno K, Okamatsu K, Yokoyama S, Ohba T, and Sakai S. Mechanical and structural characteristics of vulnerable plaques: analysis by coronary angioscopy and intravascular ultrasound. *J Am Coll Cardiol* 2001; 38: 99–104.

33. Loree HM, Kamm RD, Stringfellow RG, and Lee RT. Effects of fibrous cap thickness on peak circumferential stress in model atherosclerotic vessels. *Circ Res* 1992; 71: 850–858.

34. Varnava AM, Mills PG, and Davies MJ. Relationship between coronary artery remodeling and plaque vulnerability. *Circulation* 2002; 105: 939–943.

35. Guyton JR and Klemp KF. Development of the lipid-rich core in human atherosclerosis. *Arterioscler Thromb Vasc Biol* 1996; 16: 4–11.

36. Richardson PD, Davies MJ, and Born GV. Influence of plaque configuration and stress distribution on fissuring of coronary atherosclerotic plaques. *Lancet* 1989; 2: 941–944.

37. Davies MJ, Richardson PD, Woolf N, Katz DR, and Mann J. Risk of thrombosis in human atherosclerotic plaques: role of extracellular lipid, macrophage, and smooth muscle cell content. *Br Heart J* 1993; 69: 377–381.

38. Felton CV, Crook D, Davies MJ, and Oliver MF. Relation of plaque lipid composition and morphology to the stability of human aortic plaques. *Arterioscler Thromb Vasc Biol* 1997; 17: 1337–1345.

39. Burleigh MC, Briggs AD, Lendon CL, Davies MJ, Born GV, and Richardson PD. Collagen types I and III, collagen content, GAGs and mechanical strength of human atherosclerotic plaque caps: span-wise variations. *Atherosclerosis* 1992; 96: 71–81.

40. Moreno PR, Falk E, Palacios IF, Newell JB, Fuster V, and Fallon JT. Macrophage infiltration in acute coronary syndromes: implications for plaque rupture. *Circulation* 1994; 90: 775–778.

41. Moreno PR, Bernardi VH, Lopez-Cuellar J, et al. Macrophages, smooth muscle cells, and tissue factor in unstable angina: implications for cell-mediated thrombogenicity in acute coronary syndromes. *Circulation* 1996; 94: 3090–3097.

42. Lendon CL, Davies MJ, Born GV, and Richardson PD. Atherosclerotic plaque caps are locally weakened when macrophages density is increased. *Atherosclerosis* 1991; 87: 87–90.

43. Depre C, Havaux X, and Wijns W. Neovascularization in human coronary atherosclerotic lesions. *Cathet Cardiovasc Diagn* 1996; 39: 215–220.

44. Tenaglia AN, Peters KG, Sketch MH, Jr., and Annex BH. Neovascularization in atherectomy specimens from patients with unstable angina: implications for pathogenesis of unstable angina. *Am Heart J* 1998; 135: 10–14.

45. Feng B, Yao PM, Li Y, Devlin CM, et al. The endoplasmic reticulum is the site of cholesterol-induced cytotoxicity in macrophages. *Nat Cell Biol* 2003; 5: 781–792.

46. Kolodgie FD, Gold HK, Burke AP, Fowler DR, et al. Intraplaque hemorrhage and progression of atheroma. *New Engl J Med* 2003; 349: 2316–2325.

47. Cheng GC, Loree HM, Kamm RD, Fishbein MC, and Lee RT. Distribution of circumferential stress in ruptured and stable atherosclerotic lesions: a structural analysis with histopathological correlation. *Circulation* 1993; 87: 1179–1187.

48. Loree HM, Tobias BJ, Gibson LJ, Kamm RD, et al. Mechanical properties of model atherosclerotic lesion lipid pools. *Arterioscler Thromb* 1994; 14: 230–234.

49. Huang H, Virmani R, Younis H, Burke AP, et al. The impact of calcification on the biomechanical stability of atherosclerotic plaques. *Circulation* 2001; 103: 1051–1056.

50. Faber BC, Cleutjens KB, Niessen RL, et al. Identification of genes potentially involved in rupture of human atherosclerotic plaques. *Circ Res* 2001; 89: 547–554.

51. Essler M, Retzer M, Bauer M, Zangl KJ, et al. Stimulation of platelets and endothelial cells by mildly oxidized LDL proceeds through activation of lysophosphatidic acid receptors and the Rho/Rho-kinase pathway: inhibition by lovastatin. *Ann NY Acad Sci* 2000; 905: 282–286.

52. Toschi V, Gallo R, Lettino M, et al. Tissue factor modulates the thrombogenicity of human atherosclerotic plaques. *Circulation* 1997; 95: 594–599.

53. Mallat Z, Hugel B, Ohan J, Leseche G, et al. Shed membrane microparticles with procoagulant potential in human atherosclerotic plaques: a role for apoptosis in plaque thrombogenicity. *Circulation* 1999; 99: 348–353.

54. Badimon JJ, Lettino M, Toschi V, et al. Local inhibition of tissue factor reduces the thrombogenicity of disrupted human atherosclerotic plaques: effects of tissue factor pathway inhibitor on plaque thrombogenicity under flow conditions. *Circulation* 1999; 99: 1780–1787.

55. Fernandez-Ortiz A, Badimon JJ, Falk E, et al. Characterization of the relative thrombogenicity of atherosclerotic plaque components: implications for consequences of plaque rupture. *J Am Coll Cardiol* 1994; 23: 1562–1569.

56. van der Wal AC, Becker AE, van der Loos CM, and Das PK. Site of intimal rupture or erosion of thrombosed coronary atherosclerotic plaques is characterized by an inflammatory process irrespective of the dominant plaque morphology. *Circulation* 1994; 89: 36–44.

57. Kovanen PT. The mast cell — a potential link between inflammation and cellular cholesterol deposition in atherogenesis. *Eur Heart J* 1993; 14 Suppl K: 105–117.

58. Kovanen PT, Kaartinen M, and Paavonen T. Infiltrates of activated mast cells at the site of coronary atheromatous erosion or rupture in myocardial infarction. *Circulation* 1995; 92: 1084–1088.

59. Kaartinen M, van der Wal AC, van der Loos CM, et al. Mast cell infiltration in acute coronary syndromes: implications for plaque rupture. *J Am Coll Cardiol* 1998; 32: 606–612.

60. Laine P, Kaartinen M, Penttila A, Panula P, et al. Association between myocardial infarction and the mast cells in the adventitia of the infarct-related coronary artery. *Circulation* 1999; 99: 361–369.

61. Libby P. Inflammation in atherosclerosis. *Nature* 2002; 420: 868–874.

62. Barger AC, Beeuwkes R, 3rd, Lainey LL, and Silverman KJ. Hypothesis: vasa vasorum and neovascularization of human coronary arteries: a possible role in the pathophysiology of atherosclerosis. *New Engl J Med* 1984; 310: 175–177.

63. Kamat BR, Galli SJ, Barger AC, Lainey LL, and Silverman KJ. Neovascularization and coronary atherosclerotic plaque: cinematographic localization and quantitative histologic analysis. *Hum Pathol* 1987; 18: 1036–1042.

64. Barger AC and Beeuwkes R, 3rd. Rupture of coronary vasa vasorum as a trigger of acute myocardial infarction. *Am J Cardiol* 1990; 66: 41G-43G.

65. Heistad DD and Armstrong ML. Blood flow through vasa vasorum of coronary arteries in atherosclerotic monkeys. *Arteriosclerosis* 1986; 6: 326–331.

66. Williams JK and Heistad DD. The vasa vasorum of the arteries. *J Mal Vasc* 1996; 21: 266–269.

67. Kwon HM, Sangiorgi G, Ritman EL, et al. Enhanced coronary vasa vasorum neovascularization in experimental hypercholesterolemia. *J Clin Invest* 1998; 101: 1551–1556

68. Gojova A, Brun V, Bruno E, Cottrez F, et al. Specific abrogation of transforming growth factor beta signaling in T cells alters atherosclerotic lesion size and composition in mice. *Blood* 2003; 102: 4052–4058.

69. Robertson AL, Rudling M, Zhore X, Gorelik L, et al. Disruption of TGF-beta signaling in T-cells accelerates atherosclerosis. *J Clin Invest* 2003; 112: 1342–1350.

70. Tedgui A and Mallat Z. Anti-inflammatory mechanisms in the vascular wall. *Circulation Res* 200; 88: 877–887.

71. Henney AM, Wakeley PR, Davies MJ, et al. Localization of stromelysin gene expression in atherosclerotic plaques by *in situ* hybridization. *Proc Natl Acad Sci USA* 1991; 88: 8154–8158.

72. Galis ZS, Sukhova GK, Lark MW, and Libby P. Increased expression of matrix metalloproteinases and matrix degrading activity in vulnerable regions of human atherosclerotic plaques. *J Clin Invest* 1994; 94: 2493–2503.

73. Brown DL, Hibbs MS, Kearney M, Loushin C, and Isner JM. Identification of 92-kD gelatinase in human coronary atherosclerotic lesions: association of active enzyme synthesis with unstable angina. *Circulation* 1995; 91: 2125–2131.

74. Nikkari ST, O'Brien KD, Ferguson M, et al. Interstitial collagenase (MMP-1) expression in human carotid atherosclerosis. *Circulation* 1995; 92: 1393–1398.

75. Li Z, Li LL, Zielke HR, et al. Increased expression of 72-kd type IV collagenase (MMP-2) in human aortic atherosclerotic lesions. *Am J Pathol* 1996; 148: 121–128.

76. Galis ZS, Sukhova GK, and Libby P. Microscopic localization of active proteases *by in situ* zymography: detection of matrix metalloproteinase activity in vascular tissue. *FASEB J* 1995; 9: 974–980.

77. Xu XP, Meisel SR, and Ong JM, et al. Oxidized low-density lipoprotein regulates matrix metalloproteinase-9 and its tissue inhibitor in human monocyte-derived macrophages. *Circulation* 1999; 99: 993–998.

78. Rajavashisth TB, Xu XP, Jovinge S, et al. Membrane type 1 matrix metalloproteinase expression in human atherosclerotic plaques: evidence for activation by proinflammatory mediators. *Circulation* 1999; 99: 3103–3109.

79. Rajavashisth TB, Liao JK, Galis ZS, et al. Inflammatory cytokines and oxidized low density lipoproteins increase endothelial cell expression of membrane type 1-matrix metalloproteinase. *J Biol Chem* 1999; 274: 11924–11929.

80. Herman MP, Sukhova GK, Libby P, et al. Expression of neutrophil collagenase (matrix metalloproteinase-8) in human atheroma: a novel collagenolytic pathway suggested by transcriptional profiling. *Circulation* 2001; 104: 1899–1904.

81. Shah PK, Falk E, Badimon JJ, et al. Human monocyte-derived macrophages induce collagen breakdown in fibrous caps of atherosclerotic plaques: potential role of matrix-degrading metalloproteinases and implications for plaque rupture. *Circulation* 1995; 92: 1565–1569.

82. Shah PK. Role of inflammation and metalloproteinases in plaque disruption and thrombosis. *Vasc Med* 1998; 3: 199–206.

83. Sukhova GK, Schonbeck U, Rabkin E, et al. Evidence for increased collagenolysis by interstitial collagenases-1 and -3 in vulnerable human atheromatous plaques. *Circulation* 1999; 99: 2503–2509.

84. Lee RT, Schoen FJ, Loree HM, Lark MW, and Libby P. Circumferential stress and matrix metalloproteinase 1 in human coronary atherosclerosis: implications for plaque rupture. *Arterioscler Thromb Vasc Biol* 1996; 16: 1070–1073.

85. Galis ZS, Muszynski M, Sukhova GK, Simon-Morrissey E, and Libby P. Enhanced expression of vascular matrix metalloproteinases induced *in vitro* by cytokines and in regions of human atherosclerotic lesions. *Ann NY Acad Sci* 1995; 748: 501–507.

86. Galis ZS, Sukhova GK, Kranzhofer R, Clark S, and Libby P. Macrophage foam cells from experimental atheroma constitutively produce matrix-degrading proteinases. *Proc Natl Acad Sci USA* 1995; 92: 402–406.

87. Kol A, Sukhova GK, Lichtman AH, and Libby P. Chlamydial heat shock protein 60 localizes in human atheroma and regulates macrophage tumor necrosis factor-alpha and matrix metalloproteinase expression. *Circulation* 1998; 98: 300–307.

88. Mach F, Schonbeck U, Fabunmi RP, et al. T lymphocytes induce endothelial cell matrix metalloproteinase expression by a CD40L-dependent mechanism: implications for tubule formation. *Am J Pathol* 1999; 154: 229–238.

89. Schonbeck U, Mach F, Sukhova GK, et al. Regulation of matrix metalloproteinase expression in human vascular smooth muscle cells by T lymphocytes: a role for CD40 signaling in plaque rupture? *Circ Res* 1997; 81: 448–454.

90. Wallner K, Li C, Shah PK, et al. Tenascin-C is expressed in macrophage-rich human coronary atherosclerotic plaque. *Circulation* 1999; 99: 1284–1289.

91. Sukhova GK, Shi GP, Simon DI, Chapman HA, and Libby P. Expression of the elastolytic cathepsins S and K in human atheroma and regulation of their production in smooth muscle cells. *J Clin Invest* 1998; 102: 576–583.

92. Shi GP, Sukhova GK, Grubb A, et al. Cystatin C deficiency in human atherosclerosis and aortic aneurysms. *J Clin Invest* 1999; 104: 1191–1197.

93. Bennett MR, Evan GI, and Schwartz SM. Apoptosis of human vascular smooth muscle cells derived from normal vessels and coronary atherosclerotic plaques. *J Clin Invest* 1995; 95: 2266–2274.

94. Bjorkerud S and Bjorkerud B. Apoptosis is abundant in human atherosclerotic lesions, especially in inflammatory cells (macrophages and T cells), and may contribute to the accumulation of gruel and plaque instability. *Am J Pathol* 1996; 149: 367–380.

95. Kockx MM and Knaapen MW. The role of apoptosis in vascular disease. *J Pathol* 2000; 190: 267–280.

96. Ihling C, Haendeler J, Menzel G, et al. Co-expression of p53 and MDM2 in human atherosclerosis: implications for the regulation of cellularity of atherosclerotic lesions. *J Pathol* 1998; 185: 303–312.

97. Crisby M, Kallin B, Thyberg J, et al. Cell death in human atherosclerotic plaques involves both oncosis and apoptosis. *Atherosclerosis* 1997; 130: 17–27.

98. Bennett MR. Apoptosis of vascular smooth muscle cells in vascular remodelling and atherosclerotic plaque rupture. *Cardiovasc Res* 1999; 41: 361–368.

99. Galle J, Heermeier K, and Wanner C. Atherogenic lipoproteins, oxidative stress, and cell death. *Kidney Int Suppl* 1999; 71: S62–S65.

100. Vieira O, Escargueil-Blanc I, Jurgens G, et al. Oxidized LDLs alter the activity of the ubiquitin–proteasome pathway: potential role in oxidized LDL-induced apoptosis. *FASEB J* 2000; 14: 532–542.

101. Rossig L, Dimmeler S, and Zeiher AM. Apoptosis in the vascular wall and atherosclerosis. *Basic Res Cardiol* 2001; 96: 11–22.

102. Geng YJ, Wu Q, Muszynski M, Hansson GK, and Libby P. Apoptosis of vascular smooth muscle cells induced by *in vitro* stimulation with interferon-gamma, tumor necrosis factor-alpha, and interleukin-1-beta. *Arterioscler Thromb Vasc Biol* 1996; 16: 19–27.

103. Geng YJ, Henderson LE, Levesque EB, Muszynski M, and Libby P. Fas is expressed in human atherosclerotic intima and promotes apoptosis of cytokine-primed human vascular smooth muscle cells. *Arterioscler Thromb Vasc Biol* 1997; 17: 2200–2208.

104. Mallat Z and Tedgui A. Apoptosis in the vasculature: mechanisms and functional importance. *Br J Pharmacol* 2000; 130: 947–962.

104a. Wallner K, Shah PK, Wu KJ, Schwartz SM, and Sharifi BG. EGF-like domain of tenascin-C is pro-apoptotic for cultured smooth muscle cells. *Arteriosclerosis Thromb. Vasc. Biol.* (in press).

105. Kolmakova A, Kwiterovich P, Virgil D, Alaupovic P, et al. Apolipoprotein C-1 induces apoptosis in human aortic smooth muscle cells via recruiting neutral sphingomyelinase. *Arterioscler Thromb Vasc Biol.* 2004; 24: 264–269.

106. Abela GS, Picon PD, Friedl SE, et al. Triggering of plaque disruption and arterial thrombosis in an atherosclerotic rabbit model. *Circulation* 1995; 91: 776–784.

107. Rekhter MD, Hicks GW, Brammer DW, et al. Animal model that mimics atherosclerotic plaque rupture. *Circ Res* 1998; 83: 705–713.

108. Caligiuri G, Levy B, Pernow J, Thoren P, and Hansson GK. Myocardial infarction mediated by endothelin receptor signaling in hypercholesterolemic mice. *Proc Natl Acad Sci USA* 1999; 96: 6920–6924.

109. Rosenfeld ME, Polinsky P, Virmani R, Kauser K, et al. Advanced atherosclerotic lesions in the innominate artery of the ApoE knockout mouse. *Arterioscler Thromb Vasc Biol* 2000; 20: 2587–2592.

110. Johnson JL and Jackson CL. Atherosclerotic plaque rupture in the apolipoprotein E knockout mouse. *Atherosclerosis* 2001; 154: 399–406.

111. Lemaitre V, O'Byrne TK, Borczuk AC, Okada Y, Tall AR, and D'Armiento J. ApoE knockout mice expressing human matrix metalloproteinase-1 in macrophages have less advanced atherosclerosis. *J Clin Invest* 2001; 107: 1227–1234.

112. Calara F, Silvestre M, Casanada F, Yuan N, Napoli C, and Palinski W. Spontaneous plaque rupture and secondary thrombosis in apolipoprotein E-deficient and LDL receptor-deficient mice. *J Pathol* 2001; 195: 257–263.

113. Von der Thusen JH, Van Vlijmen BJ, Hoeben RC, Kockx MM, and Van Berkel TJ. *Circulation* 2001: 117 [abstr].

114. Muller JE, Tofler GH, and Stone PH. Circadian variation and triggers of onset of acute cardiovascular disease. *Circulation* 1989; 79: 733–743.
115. Muller JE. Morning increase of onset of myocardial infarction: implications concerning triggering events. *Cardiology* 1989; 76: 96–104.
116. Muller JE and Tofler GH. Triggering and hourly variation of onset of arterial thrombosis. *Ann Epidemiol* 1992; 2: 393–405.
117. Willich SN, Jimenez AH, Tofler GH, DeSilva RA, and Muller JE. Pathophysiology and triggers of acute myocardial infarction: clinical implications. *Clin Invest* 1992; 70: S73–S78.
118. Willich SN, Maclure M, Mittleman M, Arntz HR, and Muller JE. Sudden cardiac death: support for a role of triggering in causation. *Circulation* 1993; 87: 1442–1450.
119. Peters A, Dockery DW, Muller JE, and Mittleman MA. Increased particulate air pollution and the triggering of myocardial infarction. *Circulation* 2001; 103: 2810–2815.
120. Mittleman MA, Lewis RA, Maclure M, Sherwood JB, and Muller JE. Triggering myocardial infarction by marijuana. *Circulation* 2001; 103: 2805–2809.
121. Muller JE. Circadian variation and triggering of acute coronary events. *Am Heart J* 1999; 137: S1–S8.
122. Muller JE. Triggering of cardiac events by sexual activity: findings from a case crossover analysis. *Am J Cardiol* 2000; 86: 14F–18F.
123. Goldstein JA, Demetriou D, Grines CL, Pica M, Shoukfeh M, and O'Neill WW. Multiple complex coronary plaques in patients with acute myocardial infarction. *New Engl J Med* 2000; 343: 915–922.
124. Matetzky S, Tani S, Kangavari S, et al. Smoking increases tissue factor expression in atherosclerotic plaques: implications for plaque thrombogenicity. *Circulation* 2000; 102: 602–604.
125. Burke AP, Kolodgie FD, Farb A, et al. Healed plaque ruptures and sudden coronary death: evidence that subclinical rupture has a role in plaque progression. *Circulation* 2001; 103: 934–940.
126. Burke AP, Farb A, Malcom GT, Liang YH, Smialek J, and Virmani R. Coronary risk factors and plaque morphology in men with coronary disease who died suddenly. *New Engl J Med* 1997; 336: 1276–1282.
127. Farb A, Burke AP, Tang AL, et al. Coronary plaque erosion without rupture into a lipid core: a frequent cause of coronary thrombosis in sudden coronary death. *Circulation* 1996; 93: 1354–1363.
128. Rauch U, Bonderman D, Bohrmann B, et al. Transfer of tissue factor from leukocytes to platelets is mediated by CD15 and tissue factor. *Blood* 2000; 96: 170–175.
129. Mallat Z, Benamer H, Hugel B, et al. Elevated levels of shed membrane microparticles with procoagulant potential in the peripheral circulating blood of patients with acute coronary syndromes. *Circulation* 2000; 101: 841–843.
130. Laszik ZG, Zhou XJ, Ferrell GL, Silva FG, and Esmon CT. Down-regulation of endothelial expression of endothelial cell protein C receptor and thrombomodulin in coronary atherosclerosis. *Am J Pathol* 2001; 159: 797–802.
131. Schwartz CJ, Valente AJ, Sprague EA, Kelley JL, Cayatte AJ, and Mowery J. Atherosclerosis: potential targets for stabilization and regression. *Circulation* 1992; 86: 117–123.
132. Waters D. Plaque stabilization: a mechanism for the beneficial effect of lipid-lowering therapies in angiography studies. *Prog Cardiovasc Dis* 1994; 37: 107–120.
133. Shah PK. Pathophysiology of plaque rupture and the concept of plaque stabilization. *Cardiol Clin* 2003; 21: 303–314.

134. Shah PK. Mechanisms of plaque vulnerability and rupture. *J Am Coll Cardiol* 2003; 41: 15S-22S.
135. Kullo IJ, Edwards WD, and Schwartz RS. Vulnerable plaque: pathobiology and clinical implications. *Ann Intern Med* 1998; 129: 1050–1060.
136. Lee RT. Plaque stabilization: the role of lipid lowering. *Int J Cardiol* 2000; 74 Suppl 1: S11–S15.
137. Aikawa M, Rabkin E, Okada Y, et al. Lipid lowering by diet reduces matrix metalloproteinase activity and increases collagen content of rabbit atheroma: a potential mechanism of lesion stabilization. *Circulation* 1998; 97: 2433–2444.
138. Aikawa M and Libby P. Lipid lowering reduces proteolytic and prothrombotic potential in rabbit atheroma. *Ann NY Acad Sci* 2000; 902: 140–152.
139. Aikawa M, Rabkin E, Sugiyama S, et al. An HMG-CoA reductase inhibitor, cerivastatin, suppresses growth of macrophages expressing matrix metalloproteinases and tissue factor *in vivo* and *in vitro*. *Circulation* 2001; 103: 276–283.
140. Fukumoto Y, Libby P, Rabkin E, et al. Statins alter smooth muscle cell accumulation and collagen content in established atheroma of Watanabe heritable hyperlipidemic rabbits. *Circulation* 2001; 103: 993–999.
141. Ameli S, Hultgardh-Nilsson A, Cercek B, et al. Recombinant apolipoprotein A-I Milano reduces intimal thickening after balloon injury in hypercholesterolemic rabbits. *Circulation* 1994; 90: 1935–1941.
142. Shah PK, Nilsson J, Kaul S, et al. Effects of recombinant apolipoprotein A-I (Milano) on aortic atherosclerosis in apolipoprotein E-deficient mice. *Circulation* 1998; 97: 780–785.
143. Shah PK, Yano J, Reyes O, et al. High-dose recombinant apolipoprotein A-I (Milano) mobilizes tissue cholesterol and rapidly reduces plaque lipid and macrophage content in apolipoprotein e-deficient mice: potential implications for acute plaque stabilization. *Circulation* 2001; 103: 3047–3050.
144. Crisby M, Nordin-Fredriksson G, Shah PK, Yano J, Zhu J, and Nilsson J. Pravastatin treatment increases collagen content and decreases lipid content, inflammation, metalloproteinases, and cell death in human carotid plaques: implications for plaque stabilization. *Circulation* 2001; 103: 926–933.
145. Shah PK, Kaul S, Nilsson J, and Cercek B. Exploiting the vascular protective effects of high-density lipoprotein and its apolipoproteins: an idea whose time for testing is coming, Part I. *Circulation* 2001; 104: 2376–2383.
146. Shah PK, Kaul S, Nilsson J, and Cercek B. Exploiting the vascular protective effects of high-density lipoprotein and its apolipoproteins: an idea whose time for testing is coming, Part II. *Circulation* 2001; 104: 2498–2502.
147. Claudel T, Leibowitz MD, Fievet C, et al. Reduction of atherosclerosis in apolipoprotein E knockout mice by activation of the retinoid X receptor. *Proc Natl Acad Sci USA* 2001; 98: 2610–2615.

2 Apoptosis and Plaque Vulnerability

Martin R. Bennett

CONTENTS

2.1 INTRODUCTION

The atherosclerotic plaque is composed largely of vascular smooth muscle cells (VSMCs), macrophages and T lymphocytes surrounding a lipid core.[1] Plaque rupture or erosion may lead to coronary artery occlusion resulting in myocardial infarction or, if repaired successfully, plaque growth. Work performed in the 1980s and 1990s identified a "typical" plaque associated with clinical events — the so-called vulnerable plaque.[2-4]

In general, plaques that rupture have low contents of VSMCs and high inflammatory cell contents, and they demonstrate apoptosis of both VSMCs and macrophages (see Walsh et al.[5]). The fibrous cap overlying the lipid-rich core is rich in VSMCs and loss of these cells at the plaque shoulders may contribute to rupture via loss of mechanical integrity. Consistent with this, increased VSMC apoptosis has been detected in unstable compared with stable angina lesions.[6] Apoptosis of vascular cells is also the basis for the generation of microparticles within the circulation that act as potent procoagulant substrates both locally and systemically.[7,8] These particles are increased in patients with unstable coronary disease, and account for the vast proportion of the pro-coagulant activity of the plaque. However, the majority of apoptotic cells at the site of rupture are macrophages,[9] implicating macrophage apoptosis in plaque rupture.

It is not clear whether loss of VSMCs or macrophages is the primary cause of rupture or whether VSMCs and macrophages act in concert to destabilize the plaque. In addition, the death of vascular endothelial cells is also seen downstream of the lesion and may contribute to both atherogenesis and progression of the athero-sclerotic lesion.[10] Thus, considerable circumstantial evidence implicates apoptosis of vascular cells in plaque rupture. More importantly, direct evidence of causality has recently emerged that, together with increasing knowledge of apoptosis regula-tion in the vasculature, may lead to novel therapies for improving plaque stability.[11]

2.2 EVIDENCE FOR APOPTOSIS IN THE VASCULATURE

Vascular smooth muscle cells within the vessel walls are able to proliferate, migrate, synthesize, and degrade extracellular matrices upon receiving appropriate stimuli. In undiseased walls, cells are parties to all the normal controls that govern cell proliferation and death, such as the presence of survival factors and mitogens, cell-to-cell contact inhibition, and cell–matrix interactions. The normal adult artery shows very low levels of VSMC turnover; thus apoptotic and mitotic indices are low in this tissue.[12]

In diseased tissue, additional factors are present both locally (e.g., inflammatory cytokines, inflammatory cells, and modified cholesterol) and systemically (e.g., blood pressure and blood flow). These factors can substantially alter the normal balance of cell proliferation and apoptosis, although the degree to which they are altered is dependent upon the vascular disease under study. Apoptosis of cells has been found in a variety of both physiological and disease states, including remod-elling, arterial injury, aneurysm formation, and atherosclerosis.

2.2.1 REMODELLING

Vessel wall remodelling is a condition in which alterations in luminal size can occur through processes that do not necessarily require large changes in overall cell number or tissue mass. Thus, redistribution of cells toward or away from the lumen through processes such as selective cell proliferation and apoptosis or matrix synthesis and degradation can significantly alter lumen dimensions. Physiological remodelling occurs in closure of the ductus arteriosus due to a reduction in blood flow[13] and reduction in lumen size of infra-umbilical arteries after birth.[14,15] Surgical reduction in flow also results in compensatory reduction in VSMC numbers by apoptosis.[16,17] Remodelling also occurs in primary atherosclerosis, after angioplasty and in angio-plasty restenosis. Although apoptosis undoubtedly occurs in all of these conditions (see below), the role of VSMC apoptosis in determining the outcome of remodelling is unclear.

A further example of vessel remodelling accompanied by VSMC apoptosis comes from studies examining both development and regression of vessel hypertrophy and hyperplasia in hypertension. Hypertension is associated with VSMC apoptosis in cells from SHR rats[18] and in SHR rats as hypertension develops.[19,20] In addition, relief of systemic or pulmonary hypertension results in apoptosis of VSMCs in the affected artery, with evidence that some antihypertensives are more potent than others.[20-22] In particular, angiotensin-converting enzyme inhibitors, angiotensin II receptor antagonists, and calcium channel blockers can also modify the contribution of apoptosis, independently of the blood pressure fall.[20,21]

2.2.2 ARTERIAL INJURY

Acute arterial injury, such as that occurring at angioplasty, is followed by rapid induction of medial cell apoptosis, at least in animal models. Thus, in rat or rabbit vessels, balloon over-stretch injury results in medial cell apoptosis from 30 min to 4 hr after injury.[23-25] In pigs, apoptotic cells appear within the media at 6 hr with peaks in the media, adventitia, and neointima at 6 hr, 18 hr, and 7 days after PTCA, respectively.[26]

Although we have no direct evidence, the consistency of this response in animal models suggests that human vessels may behave similarly. Repair of a vessel after injury is also associated with VSMC apoptosis, both in the media and in the intima, and in rats occurs 8 to 21 days after injury.[27] In humans, restenosis after angioplasty has been reported to be associated with either an increase[28] or decrease[29] in VSMC apoptosis. The role of VSMC apoptosis in the initial injury or the remodelling process in restenosis is still unclear in human vessels.

2.2.3 ANEURYSM FORMATION

The commonest form of arterial aneurysm in humans is associated with advanced atherosclerosis and is characterised by a loss of VSMCs from the vessel media, with fragmentation of elastin and matrix degradation, leading to progressive dilatation and eventually rupture. Apoptosis of VSMCs is increased in aortic aneurysms[30-32] compared with normal aorta and is associated with an increase in expression of a number of pro-apoptotic molecules such as death receptors and p53.[30,32] Macrophages and T lymphocytes are found in aneurysmal lesions, suggesting that inflammatory mediators released by these cells may increase the loss of cells from these areas. Moreover, the production of tissue metalloproteinases by macrophages may accelerate cell death by degrading the extracellular matrix from which VSMCs derive survival signals (see below).

2.2.4 ATHEROSCLEROSIS

Rupture of atherosclerotic plaques is associated with a thinning of the VSMC-rich fibrous cap overlying the core. Rupture occurs particularly at the shoulder regions of plaques, which are noted for their lack of VSMCs and the presence of macrophages and other inflammatory cells. Not surprisingly, apoptotic VSMCs are evident in advanced human plaques,[28,33,34] including the shoulder regions, prompting the suggestion that VSMC apoptosis may hasten plaque rupture. Indeed, there is evidence of increased VSMC apoptosis in unstable versus stable angina lesions.[29] However, there is no direct evidence of the effect of apoptosis per se in the advanced human lesion. Most apoptotic cells in histological sections are found in advanced lesions next to the lipid cores[35] and it is still not clear how many of these apoptotic cells are macrophages or VSMCs.

Loss of macrophages from atherosclerotic lesions is likely to promote plaque stability rather than rupture because macrophages can promote VSMC apoptosis by both direct interaction[36] and by release of cytokines.[37] Apoptosis also occurs in early stages of atherosclerosis induced by cholesterol feeding in animals, at the fatty streak stage, before morphological evidence of lesion formation appears.[38] Again, the effect of apoptosis at this early stage of lesion development is unknown.

2.3 EFFECT OF VSMC APOPTOSIS

The effect of VSMC apoptosis is clearly context-dependent. Thus, VSMC apoptosis in advanced atherosclerotic plaques would be expected to promote plaque rupture and medial atrophy in aneurysm formation. In neointima formation post-injury, VSMC apoptosis of both the intima and media can limit neointimal formation[24,25,39] at a defined time point (although long term studies have not been performed to ensure that the neointima is not simply delayed). It is not yet known whether such inhibition of neointimal formation by apoptosis in an animal model can translate into suppression of restenosis following angioplasty or stenting. However, the recent success of anti-proliferative therapy to inhibit restenosis after stenting suggests that this approach is feasible.

Therapeutic induction of apoptosis in the vessel wall may also be limited by important sequelae. In contrast to the prevailing notion that apoptotic deaths are effectively silent (that is, they do not elicit an immune response), a number of deleterious effects of apoptotic cells have emerged within the vasculature. First, the phosphatidylserine on the surfaces of apoptotic cells provides a potent substrate for the generation of thrombin and activation of the coagulation cascade.[40,41] Apoptotic cells release membrane-bound microparticles that remain pro-coagulant into the circulation; they are increased in patients with unstable versus stable coronary syndromes.[7,8]

Although apoptotic cells are not the only sources of circulating microparticles, such microparticles may contribute to the increased pro-coagulant state in these syndromes. Apoptotic VSMCs can also release both mitogens (bFGFs) and pro-inflammatory cytokines such as MCP-1 resulting in recruitment of monocytes,[42] both of which may abrogate any direct reduction in neointima formation. Indeed, in some studies, massive induction of apoptosis in intimal VSMCs may reduce cell density but not overall neointimal size or increase lumen dimensions.[42] The demonstration that apoptosis releases active molecules somewhat negates the idea of apoptosis as a "silent" mechanism of deleting cells. However, apoptotic cells that are not rapidly phagocytosed will begin to release inflammatory cytokines as they undergo secondary necrosis.

This release of inflammatory cytokines will result in the recruitment of mono-cytes and macrophages to the surrounding area. This may well occur to allow phagocytosis of a large number of apoptotic cells that cannot be efficiently disposed of by surrounding healthy smooth muscle cells.[43] In atherosclerosis, inefficient phagocytosis of dead cells may occur due to the presence of modified LDL, which hampers phagocytosis of apoptotic cells.[44] Thus, it may be that death is initially silent in atherosclerotic lesions but as cell corpses mount and professional phagocytes are impeded by modified LDL, more inflammatory cells maybe recruited. Moreover, soluble death ligands such as Fas-L are released from the surfaces of monocytes and macrophages as they phagocytose, resulting in bystander deaths of adjacent neutrophils or monocytes,[45] enhancing the deficit of professional phagocytic cells. Thus there exists the potential for the deaths and subsequent phagocytoses of apo-ptotic cells in atherosclerotic plaques to trigger further apoptosis, setting up a positive feedback loop.

2.4 MECHANISM OF APOPTOSIS IN THE VASCULATURE

The intracellular signalling pathways that regulate apoptosis have been elucidated in many cell types and very similar pathways exist in vascular cells (see Geng and Libby[1] and references therein). Basically two types of signalling pathways regulate cellular apoptosis (Figure 2.1 and Figure 2.2). First, binding of specific death ligands to their respective cell surface receptors activates many downstream pathways through the recruitment of adapter molecules. These adapter molecules recruit a cysteine protease (e.g., caspase-8) that in turn cleaves further caspases. The down-stream caspases are responsible for cleavage of various intracellular substrates and the activation of targets involved in DNA degradation (Figure 2.1).

A parallel pathway that does not require activation of cell surface death receptors is also present. This second pathway is dependent on the release of cytochrome C and other pro-apoptotic molecules (e.g., Smac/DIABLO) into the cytoplasm. The association of cytochrome C with an adapter molecule, Apaf1, and caspase-9 in the cytoplasm activates the latter that in turn activates downstream caspases (Figure 2.2). Although the intracellular triggers causing loss of mitochondrial integrity are varied and often difficult to identify, it is clear that the release of cytochrome C (and presumably other pro-apoptotic molecules) in response to these triggers is ultimately mediated by the relative expression and/or activity of members of the Bcl-2 family that regulate the permeability of the mitochondrial membrane. Although the "death receptor" and "mitochondrial" pathways are distinct, considerable cross-talk is exchanged between them. For example, activated caspase-8 in response to tumor necrosis factor alpha (TNF-) can cleave Bid (one of the Bcl-2 family members), thereby converting it into a pro-apoptotic molecule that can promote cytochrome C release. Nonetheless, this "mitochondrial amplification loop" is not always necessary since cytochrome C release is not always observed.[46]

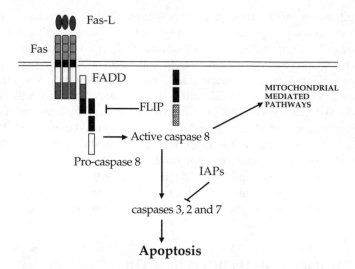

FIGURE 2.1 Fas death signalling pathways. Fas, the prototypic member of the tumor necrosis factor death receptor family, binds to its cognate ligand. Recruitment of the adapter molecule FADD and procaspase-8 results in activation of the latter. Caspase-8 activation directly activates downstream caspases (-3, -6, and -7) and results in DNA fragmentation and cleavage of cellular proteins. This pathway is thought to occur in type I cells and does not involve mitochondrial pathways. Caspase-8 activation also results in cleavage of Bid, which translocates and interacts with other Bcl-2 family members (see Figure 2.2).

2.5 APOPTOSIS OF VSMCs

VSMCs in normal vessel walls demonstrate little if any basal cell proliferation or apoptosis. However, in plaque tissue, additional factors such as the presence of inflammatory cells, cytokines, and modified low density lipoprotein (LDL) cholesterol may promote apoptosis. For example, VSMCs derived from plaque tissue exhibit both reduced proliferative capacity[47] and increased sensitivity to apoptosis[48] compared to cells from normal vessels. Moreover, neointimal VSMCs show increased apoptosis compared with medial cells.[49]

Evidence suggests that VSMC death *in vitro* can be triggered by interaction with inflammatory cells that express cell surface death ligands or secrete pro-apoptotic cytokines such as TNF-.[46,50,51] Moreover, exposure to altered lipid composition (e.g., predominantly oxidized LDL) and external mechanical stress (e.g., shear stress or nitric oxide as a result of alterations in blood flow) can also trigger the deaths of these cells.[52–56] Activation of receptors other than those of the death receptor superfamily can also affect VSMC apoptosis. For example, mice that lack the neurotrophin receptor (p75 NTR) demonstrate changes in the regulation of apoptosis following ligation of the left carotid artery. p75 NTR-deficient mice exhibit decreased apoptosis in neointimal smooth muscle cells and three- to fourfold increased development of stenosis when compared with wild type animals.[57] Thus, apoptosis regulated via p75 NTR may suppress neointima formation in this model.

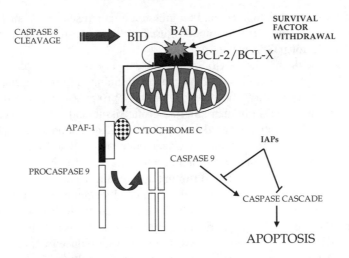

FIGURE 2.2 Mitochondrial death signalling pathways. Anti-apoptotic members of the Bcl-2 family, such as Bcl-2 and Bcl-X are located on the mitochondrial outer membranes where they act to prevent the release of apoptogenic factors from the inner mitochondrial space. Binding of the pro-apoptotic proteins Bid (after cleavage by caspase-8) or Bad (after dephosphorylation) to Bcl-2 mitigates the protective effect of Bcl-2 and triggers release of cytochrome C. Cytochrome C, in concert with the adapter protein apaf-1 and caspase-9, activates caspase-3 and the downstream caspase cascade. Stimuli such as growth factor withdrawal, deregulated oncogene (c-*myc*, E1A) expression, activation of p53, and Fas activation in type II cells act through this mitochondrial pathway.

A recurrent theme in apoptosis regulation is the coupling of apoptosis and control of cell proliferation. For example, activation of the angiotensin II type 2 receptor (AT2) exerts anti-proliferative and pro-apoptotic effects on VSMCs during neointimal formation after vascular injuries in mice.[58,59] Thus, AT2-deficient mice exhibit increased DNA synthesis and neointimal formation, suggesting that the AT2 receptor normally functions to repress VSMC proliferation.[58] In contrast, AT1 knockout animals exhibit decreased neointima formation after injury.

These results are consistent with *in vitro* studies, indicating that angiotensin II type 1 (AT1) and type 2 (AT2) receptors exert opposite effects on vasoconstriction, natriuresis, and proliferation. Furthermore, reverse transcriptase polymerase chain reaction (RT-PCR) and immunohistochemical data suggest that AT1 and AT2 exert different effects on the expression of Bax, Bcl2, and Bcl-X_L, which may explain their contrasting effects on VSMCs.[58] Despite a lack of direct evidence for the release of cytochrome C, these data suggest that AT2 activation promotes cell death via effects on the mitochondrial-mediated pathway of apoptosis.

The release of cytochrome C from mitochondria is also implicated in apoptosis of VSMCs in response to oxidized LDL (OxLDL), mechanical stress, reactive oxygen species, and reduction in the local concentration of survival factors [notably insulin-like growth factor-1 (IGF-1)].[48,60–62] Regulation of cytochrome C release is influenced by the tumor suppressor gene p53 in response to stress and DNA damage (for example, elicited by reactive oxygen species[55]). Elevated p53 expression has been linked with the development and progression of atherosclerotic lesions. Indeed, the sensitivity of plaque-derived smooth muscle cells to p53-induced apoptosis has suggested a role for p53 in plaque rupture.[63]

Consistent with this, adenoviral-mediated delivery of ectopic p53 to smooth muscle cell-rich plaque caps resulted in a marked thinning of the cap, a characteristic feature of plaque instability, and plaque rupture.[64,65] Expression of the p73 related protein is also increased in human atherosclerotic tissue and ectopic expression in VSMCs *in vitro* results in decreased cell cycle transit and apoptosis independent of p53.[66] These studies represent an important concept — that local induction of apoptosis may reduce neointima formation after injury, but may promote ultimate atherosclerotic plaque growth due to rupture and repair of plaques.

VSMC apoptosis *in vitro* is negatively regulated by a number of survival factors including IGF-1 and platelet-derived growth factor (PDGF). IGF-1 protects VSMCs by activation of the PI3 kinase–pyruvate dehydrogenase kinase (PDK)–Akt/protein kinase B (PKB) pathway. Plaque VSMCs demonstrate reduced expression of cell surface IGF-1 receptor and intracellular signalling,[48,60] resulting in defective IGF-1-mediated survival. In contrast, the protective effect of PDGF-AB appears to be mediated by survivin,[67] a member of the inhibitor-of-apoptosis (IAP) family. However, PDGF-AB-dependent survival is limited to proliferating VSMCs *in vitro*. Since VSMCs in the advanced plaques are non-proliferating, PDGF-AB-mediated survival may only be significant in neointimal formation rather than plaque rupture, even though expression of survivin persists in the neointimas of injured vessels.[67]

Finally, gene array technology has identified expression profiles of apoptosis-related genes in human atherosclerosis.[68] Consistent with other observations, TNFRII, caspase-1 and Bax are all up-regulated (approximately threefold) in carotid endarterectomy specimens compared with non-atherosclerotic mammary arteries. The largest increase was in the expression of death-associated protein (DAP) kinase, which participates in IFN-, TNF-, and Fas-induced death. Immunohistochemical analysis indicates that DAP kinase expression is located primarily in foam cells of smooth muscle cell origin.[68] Consistent with other data,[48,60] IGF-1R is down-regulated in plaque cells. While many of the usual apoptosis-regulating proteins were identified, this technology will undoubtedly play a major role in identifying candidate targets for therapeutic intervention.

2.6   APOPTOSIS OF MACROPHAGES

Although apoptotic macrophages are frequently observed in atherosclerotic lesions, notably at the sites of plaque ruptures,[9] the factors that regulate the deaths of macrophages within lesions are unknown. A number of *in vitro* studies have implicated cytokines in the activation and apoptosis of macrophages, the major players appearing to be oxidized lipids and inflammatory cytokines. Altered LDLs (e.g., oxidized forms) are able to induce apoptosis in all the major cell types present in the lesions[69–71] (reviewed in Salvayre et al.[61]).

Experimental models of atherosclerosis implicate oxidative DNA damage (which promotes apoptosis) as the pathway through which OxLDL exerts its pro-apoptotic effect, and this effect is reversed by lipid lowering.[55] In addition, IFN-γ, a cytokine secreted by T helper lymphocytes, induces THP-1 macrophages *in vitro* to generate monocyte chemoattractant protein (MCP-1) and undergo apoptosis.[72] The ability of antibodies to TNF-α to inhibit IFN-γ-induced macrophage apoptosis suggests that autocrine or paracrine TNF-α released or displayed on macrophages or surrounding VSMCs may have a role to play. In addition, macrophage survival depends upon expression and activation of protective proteins. For example, monocytes differentiating to macrophages up-regulate FLIP, an inhibitor of caspase-8 activation[73] and are also dependent upon Akt and Mcl-1 for their survival.[74]

2.7 APOPTOSIS OF ENDOTHELIAL CELLS

Apoptosis of endothelial cells within atherosclerotic lesions may also contribute to plaque instability. Recent data demonstrate that serum from patients with acute coronary syndromes increases apoptosis of human umbilical vein endothelial cells (HUVECs) *in vitro* compared to serum from patients with stable angina or healthy individuals, respectively.[75] This suggests the existence of circulating apoptotic triggers of endothelial cell death. Serum levels of TNF-α, its soluble receptors (sTNFR-I and sTNFR-II), IL-6, and the IL-1 receptor (IL-1Ra) are all elevated in patients with acute coronary syndromes. However, pre-incubation of the serum with antibodies to TNF-α and IL-6 had no effect, suggesting that the pro-apoptotic effect of these sera on HUVECs is not mediated by these agents.

Like TNF-α, FasL and TGF-β are also released by inflammatory cells at the sites of lesions. Although no data were available on the levels and effect of FasL or TGF-β in the sera used in this study, evidence implicates both FasL and TGF-β in apoptosis of vascular endothelial cells.[76,77] For example, adenovirus-mediated overexpression of soluble Fas (sFas) which blocks the Fas–FasL interaction by sequestering FasL can inhibit monocyte-induced apoptosis of vascular endothelial cells *in vitro*.[76] The authors also showed that sFas expression suppresses intimal formation and inhibits apoptosis in a rat aortic allograft model, suggesting that Fas-mediated apoptosis of vascular cells may promote graft disease. This also raises the possibility that FasL may act as a proliferative stimulus for vascular cells in certain circumstances.

A similar role for FasL has been reported in other cell types.[78,79] In addition, others have demonstrated an OxLDL-dependent trafficking of Fas to the cell surface.[71] In contrast, both TGF- and lysophosphatidylcholine (a specific component of OxLDL)-induced apoptosis of HUVECs may be mediated primarily by the p38 mitogen-activated protein kinase (MAPK) pathway[77,80] rather than via Fas.

In addition to the effects of pro-apoptotic cytokines, endothelial cell apoptosis is determined by the expression of protective cytokines. For example, hepatocyte growth factor (HGF) exhibits a potent anti-apoptotic effect on HUVECs *in vitro* and HGF localizes within atherosclerotic lesions in humans.[81] Clearly, the death or survival of these cells is governed by the net signalling from a complex combination of pro- and anti-apoptotic molecules.

2.8 SUICIDE OR MURDER?

While cell death is apparent in all the major types of cells within atherosclerotic lesions, the contributions of apoptosis of different cell types to the progression of the lesions are unclear. In addition to uncertainties about the role of vascular cell apoptosis, the triggers for death of each cell type are mostly unknown. Macrophages, vascular smooth muscle cells, and endothelial cells all undergo apoptosis in response to certain extracellular factors.

Many of these factors, their effects on different cell types *in vitro*, and their presence in lesions have been characterized in recent years. However, it has proven difficult to establish which factors are important in the complex lesions present *in vivo*, not least because the sources of these factors, both pro- and anti-apoptotic, are often the very same cells. Although growth factors and cytokines regulate apoptosis, *in vivo* the major inducers of apoptosis are likely to be oxidized lipids. Altered LDLs (e.g., oxidized forms) are able to induce apoptosis in all the major cell types present in the lesions[69–71] (reviewed in Salvayre et al.[61]). In addition, lipids induce monocytes and macrophages to express death ligands and secrete cytokines that induce local VSMC and EC apoptosis.[50]

Membrane vesicles from ECs also contain oxidized lipids that can stimulate ECs to specifically bind monocytes,[82] further promoting monocyte recruitment and subsequent lipid oxidation. In advanced atherosclerosis, macrophages also accumulate large amounts of unesterified cholesterol that lead to a failure of lipid homeostasis.[83,84] The reduction in cholesterol and phospholipid efflux as a result of downregulation of the ABCA1 adenosine triphosphate (ATP)-binding cassette transporter[84] ultimately leads to a breakdown of membrane integrity and cell death. Intriguingly, expression of the short, anti-apoptotic isoform of caspase-2 has been detected specifically in macrophage foam cells located around the necrotic cores of advanced human atherosclerotic plaques,[85] suggesting that distinct populations of macrophages within the lesions may undergo apoptosis. Nonetheless, lipid-induced death of macrophage-derived foam cells is likely to be a major source of pro-inflammatory molecules.

The complex interactions between macrophages, vascular smooth muscle cells, and endothelial cells suggest a coordinated apoptotic response to vascular injury. Coordinated apoptosis may be the result of a "suicide pact" (individual cell types regulate their own demises) in response to a single stimulus (e.g., oxidized lipids) or murder akin to mutually assured destruction (one cell type destroys another) or, more likely, a combination of both. Whatever the trigger, apoptosis promotes ongoing inflammation, calcification, thrombosis, and plaque rupture, the major sequelae of advanced atherosclerosis.

2.9 CONCLUSIONS

Apoptosis is a central process in advanced atherosclerosis, present in all cellular compartments, and good experimental evidence has identified the triggers that induce apoptosis in plaques. Since many of these experiments are based on *in vitro* models it is, however, dangerous to extrapolate the observations to the disease process *in vivo*.

In contrast, recent work has shown that VSMC apoptosis can trigger plaque rupture in animal models of advanced atherosclerosis. We are now entering the phase where we can dissect the intracellular pathways regulating apoptosis *in vivo* in animal models with the aim of experimentally (and perhaps ultimately, therapeutically) manipulating these events.

ACKNOWLEDGMENTS

MRB is supported by a British Heart Foundation Professorship grant.

REFERENCES

1. Geng YJ and Libby P. Progression of atheroma: a struggle between death and pro-creation. *Arterioscler Thromb Vasc Biol* 2002, 22: 1370–1380.
2. Davies MJ. Anatomic features in victims of sudden coronary death: coronary artery pathology. *Circulation* 1992, 85 (1 Suppl): 119–124.
3. Davies MJ, Richardson PD, Woolf N, Katz DR, and Mann J. Risk of thrombosis in human atherosclerotic plaques: role of extracellular lipid, macrophage, and smooth-muscle cell content. *Br Heart J* 1993, 69: 377–381.
4. Davies MJ. Acute coronary-thrombosis: the role of plaque disruption and its initiation and prevention. *Eur Heart J* 1995, 16: 3–7.
5. Walsh K, Smith RC, and Kim HS. Vascular cell apoptosis in remodeling, restenosis, and plaque rupture. *Circ Res* 2000, 87: 184–188.
6. Bauriedel G, Hutter R, Welsch U, Bach R, Sievert H, and Luderitz B. Role of smooth muscle cell death in advanced coronary primary lesions: implications for plaque instability. *Cardiovasc Res* 1999, 41: 480–488.
7. Mallat Z, Hugel B, Ohan J, Leseche G, Freyssinet JM, and Tedgui A. Shed membrane microparticles with procoagulant potential in human atherosclerotic plaques: a role for apoptosis in plaque thrombogenicity. *Circulation* 1999, 99: 348–353.
8. Mallat Z, Benamer H, Hugel B, Benessiano P, Steg P, Freyssinet J, and Tedgui A. Elevated levels of shed membrane microparticles with procoagulant potential in the peripheral circulating blood of patients with acute coronary syndromes. *Circulation* 2000, 101: 841–843.
9. Kolodgie FD, Narula J, Burke AP, Haider N, Farb A, Hui-Liang Y, Smialek J, and Virmani R. Localization of apoptotic macrophages at the site of plaque rupture in sudden coronary death. *Am J Pathol* 2000, 157: 1259–1268.
10. Tricot O, Mallat Z, Heymes C, Belmin J, Leseche G, and Tedgui A. Relation between endothelial cell apoptosis and blood flow direction in human atherosclerotic plaques. *Circulation* 2000, 101: 2450–2453.
11. Libby P. Inflammation in atherosclerosis. *Nature* 2002, 420: 868–874.
12. Gordon D, Reidy MA, Benditt EP, and Schwartz SM. Cell proliferation in human coronary arteries. *Proc Natl Acad Sci USA* 1990, 87: 4600–4604.
13. Slomp J, GittenbergerdeGroot AC, Glukhova MA, vanMunsteren JC, Kockx MM, Schwartz SM, and Koteliansky VE. Differentiation, dedifferentiation, and apoptosis of smooth muscle cells during the development of the human ductus arteriosus. *Arterioscler Thromb Vasc Biol* 1997, 17: 1003–1009.
14. Cho A and Langille BL. Arterial smooth-muscle cell turnover during the postnatal period in lambs. *FASEB J* 1993, 7: A756–A766.

15. Cho A, Courtman D, and Langille L. Apoptosis (programmed cell death) in arteries of the neonatal lamb. *Circ Res* 1995, 76: 168–175.

16. Cho A, Mitchell L, Koopmans D, and Langille BL. Effects of changes in blood flow rate on cell death and cell proliferation in carotid arteries of immature rabbits. *Circ Res* 1997, 81: 328–337.

17. Kumar A and Lindner V. Remodeling with neointima formation in the mouse carotid artery after cessation of blood flow. *Arterioscler Thromb Vasc Biol* 1997, 17: 2238–2244.

18. Vega F, Panizo A, Toledo G, Diaz L, Diez J, and Pardo-Mindan FJ. Susceptibility to apoptosis of vascular smooth muscle cells of adult spontaneously hypertensive rats. *Lab Invest* 1998, 78: 187–197.

19. Hamet P, Richard L, Dam T, Teiger E, Orlov S, Gaboury L, Gossard F, and Tremblay J. Apoptosis in target organs of hypertension. *Hypertension* 1995, 26: 642–648.

20. Sharifi AM, Schiffrin EL, Iwashina M, Shichiri M, Marumo F, and Hirata Y. Apoptosis in vasculature of spontaneously hypertensive rats: effect of an angiotensin-converting enzyme inhibitor and a calcium channel antagonist: transfection of inducible nitric oxide synthase gene causes apoptosis in vascular smooth muscle cells. *Am J Hypertension* 1998, 11: 1108–1116.

21. deBlois D, Tea BS, Dam TV, Tremblay J, and Hamet P. Smooth muscle apoptosis during vascular regression in spontaneously hypertensive rats. *Hypertension* 1997, 29: 340–349.

22. Cowan KN, Jones PL, and Rabinovitch M. Serine elastase and matrix metalloproteinase (MMP) inhibition induces pulmonary artery (PA) smooth muscle cell (SMC) apoptosis leading to regression of vascular hypertrophy. *Mol Biol Cell* 1997, 8: 1661–1671.

23. Perlman H, Maillard L, Krasinski K, and Walsh K. Evidence for the rapid onset of apoptosis in medial smooth muscle cells after balloon injury. *Circulation* 1997, 95: 981–987.

24. Pollman MJ, Hall JL, Mann MJ, Zhang LN, and Gibbons GH. Inhibition of neointimal cell bcl-x expression induces apoptosis and regression of vascular disease. *Nat Med* 1998, 4: 222–227.

25. Pollman MJ, Hall JL, and Gibbons GH. Determinants of vascular smooth muscle cell apoptosis after balloon angioplasty injury: influence of redox state and cell phenotype. *Circ Res* 1999, 84: 113–121.

26. Malik N, Francis SE, Holt CM, Gunn J, Thomas GL, Shepherd L, Chamberlain J, Newman CMH, Cumberland DC, and Crossman DC. Apoptosis and cell proliferation after porcine coronary angioplasty. *Circulation* 1998, 98: 1657–1665.

27. Bochatonpiallat M, Gabbiani F, Redard M, Desmouliere A, and Gabbiani G. Apoptosis participates in cellularity regulation during rat aortic intimal thickening. *Am J Path* 1995, 146: 1059–1064.

28. Isner J, Kearney M, Bortman S, and Passeri J. Apoptosis in human atherosclerosis and restenosis. *Circulation* 1995, 91: 2703–2711.

29. Bauriedel G, Schluckebier S, Hutter R, Welsch U, Kandoff R, Lüderitz B, and Prescott M. Apoptosis in restenosis versus stable-angina atherosclerosis. *Arterioscler Thromb Vasc Biol* 1998, 18: 1132–1139.

30. Lopez-Candales A, Holmes DR, Liao SX, Scott MJ, Wickline SA, and Thompson RW. Decreased vascular smooth muscle cell density in medial degeneration of human abdominal aortic aneurysms. *Am J Pathol* 1997, 150: 993–1007.

31. Thompson RW, Liao SX, and Curci JA. Vascular smooth muscle cell apoptosis in abdominal aortic aneurysms. *Cor Art Dis* 1997, 8: 623–631.

32. Henderson EL, Gang YJ, Sukhova GK, Whittemore AD, Knox J, and Libby P. Death of smooth muscle cells and expression of mediators of apoptosis by T lymphocytes in human abdominal aortic aneurysms. *Circulation* 1999, 99: 96–104.

33. Han D, Haudenschild C, Hong M, Tinkle B, Leon M, and Liau G. Evidence for apoptosis in human atherosclerosis and in a rat vascular injury model. *Am J Pathol* 1995, 147: 267–277.

34. Geng Y and Libby P. Evidence for apoptosis in advanced human atheroma: colocalization with interleukin-1b converting enzyme. *Am J Pathol* 1995, 147: 251–266.

35. Kockx MM. Apoptosis in the atherosclerotic plaque: quantitative and qualitative aspects. *Arterioscler Thromb Vasc Biol* 1998, 18: 1519–1522.

36. Boyle J, Bowyer D, Weissberg P, and Bennett M. Human blood-derived macrophages induce apoptosis in human plaque-derived vascular smooth muscle cells by Fas ligand/Fas interactions. *Art Thromb Vasc Biol* 2001, 21: 1402–1407.

37. Boyle JJ, Weissberg PL, and Bennett MR. Human macrophage-induced vascular smooth muscle cell apoptosis requires NO enhancement of Fas/Fas-L interactions. *Arterioscler Thromb Vasc Biol* 2002, 22: 1624–1630.

38. Hasdai D, Sangiorgi G, Spagnoli L, Simari R, Holmes Jr D, Kwon H, Carlson P, Schwartz R, and Lerman A. Coronary artery apoptosis in experimental hypercholesterolaemia. *Atherosclerosis* 1999, 142: 317–325.

39. Sata M, Perlman HR, Muruve DA, Silver M, Ikebe M, Libermann TA, Oettgen P, and Walsh K. Fas ligand gene transfer to the vessel wall inhibits neointima formation and overrides the adenovirus-mediated T cell response. *Proc Natl Acad Sci USA* 1998, 95: 1213–1217.

40. Flynn P, Byrne C, Baglin T, Weissberg P, and Bennett M. Thrombin generation by apoptotic vascular smooth muscle cells. *Blood* 1997, 89: 4373–4384.

41. Bombeli T, Karsan A, Tait JF, and Harlan JM. Apoptotic vascular endothelial cells become procoagulant. *Blood* 1997, 89: 2429–2442.

42. Schaub FJ, Han DK, Conrad Liles W, Adams LD, Coats SA, Ramachandran RK, Seifert RA, Schwartz SM, and Bowen-Pope DF. Fas/FADD-mediated activation of a specific program of inflammatory gene expression in vascular smooth muscle cells. *Nat Med* 2000, 6: 790–796.

43. Savill J. Recognition and phagocytosis of cells undergoing apoptosis. *Br Med Bull* 1997, 53: 491–508.

44. Sambrano GR and Steinberg D. Recognition of oxidatively damaged and apoptotic cells by an oxidised low density lipoprotein receptor on mouse peritoneal macrophages: role of membrane phosphatidylserine. *Proc Natl Acad Sci USA* 1995, 92: 1396–1400.

45. Brown SB and Savill J. Phagocytosis triggers macrophage release of Fas ligand and induces apoptosis of bystander leukocytes. *J Immunol* 1999, 162: 480–485.

46. Kim HH and Kim K. Enhancement of TNF-alpha-mediated cell death in vascular smooth muscle cells through cytochrome C-independent pathway by the proteasome inhibitor. *FEBS Lett* 2003, 535: 190–194.

47. O'Sullivan M, Scott S, McCarthy N, Shapiro LM, and Kirkpatrick PJ, and Bennett, MR. Differential cyclin E expression in human in stent stenosis vascular smooth muscle cells identifies targets for selective anti-restenotic therapy. *Cardiovasc Res* 2003, 60: 673–683.

48. Patel VA, Zhang QJ, Siddle K, Soos MA, Goddard M, Weissberg PL, and Bennett MR. Defect in insulin-like growth factor-1 survival mechanism in atherosclerotic plaque-derived vascular smooth muscle cells is mediated by reduced surface binding and signaling. *Circ Res* 2001, 88: 895–902.

49. Niemann-Jonsson A, Ares MP, Yan ZQ, Bu DX, Fredrikson GN, Branen L, Porn-Ares I, Nilsson AH, and Nilsson J. Increased rate of apoptosis in intimal arterial smooth muscle cells through endogenous activation of TNF receptors. *Arterioscler Thromb Vasc Biol* 2001, 21: 1909–1914.

50. Boyle J, Weissberg P, and Bennett M. Tumour necrosis factor promotes macrophage-induced vascular smooth muscle cell apoptosis by direct and autocrine mechanisms. *Arterioscl Thromb Vasc Biol* 2003, 23: 1553–1558.

51. Seshiah PN, Kereiakes DJ, Vasudevan SS, Lopes N, Su BY, Flavahan NA, and Goldschmidt-Clermont PJ. Activated monocytes induce smooth muscle cell death: role of macrophage colony-stimulating factor and cell contact. *Circulation* 2002, 105: 174–180.

52. Taguchi S, Oinuma T, and Yamada T. A comparative study of cultured smooth muscle cell proliferation and injury, utilizing glycated low density lipoproteins with slight oxidation, auto-oxidation, or extensive oxidation. *J Atheroscler Thromb* 2000, 7: 132–137.

53. Mayr M and Xu Q. Smooth muscle cell apoptosis in arteriosclerosis. *Exp Gerontol* 2001, 36: 969–987.

54. Kataoka H, Kume N, Miyamoto S, Minami M, Morimoto M, Hayashida K, Hashimoto N, and Kita T. Oxidized LDL modulates Bax/Bcl-2 through the lectinlike Ox-LDL receptor-1 in vascular smooth muscle cells. *Arterioscler Thromb Vasc Biol* 2001, 21: 955–960.

55. Martinet W, Knaapen MW, De Meyer GR, Herman AG, and Kockx MM. Oxidative DNA damage and repair in experimental atherosclerosis are reversed by dietary lipid lowering. *Circ Res* 2001, 88: 733–739.

56. Berceli SA, Davies MG, Kenagy RD, and Clowes AW. Flow-induced neointimal regression in baboon polytetrafluoroethylene grafts is associated with decreased cell proliferation and increased apoptosis. *J Vasc Surg* 2002, 36: 1248–1255.

57. Kraemer R. Reduced apoptosis and increased lesion development in the flow-restricted carotid artery of p75(NTR)-null mutant mice. *Circ Res* 2002, 91: 494–500.

58. Suzuki J, Iwai M, Nakagami H, Wu L, Chen R, Sugaya T, Hamada M, Hiwada K, and Horiuchi M. Role of angiotensin II-regulated apoptosis through distinct AT1 and AT2 receptors in neointimal formation. *Circulation* 2002, 106: 847–853.

59. Henrion D, Kubis N, and Levy BI. Physiological and pathophysiological functions of the AT(2) subtype receptor of angiotensin II: from large arteries to the microcirculation. *Hypertension* 2001, 38: 1150–1157.

60. Okura Y, Brink M, Zahid AA, Anwar A, and Delafontaine P. Decreased expression of insulin-like growth factor-1 and apoptosis of vascular smooth muscle cells in human atherosclerotic plaque. *J Mol Cell Cardiol* 2001, 33: 1777–1789.

61. Salvayre R, Auge N, Benoist H, and Negre-Salvayre A. Oxidized low-density lipoprotein-induced apoptosis. *Biochim Biophys Acta* 2002, 1585: 213–221.

62. Olinski R, Gackowski D, and Foksinski MEA. Oxidative DNA damage: assessment of the role in carcinogenesis, atherosclerosis and acquired immune deficiency syndrome. *Free Radical Biol Med* 2002, 33: 192–200.

63. Bennett MR, Littlewood TD, Schwartz SM, and Weissberg PL. Increased sensitivity of human vascular smooth muscle cells from atherosclerotic plaque to p53-mediated apoptosis. *Circ Res* 1997, 81: 591–599.

64. von der Thusen JH, van Vlijmen BJ, Hoeben RC, Kockx MM, Havekes LM, van Berkel TJ, and Biessen EA. Induction of atherosclerotic plaque rupture in apolipoprotein E–/– mice after adenovirus-mediated transfer of p53. *Circulation* 2002, 105: 2064–2070.

65. Majesky MW. Mouse model for atherosclerotic plaque rupture. *Circulation* 2002, 105: 2010–2011.
66. Davis BB, Dong Y, and Weiss RH. Overexpression of p73 causes apoptosis in vascular smooth muscle cells. *Am J Physiol Cell Physiol* 2003, 284: C16–C23.
67. Blanc-Brude OP, Yu J, Simosa H, Conte MS, Sessa WC, and Altieri DC. Inhibitor of apoptosis protein survivin regulates vascular injury. *Nat Med* 2002, 8: 987–994.
68. Martinet W, Schrijvers DM, De Meyer GR, Thielemans J, Knaapen MW, Herman AG, and Kockx MM. Gene expression profiling of apoptosis-related genes in human atherosclerosis: upregulation of death-associated protein kinase. *Arterioscler Thromb Vasc Biol* 2002, 22: 2023–2029.
69. Li DY, Chen HJ, Staples ED, Ozaki K, Annex B, Singh BK, Vermani R, and Mehta JL. Oxidized low-density lipoprotein receptor LOX-1 and apoptosis in human atherosclerotic lesions. *J Cardiovasc Pharmacol Ther* 2002, 7: 147–153.
70. Kontush A, Chancharme L, Escargueil-Blanc I, Therond P, Salvayre R, Negre-Salvayre A, and Chapman MJ. Mildly oxidized LDL particle subspecies are distinct in their capacity to induce apoptosis in endothelial cells: role of lipid hydroperoxides. *FASEB J* 2003, 17: 88–90.
71. Imanishi T, Han DK, Hofstra L, Hano T, Nishio I, Conrad Liles W, Gown AM, Schwartz SM, and Gorden AM. Apoptosis of vascular smooth muscle cells is induced by Fas ligand derived from monocytes/macrophage. *Atherosclerosis* 2002, 161: 143–151.
72. Inagaki Y, Yamagishi S, Amano S, Okamoto T, Koga K, and Makita Z. Interferon-gamma-induced apoptosis and activation of THP-1 macrophages. *Life Sci* 2002, 71: 2499–2508.
73. Perlman H, Pagliari L, Georganas C, Mano T, Walsh K, and Pope R. FLICE-inhibitory protein expression during macrophage differentiation confers resistance to Fas-mediated apoptosis. *J Exp Med* 1999, 190: 1679–1688.
74. Liu H, Perlman H, Pagliari LJ, and Pope RM. Constitutively activated Akt-1 is vital for the survival of human monocyte-differentiated macrophages: role of Mcl-1, independent of nuclear factor (NF)-kappaB, Bad, or caspase activation. *J Exp Med* 2001, 194: 113–126.
75. Valgimigli M, Agnoletti L, Curello S, et al. Serum from patients with acute coronary syndromes displays a proapoptotic effect on human endothelial cells: a possible link to pan-coronary syndromes. *Circulation* 2003, 107: 264–270.
76. Wang T, Dong C, Stevenson SC, Herderick EE, Marshall-Neff J, Vasudevan SS, Moldovan NI, Michler RE, Movva NR, and Goldschmidt-Clermont PJ. Overexpression of soluble Fas attenuates transplant arteriosclerosis in rat aortic allografts. *Circulation* 2002, 106: 1536–1542.
77. Hyman KM, Seghezzi G, Pintucci G, Stellari G, Kim JH, Grossi EA, Galloway AC, and Mignatti P. Transforming growth factor-beta1 induces apoptosis in vascular endothelial cells by activation of mitogen-activated protein kinase. *Surgery* 2002, 132: 173–179.
78. Hua ZC, Sohn SJ, Kang C, Cado D, and Winoto A. A function of Fas-associated death domain protein in cell cycle progression localized to a single amino acid at its C-terminal region. *Immunity* 2003, 18: 513–521.
79. Freiberg RA, Spencer DM, Choate KA, Duh HJ, Schreiber SL, Crabtree GR, and Khavari PA. Fas signal transduction triggers either proliferation or apoptosis in human fibroblasts. *J Invest Dermatol* 1997, 108: 215–219.

80. Takahashi M, Okazaki H, Ogata Y, Takeuchi K, Ikeda U, and Shimada K. Lysophos-phatidylcholine induces apoptosis in human endothelial cells through a p38-mitogen-activated protein kinase-dependent mechanism. *Atherosclerosis* 2002, 161: 387–394.

81. Ma H, Calderon TM, Fallon JT, and Berman JW. Hepatocyte growth factor is a survival factor for endothelial cells and is expressed in human atherosclerotic plaques. *Atherosclerosis* 2002, 164: 79–87.

82. Huber J, Vales A, Mitulovic G, Blumer M, Schmid R, Witztum JL, Binder BR, and Leitinger N. Oxidized membrane vesicles and blebs from apoptotic cells contain biologically active oxidized phospholipids that induce monocyte-endothelial interactions. *Arterioscler Thromb Vasc Biol* 2002, 22: 101–107.

83. Schmitz G and Kaminski WE. ATP-binding cassette (ABC) transporters in athero-sclerosis. *Curr Atheroscler Rep* 2002, 4: 243–251.

84. Feng B and Tabas I. ABCA1-mediated cholesterol efflux is defective in free choles-terol-loaded macrophages: mechanism involves enhanced ABCA1 degradation in a process requiring full NPC1 activity. *J Biol Chem* 2002, 277: 43271–43280.

85. Martinet W, Knaapen MW, De Meyer GR, Herman AG, and Kockx MM. Overexpres-sion of the anti-apoptotic caspase-2 short isoform in macrophage-derived foam cells of human atherosclerotic plaques. *Am J Pathol* 2003, 162: 731–736.

3 Animal Models of Vulnerable Plaque

Harry C. Lowe, Levon M. Khachigian,
Leonard Kritharides, and Jason L. Johnson

CONTENTS

3.1 INTRODUCTION

Atherosclerotic cardiovascular disease remains the leading cause of death in the industrialized world. Most deaths are the results of acute coronary syndromes including unstable angina pectoris, acute myocardial infarction, and sudden death.[1-4] Coronary syndromes are largely the results of acute coronary thrombosis, itself most commonly the result of disruption or rupture of the fibrous cap of a lipid-laden — so called vulnerable — atherosclerotic plaque.[3,5,6] Despite the prevalence of atherosclerotic disease, we have no established animal models of vulnerable plaque (VP) and plaque rupture. Whilst animal models have provided key insights into the processes of restenosis, atherosclerosis development, and myocardial ischemia, models of VP have only recently been proposed.[7]

A wide variety of models are presently under development in a number of animal species — an indication that no model developed to date is entirely optimal. The following analysis, therefore, first discusses the terminology and definitions of VP and relevant clinical aspects. The animal models of VP are then discussed in relation to what is becoming a dynamic area of change in cardiovascular investigation.

3.2 DEFINITIONS OF VULNERABLE PLAQUE AND PLAQUE RUPTURE

Originally proposed in 1992,[8] the term *vulnerable plaque* (VP) was redefined as any atherosclerotic lesion subsequently resulting in coronary thrombosis.[9] Three principal types of VP have been described.[9] The most common type is thin cap fibroatheroma, an eccentric lesion composed of a lipid-rich core with a thin (<65 μm) fibrous cap and macrophage infiltration (>25 macrophages per 0.3 mm diameter microscope field).[10] Plaque rupture is defined as fibrous cap disruption whereby the overlying thrombus is in continuity with the lipid core.[11] This overlying thrombus may then lead to luminal thrombus extension.[9,11] This definition distinguishes plaque rupture from intraplaque hemorrhage, which may occur independently of plaque rupture and is defined simply as the deposition of blood products within plaque by whatever means.[12,13] While these differences in definition may appear subtle, they have clear implications as to pathogenesis, and become important in describing and understanding proposed animal models.

Two other types of VP are described pathologically: eroded plaques and calcified nodules.[9] Plaque erosion is defined when a thrombosed artery fails to show evidence of rupture and the endothelium is absent at the site of erosion.[2] The calcified nodule is typified by a predominantly fibrotic lesion with superficial calcification.[11] These superficial calcifications may have the appearance of nodules and may form the nidus for thrombus formation.[11] In the setting of acute myocardial infarction (AMI), 70 to 80% of coronary thrombi are associated with plaque rupture, and 20 to 30% with plaque erosion or calcified nodules.[2,9,14] However, since little is known of the pathogenesis of these two lesions, they are not discussed further. In the discussion that follows, in line with much of the current literature and for reasons of simplicity, the terms *vulnerable plaque* and *thin cap fibroatheroma* are used synonymously, although further changes to these terms have been proposed.[15–17]

3.3 HISTOPATHOLOGY AND PATHOGENESIS OF VULNERABLE PLAQUE AND PLAQUE RUPTURE

The histopathology and pathogenesis of VP and plaque rupture are described in detail in Chapters 1, 2, 4, and 10. Important to any description of individual animal models, in addition to the defining histopathological characteristics listed above, lesions of VP possess a number of other key features summarized in Table 3.1. Plaques that rupture have significant plaque volume but maintain relatively preserved

TABLE 3.1
Histopathologic Characteristics of Vulnerable Plaque

Characteristic	Reference
Increased volume	15
Positive remodeling	10, 12
Lipid core comprising up to 60% plaque volume	18
Lipid core containing cholesterol crystals and esters, oxidized lipids, and tissue factor	3, 18, 19
Inflammatory cell infiltrate	18, 23, 92, 93
Thin cap depleted of SMCs and collagen	25
Increased neovascularity	94

Source: Modified from Shah, P.K., *Progr. Carviovasc. Dis.* 44, 357–368, 2002.

lumens by positive or outward remodeling.[9,11] The plaque has a large lipid pool component of up to 60% by area.[18] The lipid core has a number of key features. Its increased size increases plaque distensibility, causing increased circumferential stress to the plaque shoulder.

The plaque shoulder is the site of rupture in many cases.[19,20] This increased distensibility also forms the basis for certain novel methods of plaque detection. The lipid core components include free cholesterol, cholesterol esters, and cholesterol crystals in addition to a number of prothrombotic components including oxidized lipids and macrophage-derived tissue factor.[5,21,22]

Among the cellular components of VP, inflammatory cells predominate. The majority are monocytes/macrophages, although T cells and mast cells are also present.[5,18,23] A number of inflammatory mediators are involved in the recruitment of these cells including oxidized lipids, cytokines, and angiotensin II.[3,24] The fibrous cap also contains structural components including collagen, elastin, and proteoglycans, containing less ECM (collagen and proteoglycans) and fewer SMCs than caps from intact plaques.[25] Increased neovascularity is also a feature of VP and may provide a source of inflammatory cell infiltrate.[5]

The pathogenesis of acute plaque rupture can be viewed as the end result of an imbalance of factors increasing the smooth muscle cell (SMC) component responsible for structural integrity and collagen synthesis and factors decreasing SMC numbers or activities and promoting collagen degradation.[26,27] Cellular and matrix depletion in the fibrous cap are thought to be followed by cap thinning and rupture due to hemodynamic or other triggers.[5] SMC depletion occurs as a result of apoptosis, in part at least in response to oxidized low density lipoproteins (LDLs) and inflammatory cell mediators including mast cell-released chymases.[5,26,27]

A large number of cellular metabolic pathways have been implicated in this process of apoptosis, resulting in medial SMC depletion including the caspase, Bcl-2, and p53 protein families.[28] Caspases are members of a cysteine protease group of 14 cytoplasmic proteins.[28,29] Although the precise mechanisms by which caspase activation induces cell death is unclear, the caspases can be broadly considered as initiators (caspase-2 and caspase-8) or effectors (caspase-3 and caspase-6) of apoptosis.[29] The Bcl-2 family is a second group of cellular proteins involved in apoptosis regulation. Some (Bcl-2, A1) are thought to be anti-apoptotic; others (Bax, Bak) pro-apoptotic, although again, the mechanisms of action of these specific proteins are not yet understood completely.[28,30]

SMCs in vulnerable lesions also have impaired function. Collagen synthesis is reduced by interferon gamma secreted from activated T cells.[24] The resulting collagen depletion further reduces structural integrity of the fibrous cap. In addition, matrix depletion is induced by cathepsins and a number of matrix-degrading metalloproteinases (MMPs) including MMP-1, MMP-2, and MMP-13 produced by macrophages and to a lesser degree by endothelial and SMCs. MMP production is increased by a variety of mediators including oxidized lipids, CD40 ligands, and inflammatory cytokines.[27,31] Together, these and other processes result in a net imbalance of reduced matrix synthesis and increased breakdown leading to cap thinning and ultimately rupture.[27,32]

3.4 CLINICAL SEQUELAE OF VULNERABLE PLAQUE AND PLAQUE RUPTURE

An understanding of the clinical sequelae of VP and plaque rupture is key to a precise description relating to animal models. Data linking VP and plaque rupture to clinical sequelae come from two sources: direct pathologic data from postmortem findings and indirect data from *in vivo* imaging. In the setting of AMI, well documented postmortem studies have generally found coronary thrombosis in >80% of patients with AMI in hospital settings.[1,33,34] They also found that plaque rupture was a key feature of coronary thrombosis in the majority of these AMI cases.[2,11,14,33] In addition, angiographic studies have shown that the majority of coronary lesions assessed prior to AMI are <50% in severity.[1] These and other data support the notion of the nonobstructive but thrombosis-prone coronary lesion in the etiology of AMI.

In the setting of unstable angina pectoris (UAP), data are also available from *in vivo* imaging. Angiography studies in patients with UAP revealed more eccentric lesions with asymmetric or irregular borders compared to stable angina patients. This is thought to be based on ruptured plaque with partially occlusive thrombus.[35] Intravascular ultrasound (IVUS) studies demonstrated that lesions in patients with UAP and plaque rupture had larger echolucent areas consistent with lipid pools and thinner fibrous caps.[36] Angioscopic studies indicate that 70% of patients with UAP have complex lesion morphology and/or coronary thrombosis compared to the absence of complex lesions in patients with stable angina.[37]

Finally, evidence indicates that although most acute coronary syndromes are the results of plaque ruptures, many episodes of plaque rupture may go clinically unnoticed.[38] Furthermore, there is some evidence of multiple sites at risk of plaque rupture despite a single culprit lesion and that a "pan-coronary" state of heightened activation may occur.[39,40] This suggests that a focus on a single lesion of VP rather than systemic processes may be a simplistic one.[41,42] These and other data have prompted the recent suggestion of the concept of a "vulnerable patient," placing increased emphasis on overall systemic cardiovascular risk rather than exclusive focus on specific lesions of VP.[16,17]

3.5 SYSTEMIC AND LOCAL STRATEGIES FOR VULNERABLE PLAQUE STABILIZATION

With an increasing understanding of the nature of VP and its clinical sequelae has come increasing interest in the concept of plaque stabilization by systemic or local means and this is discussed in detail in Chapters 2 and 10 and in the literature.[27,43] Small and medium-sized animal models lend themselves to the investigation of systemic therapy, whereas larger animals such as pigs are likely to be used in the investigation of local strategies. For example, hydroxymethyl glutaryl coenzyme A (HMG CoA) reductase inhibitors and dietary intervention decrease macrophage accumulation and expression of MMPs, tissue factor (TF), and other inflammatory mediators in atherosclerotic lesions in Watanabe and cholesterol-fed rabbits.[44,45]

Likewise, systemic HMG CoA reductase inhibition with simvastatin reduced intraplaque hemorrhage in the brachiocephalic artery atherosclerotic lesions of apo E knockout mice.[46] Conversely, based on trials with drug-eluting stents resulting in low morbidity and restenosis rates, a pre-emptive strategy of stenting vulnerable, but not hemodynamically significant, lesions has been proposed.[15,43] The preclinical testing of such a strategy is likely to require a large animal approach.

3.6 IMAGING VULNERABLE PLAQUE

Significant advances in a number of technologies are revolutionizing the ability to image vulnerable plaque.[47] While some of these imaging modalities are catheter-based and presently available for human intracoronary use, they are also readily applicable to large animal models of VP. IVUS is capable of discerning intact and ruptured fibrous caps and lipid cores in humans[48] in limited patient numbers. The utility of IVUS may be increased if measures of plaque distensibility are used.[19] Thermography can detect temperature differences of 0.05°C and has detected temperature differences of 0.6 to 1.5°C between unstable plaques compared to normal vessels, thought to be due to increased inflammatory activity.[49,50]

Similarly, the optically based technique of near infrared (NIR) spectroscopy may allow identification of plaques containing abundant inflammatory cells.[51] The novel optical imaging technique known as optical coherence tomography (OCT) has a resolution of 10 µm, which allows visualization of fibrous cap thickness (65 µm) that defines VP. The underlying lipid pool can also be imaged with remarkable detail, a finding generating much interest.[39] Intriguingly, this technique also appears to be able to detect infiltration of macrophages (20 to 50 µm in diameter), the second defining feature of VP.[52]

The novel field of *in vivo* optical molecular imaging permits precise molecular-based imaging in a number of contexts and finds particular use in the examination of atherosclerosis in mouse models.[53] Using molecular probes to the cathepsin B proteolytic enzyme, enzyme activity can be imaged *in vivo* in the atherosclerotic aortae of apo E/endothelial NO synthase double knockout mice.[54] The same principles have also been used to image activities of a number of molecules including caspase-1, caspase-3, and MMPs, all of which are implicated in acute plaque rupture.[53,55] At present, these molecular imaging techniques are limited to use in small animals, particularly mice because of probe costs and spatial considerations. However, with suitably pertinent (small) animal models, these increasingly sophisticated imaging techniques appear poised to significantly advance our understanding of plaque vulnerability.

3.7 ASSESSMENT OF VULNERABILITY ENDPOINTS USING TRADITIONAL ANIMAL MODELS OF ATHEROSCLEROSIS

A logical and straightforward means of proposing animal models of VP has been to use existing models of atherosclerosis development and examine specific characteristics of vulnerability within those models.[56] Traditional animal models of atherosclerosis — with inherent advantages and limitations — have been well documented.[57,58] Table 3.2 lists animal models of vulnerable plaque.

Rabbits are commonly used despite the drawback that they do not develop spontaneous atheromas. They are used because they are highly responsive to dietary manipulation, although the resultant lesions exhibit important differences from human atheromas. Rats and dogs rarely develop atheromas.[56-58] Pigs and monkeys provide models closer to humans, but are limited by cost, availability, and ethical concerns.[57]

To date, the vulnerability endpoints selected by investigators have been mostly cellular and, to a lesser degree, molecular. The most generally accepted examples describe the hallmark pathogenic features of VP, for example, cap thickness and cap:lipid core ratio. Clearly, absolute measurements are species- and size-dependent, although measurements of ratios obviate these difficulties to some extent. A "vulnerability index" defined as the ratio of plaque area occupied by lipid components (macrophages and extracellular lipids) to the area occupied by fibromuscular components (SMCs and collagen) has also been proposed as a measure of lesion composition.[59]

Macrophage accumulation forms part of the definition of VP and can be readily identified. Macrophage activity can also be inferred from levels of tissue factor, largely macrophage-derived and a potent source of thrombogenicity.[60,61] SMC accumulation is considered a feature of plaque stability and processes such as apoptosis-induced SMC degradation have been proposed as markers of increased vulnerability.[62] Likewise, enzymes associated with collagen degradation, such as MMPs and cathepsins[63,64] may also be viewed as markers of increased vulnerability.[56]

The difficulty with these vulnerability endpoints is that they are essentially descriptive. Without precise correlation with more defined endpoints such as plaque rupture, their utility remains limited.

TABLE 3.2
Animal Models of Vulnerable Plaque

Animal	Type	Characteristics	Reference
Large Animals			
Rabbit	NZW	High fat diet, triggered thrombosis	65
Rabbit	NZW	High fat diet, balloon injured	66
Rabbit	NZW	Balloon embedded in aorta	68
Rabbit	Watanabe	Triggered thrombosis	67
Pig	Domestic farm	Direct lipid injection	69
Pig	Rapacz	Inherited dyslipidemia, spontaneous plaque rupture	70
Small Animals			
Mouse	Apo E KO	Aortic trauma	76
Mouse	Apo E KO	Carotid silastic collar, p53 transfection, phenylephrine induction of plaque rupture	78
Mouse	Apo E KO	High fat diet, brachiocephalic lesions	80
Mouse	Apo E KO	Mixed C57BL/6,129SvJ strain, high fat diet; brachiocephalic lesions, spontaneous plaque rupture	81
Mouse	Apo E/LDLR dKO	High fat diet, stress induced events; no plaque rupture evident	75
Mouse	Apo E/SRBI dKO	Advanced atheroma; no relation to clinical events	85
Mouse	Apo E/eNOS dKO	Aneurysms, LVH; relation to plaque rupture unclear	86, 87
Mouse	Apo E/TFPI dKO	Combines inflammatory component to model; relation to plaque rupture unclear	90
Rat	D-S CETP KO	Myocardial infarction; relation to coronary lesions unclear	70

Note: NZW = New Zealand white. Apo E = Apolipoprotein E. KO = knockout. LDLR = low density lipoprotein receptor. SRBI = scavenger receptor type BI. eNOS = e nitric oxide synthase. TFPI = tissue factor pathway inhibitor. D-S = Dahl salt-sensitive. CETP = cholesterol ester transport protein.

3.8   NOVEL LARGE ANIMAL MODELS OF VULNERABLE PLAQUE

3.8.1   MODELS OF VULNERABLE PLAQUE INDUCTION

A rabbit model of induced plaque rupture was described over 40 years ago.[65] New Zealand white rabbits developed atherosclerosis induced with cholesterol feeding. Thrombosis was then triggered by intraperitoneal injection of Russell's viper venom, an endothelial toxin and procoagulant followed by a histamine vasopressor.[65] A modification of this technique was recently described. A balloon injury of rabbit aorta was performed to speed atherosclerotic lesion development.[66] Similarly, Watanabe rabbits with heritable hyperlipidemia challenged with Russell's viper venom combined with either serotonin or angiotensin II developed acute myocardial infarction although there appeared to be no correlation with plaque rupture.[67]

Physical triggers to plaque rupture have also been proposed. After placing an inflatable balloon into the developing atherosclerotic plaque of a rabbit aorta, plaque rupture and thrombus induction can be induced by balloon inflation.[68] The inflation pressures required to induce plaque rupture have been proposed as measures of plaque tensile strength and the resultant plaque fissuring allows the resultant plaque-related thrombosis to be examined. The model also allows delivery of drug to the lesion site, a potential means of testing potential plaque-stabilizing strategies.[68] This model clearly has size limitations and limited relevance for examining the physiologic mechanisms of plaque rupture, but may permit further examination of the mechanical properties of plaque.

Other novel approaches have also been examined. One proposed method is to create lipid-rich lesions within the porcine coronary artery by direct injection of material into the media.[69] This approach has a number of potential advantages, including the fact that the site and size of lesion can be controlled. Perhaps most importantly, the lesion composition can potentially be manipulated so that the contributions to vulnerability of the various plaque components can be assessed and plaque-stabilizing therapies examined. Initial evaluation of this technique using a specially designed balloon catheter with needle injection ports (Infiltrator, IVT Technologies) suggests feasibility[69] but associated neointima formation induced by balloon inflation may limit the utility of this model (P. Keelan, personal communication). A similar approach using needle injection without balloon inflation may avoid this difficulty.

3.8.2 MODELS OF SPONTANEOUS VULNERABLE PLAQUE DEVELOPMENT

The Rapacz pig, with inherited LDL hypercholesterolemia has been known to develop spontaneous plaque ruptures and hemorrhages at the sites of coronary lesions in 39- to 54-week old animals.[70] Although this pig is in many ways an ideal large animal model, restricted availability limits their utility at a practical level. These animals are well described in the literature.[71]

3.9 NOVEL SMALL ANIMAL MODELS OF VULNERABLE PLAQUE

3.9.1 MODELS OF VULNERABLE PLAQUE INDUCTION

Small animals such as mice and rats have not generally been popular for studies of VP and plaque rupture because they are naturally relatively resistant to atherosclerosis development.[72] However, the recent ability to generate knockout (KO) strains deficient in specific genes of interest has renewed enthusiasm for these animals. Early attempts to create atherosclerosis-prone mice have not, however, resulted in reliable acute plaque rupture, leading a number of investigators to attempt induction of plaque rupture in these animals. A number of examples involving a variety of means of induction have met with varying degrees of success.[73]

The apo E KO mouse has been recognized since 1994 to spontaneously develop lesions of the thoracic aorta.[74] However, these aortic lesions have limited clinical relevance because they resemble large xanthomata with generally large central fatty masses and extensive necrosis — manifestations rarely observed in humans.[11,75] These lesions are not generally observed to undergo plaque rupture. Mechanical stress has been used to induce plaque rupture in apo E-deficient mice by applying compression pressure to the abdominal aorta at sites of atheromatous lesions simply using blunt forceps.[76]

Although this produced a number of areas of thrombosis not associated with plaque, 10 of 32 apo E-deficient animals showed evidence of thrombus-associated plaque using this technique.[76] Histological evidence indicates intraplaque hemorrhages within disrupted plaques and plaque-associated luminal thrombi,[76] although a precise demonstration of plaque rupture was not appeared to date. Physical triggers such as using a photochemical reaction to induce thrombus formation have also been employed.[77]

Another approach has been to use apo E KO mice with carotid atheromatous lesions induced by externally placed silastic collars.[78] The lesions were then transfected with the p53 tumor supressor protein which is involved in a number of processes in cell proliferation and apoptosis. One day following transfection, increased apoptosis was evident in the cell cap and increased fibrous cap thinning was seen at later time points. The thinned fibrous caps were also observed to undergo plaque rupture in 40% of animals after administration of phenylephrine.

For the most part, these mouse models of induced rupture, like similar models in large animals, have not been used widely. The varying triggering processes are not particularly robust; in the case of the last example, despite multiple means of promoting plaque vulnerablility and rupture, less than half the lesions examined showed evidence of rupture, although a number of others demonstrated intraplaque hemorrhages.[13,78] Perhaps for these reasons, efforts have continued to develop models of spontaneous development of VP and plaque rupture.

3.9.2 NOVEL TRANSGENIC MODELS OF SPONTANEOUS VULNERABLE PLAQUE DEVELOPMENT

Dahl salt-sensitive hypertensive rats, transgenic for human cholesterol ester transfer protein, have been proposed as useful models of plaque vulnerability.[79] These rats develop age-dependent hypertriglyceridemia, hypercholesterolemia, and decreased HDL levels. They are also hypertensive and develop atherosclerotic lesions in aortas and coronary vessels, myocardial infarction, and premature death. The coronary lesions have some analogy with human VP; they contain large globular lipid deposits and fibrocellular caps. Although plaque rupture has not been observed to date, this anatomic similarity and the increased incidence of myocardial infarction in these animals suggest that these lesions represent an important step in establishing a model of coronary VP.

Most other novel transgenic models of VP have been described in mice. Recent investigations have focused on the brachiocephalic arteries of apo E-deficient mice. This artery is a short (approximately 150 μm in length) communicating vessel on the right side, originating at the aorta and bifurcating into the common carotid and subclavian arteries. Unlike the aortic lesions in apo E mice, these brachiocephalic lesions more closely resemble those of human atherosclerosis, with medial atrophy and perivascular inflammation in animals aged 24 to 60 wk.[80] In studies of more mature mice aged 42 to 54 wk with C57BL/6 strain background fed a standard chow diet, some of which received supplementary estrogens, lesions with intraplaque hemorrhages were demonstrated in up to 75% of animals along with fibrotic conversions of necrotic zones and loss of the fibrous caps.[81]

Many of these lesions also demonstrated endothelial denudation or absence of endothelium and macrophage infiltration. Although fibrous cap thinning was observed, plaque rupture and thrombosis were not identified.[81] The threefold novel findings of an acellular necrotic core, erosion of this mass through to the lumen, and the presence of intraplaque hemorrhage, however, suggest a resemblance to plaque erosion with thrombosis.[82]

More recently, this model has been taken further. Apo E KO mice with a strain background of 50% C57BL/6 and 50% 129SvJ exhibited unique characteristics. These mice, fed a diet of 21% lard and 0.15% cholesterol starting at 6 to 8 wk showed progressive, pronounced atheromatous lesions within the brachiocephalic arteries evident as early as 4 wk (Figure 3.1A). The lesions were similar to human coronary vulnerable plaque lesions in that they had high lipid contents and relatively thin fibrous caps. Most intriguingly, however, and distinct from previous studies, 51 of 98 animals demonstrated evidence of acute plaque rupture, with thinning and discontinuity of the fibrous caps and intrusion of blood within the lesions.

Supportive evidence for the role of plaque rupture in this model was provided by the suggestion of increased apoptosis in the shoulder regions of these ruptured plaques, as evidenced by caspase-3 immunoreactivity (Figure 3.1B). Animals that demonstrated acute ruptures also exhibited higher numbers of buried fibrous caps within the lesions (2.66 versus 1.06). This is strongly suggestive of prior episodes of silent plaque rupture — an observation that makes this model particularly pertinent to humans.[38] The lesions exhibiting acute plaque ruptures were somewhat larger and are associated with greater rates of luminal occlusion.[83] This model of atherosclerosis development which induces lesions with many characteristics of vulnerable plaque and most importantly demonstrates acute plaque rupture is viewed as a major advance.[72]

Double KO (dKO) mice, most commonly combining apo E deficiency with other pathophysiologically relevant gene knockouts, have also provided increased insights. Hypercholesterolemic dKO (apo E, LDL receptor) mice fed a diet of 21% fat and 0.15% cholesterol and exposed to mental stress (air was forced into the holding cage and stress was recorded as increased heart rate) or hypoxia (stepwise decreases of oxygen from 21% down to 10%) underwent ischemia and myocardial infarction.[75] These effects were inhibited by endothelin A antagonists. The animals exhibited severe coronary lesions containing fibrin and cholesterol clefts.[75] Although no acute plaque ruptures or plaque-associated thrombi were described to date,[7,75] another

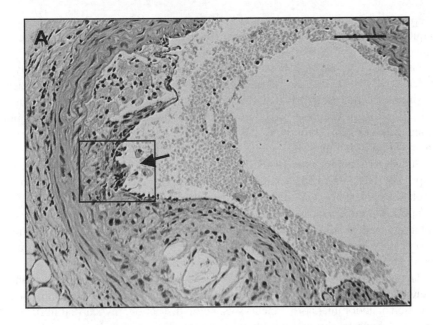

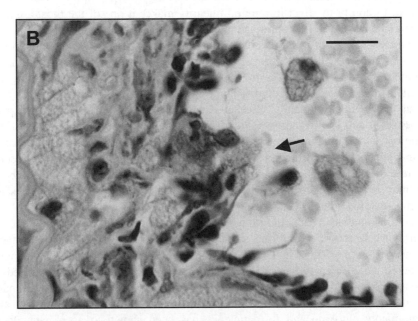

FIGURE 3.1 *(A color version of this figure follows page 112.)* Acute plaque rupture: Apo E knockout mouse, brachiocephalic artery. Cleaved caspase-3 expression in a ruptured athero-sclerotic lesion within a brachiocephalic artery of an 8-week-old, high-fat fed Apo E knockout mouse. Brown color in both panels indicates cleaved caspase-3 positive cells (apoptotic). Arrows indicate site of plaque rupture. Lower panel shows detail of insert in upper panel. Scale bars equal 100 μm (A) and 20 μm (B).

group using a separate colony of apo E/LDL receptor KO mice found evidence of plaque rupture and associated thrombosis in a minority of animals fed a variety of chow diets.[84]

Other novel transgenic models combined a genetic predisposition to hyper-lipidemia (apo E KO or LDL receptor KO) with a second pro-atherogenic tendency that promoted atherosclerosis (SRBI-KO), inflammation (influenza virus), or throm-bosis (PAI-I KO). Of these, very few models have achieved the goal of obtaining spontaneous coronary thrombosis, and even fewer have achieved the goal via clear rupture of lipid rich plaques.

Scavenger receptor type BI (SRBI) is critical for the clearance of high density lipoprotein (HDL)-derived cholesteryl ester, and thus may regulate the clearance of peripheral cholesterol via the reverse cholesterol transport pathway. The SRBI KO/apo E KO mice developed very advanced atherosclerosis, with complex lesions containing cholesterol clefts, myocardial dysfunction with fibrosis, and infarction.[85] The coronary lesions of this model did not appear to be related to plaque rupture, thus the relevance of the pathology to human disease is unclear.

The combined apo E KO/eNOS KO mouse is an interesting model that shows accelerated atherosclerosis relative to the apo E KO alone and also demonstrates formation of abdominal aortic aneurysms, aortic dissection, myocardial fibrosis, left ventricular hypertrophy and peripheral coronary disease with infarction.[86,87] How-ever, whether this model can relate to human coronary plaque rupture occurrence is unclear. Its ability to affect intramural integrity makes it one of the most attractive models of atherosclerotic complication.

The association of inflammation, both local and systemic, with acute coronary events is unequivocal, and this has led investigators to study potential inflammatory precipitants of acute plaque thrombosis. This literature is large and expanding, and excellent reviews cover chlamydia, herpes simplex, and other infections. A more recent and perhaps clinically relevant example is influenza. Vaccination against influenza is known to decrease the risk of acute coronary events. Influenza A infection can promote intra-aortic inflammation in apo E KO mice and, in one case, fibrin-rich occlusive thrombosis.[88] A better defined reproducibility of effect is required before this method can be used as a standard model of arterial thrombosis; this may require the infection of mice predisposed to both atherosclerosis and thrombosis with influenza A virus.

Among models investigating the potential for thombotic factors to interact with atherogenic factors in promoting arterial thrombosis, deficiencies of tissue factor pathway inhibitor (TFPI) and IL-10 have shown some promise. TFPI deficiency promoted atherosclerosis and arterial tissue factor expression and accelerated the time to thrombus formation following carotid injury.[89] However, the need for induc-ible injury to promote thrombus in this model is a deficiency. IL10 is an anti-inflammatory cytokine and its deficiency has been shown to accelerate athero-sclerosis development, increase systemic markers of thrombosis, increase tissue matrix metalloproteinase activity, and increase the thrombotic response to IV throm-bin in apo E KO mice.[90] This attractive model combines pro-inflammatory state with promotion of thrombosis, but still requires a critical final step — atherosclerosis-related plaque rupture — to make this model as relevant as it might be.

3.10 LIMITATIONS AND FUTURE DIRECTIONS

As is the case with the use of animal models of disease in other contexts, no single animal model of VP has proven to date to be an ideal. Available large animal models are essentially established models of atherosclerosis, with novel but merely descriptive characteristics of plaque vulnerability applied. The small animal models of induced or spontaneous plaque vulnerability and rupture are limited in that the lesions formed are in many cases located in non-coronary vessels and lesion morphology is distinct from the human process.[91] Mice also show thrombosis and thrombolysis patterns that differ distinctly from human patterns.[91] Despite these limitations, transgenic mice — particularly apo E single knockouts and double knockouts of apo E and other pertinent genes — are increasingly seen as able to address specific questions about the pathogenesis of VP and plaque rupture and are likely to see increased use.[72] While apo E KO mice have already been used to examine the effects of systemic plaque stablilizing strategies,[46] their utility in investigating local therapies for VP remains to be seen.

3.11 CONCLUDING REMARKS

Assisted by novel imaging modalities, with the ultimate aim of VP stabilization, there is a growing focus on understanding mechanisms of VP formation and acute plaque rupture. Key to this growing understanding is the appropriate use of animal models. While such models have proven of only limited utility to date, recent developments, particularly with transgenic mice, appear set to provide key breakthroughs.

REFERENCES

1. Falk E, Shah PK, and Fuster V, Coronary plaque disruption. *Circulation*, 92, 657–671, 1995.
2. Farb A, Tang AL, Burke AP, Sessums L, Liang Y, and Virmani R, Sudden coronary death: frequency of active coronary lesions, inactive coronary lesions, and myocardial infarction. *Circulation*, 92, 1701–1709, 1995.
3. Libby P, Molecular bases of the acute coronary syndromes. *Circulation*, 91, 2844–2850, 1995.
4. Shah PK, Pathophysiology of coronary thrombosis: role of plaque rupture and plaque erosion. *Progr. Card. Dis.*, 44, 357–368, 2002.
5. Shah PK, Mechanisms of plaque vulnerability and rupture. *J. Am. Coll. Card.*, 41 (Suppl.), S15–S22, 2003.
6. Davies MJ, The pathophysiology of acute coronary syndromes. *Heart*, 83, 361–366, 2000.
7. Rekhter MD, How to evaluate plaque vulnerablity in animal models of atherosclerosis. *Card. Res.*, 54, 36–41, 2002.
8. Muller JE and Tofler GH, Triggering and hourly variation of onset of arterial thrombosis. *Ann. Epidem.*, 4, 393–405, 1992.
9. Virmani R, et al., Pathology of the unstable plaque. *Progr. Card. Dis.*, 44, 349–356, 2002.

10. Burke AP, Farb A, Malcom GT, Liang YH, Smialek J, and Virmani R, Coronary risk factors and plaque morphology in men with coronary disease who died suddenly. *N. Engl. J. Med.*, 336, 1276–1282, 1997.

11. Virmani R, Kolodgie F, Burke AP, Farb A, and Schwartz SM. Lessons from sudden coronary death: a comprehensive morphological classification scheme for atherosclerotic lesions. *Arterioscl. Thromb.Vasc. Biol.*, 20, 1262–1275, 2000.

12. Stary HC, Natural and historical classification of atherosclerotic lesions: an update. *Arterioscl. Thromb. Vasc. Biol.*, 20, 1177–1178, 2000.

13. Lutgens E, van Suylen R.J, Faber BC, et al., Atherosclerotic plaque rupture: local or systemic process? *Arterioscl. Thromb. Vasc. Biol.*, 23, 2123–2130, 2003.

14. Farb A, Burke A, and Tang AL, Coronary plaque erosion without rupture into a lipid core: a frequent cause of coronary thrombosis in sudden coronary death. *Circulation*, 93, 1354–1363, 1996.

15. Kereiakes DJ, The Emperor's clothes: in search of the vulnerable plaque. *Circulation*, 107, 2076–2077, 2003.

16. Naghavi M, Libby P, Falk E, et al., From vulnerable plaque to vulnerable patient: a call for new definitions and risk assessment strategies, part I. *Circulation*, 108, 1664–1670, 2003.

17. Naghavi M, Libby P, Falk E, et al., From vulnerable plaque to vulnerable patient: a call for new definitions and risk assessment strategies, part II. *Circulation*, 108, 1772–1778, 2003.

18. Felton CV, Crook D, Davies MJ, and Oliver MF, Relation of plaque lipid composition and morphology to the stability of human aortic plaques. *Arterioscl. Thromb. Vasc. Biol.*, 17, 1337–1345, 1997.

19. Takano M, Mizuno K, Okamatsu K, Yokoyama S, Ohba T, and Sakai S, Mechanical and structural characteristics of vulnerable plaques: analysis by coronary angioscopy and intravascular ultrasound. *J. Am. Coll. Card.*, 38, 99–104, 2001.

20. Cheng GC, Loree HM, Kamm RD, Fishbein MC, and Lee RT, Distribution of circumferential stress in ruptured and stable atherosclerotic lesions: a structural analysis with histopathological correlation. *Circulation*, 87, 1179–1187, 1993.

21. Toschi V, Gallo R, Lettino M, et al., Tissue factor modulates the thrombogenicity of human atherosclerotic plaques. *Circulation*, 95, 594–599, 1993.

22. Fernandez-Ortiz A, Badimon JJ, Falk E, et al., Characterization of the relative thrombogenicity of atherosclerotic plaque components: implications for consequences of plaque rupture. *J. Am. Coll. Card.*, 23, 1562–1569, 1994.

23. Laine P, Kartinnen M, Penttila A, Panula P, Paavonen T, and Kovanen PT, Association between myocardial infarction and the mast cells in the adventitia of the infarct-related coronary artery. *Circulation*, 99, 361–369, 1999.

24. Libby P, Changing concepts of atherogenesis. *J. Intern. Med.*, 247, 349–358, 2000.

25. Burleigh MC, Briggs AD, Lendon CL, Davies MJ, Born GV, and Richardson PD, Collagen types I and III, collagen content, GAGs and mechanical strength of human atherosclerotic plaque caps: span-wise variations. *Atherosclerosis*, 96, 71–81, 1992.

26. Cullen P, Baetta R, Bellosta S, et al., Rupture of the atherosclerotic plaque: does a good animal model exist? *Arterioscl. Thromb. Vasc. Biol.*, 23, 535–542, 2003.

27. Libby P and Aikawa M, Stabilization of atherosclerotic plaques: new mechanisms and clinical targets. *Nature Medicine*, 8, 1257–1262, 2002.

28. Geng YJ and Libby P, Progression of atheroma: a struggle between death and pro-creation. *Arterioscl. Thromb. Vasc. Biol.*, 22, 1370–1380, 2002.

29. Thornberry NA and Lazebnik Y, Caspases: enemies within. *Science*, 281, 1312–1316, 1998.

30. Evan G and Littlewood T, A matter of life and death. *Science*, 281, 1317–1322, 1998.
31. Young JL, Libby P, and Schonbeck U, Cytokines in the pathogenesis of atherosclerosis. *Thromb. Haemostasis*, 88, 554–567, 2002.
32. Walsh K, Smith RC, and Kim HS, Vascular cell apoptosis in remodeling, restenosis, and plaque rupture. *Circ. Res.*, 87, 184–188, 2000.
33. Falk E, Plaque rupture with severe pre-existing stenosis precipitating coronary thrombosis: characteristics of coronary atherosclerotic plaques underlying fatal occlusive thrombi. *Br. Heart J.*, 50, 127–134, 1983.
34. Ambrose JA, Winters S, Arora RR, et al., Coronary angiographic morphology in myocardial infarction: a link between the pathogenesis of unstable angina and myocardial infarction. *J. Am. Coll. Card.*, 6, 1233–1238, 1985.
35. Ambrose JA, Winters S, Stern A, et al., Angiographic morphology and the pathogenesis of unstable angina pectoris. *J. Am. Coll. Card.*, 5, 609–616, 1985.
36. Ge J, Chirillo F, Schwedtmann J, et al., Screening of ruptured plaques in patients with coronary artery disease by intravascular ultrasound. *Heart*, 81, 621–627, 1999.
37. Sherman CT, Litvack F, Grundfest W, et al., Coronary angioscopy in patients with unstable angina pectoris. *N. Engl. J. Med.*, 315, 913–919, 1986.
38. Newby AC, Libby P, and van der Wal AC, Plaque instability—the real challenge for atherosclerosis research in the next decade? *Cardiovasc. Res.*, 41, 321–322, 1999.
39. Blake GJ and Ridker P, Inflammatory bio-markers and cardiovascular risk prediction. *J. Intern. Med.*, 252, 283–294, 2002.
40. Buffon A, Biasucci LM, Liuzzo G, D'Onofrio G, Crea F, and Maseri A, Widespread coronary inflammation in unstable angina. *N. Engl. J. Med.*, 347, 5–12, 2002.
41. Maseri A and Fuster V, Is there a vulnerable plaque? *Circulation*, 107, 2068–2071, 2003.
42. Casscells W, Naghavi M, and Willerson JT, Vulnerable atherosclerotic plaque: a multifocal disease. *Circulation*, 107, 2072–2075, 2003.
43. Popma JJ, Kuntz RE, and Baim DS, A decade of improvement in the clinical outcomes of percutaneous coronary intervention for multivessel disease. *Circulation*, 106, 1592–1594, 2002.
44. Bustos C, Hernandez.-Pressa MA, et al., HMG-CoA reductase inhibition by atorvastatin reduces neointimal inflammation in a rabbit model of atherosclerosis. *J. Am. Coll. Card.*, 32, 2057–2064, 1998.
45. Aikawa M, Rabkin E, Sugiyama S, et al., An HMG-CoA reductase inhibitor, cerivastatin, suppresses growth of macrophages expressing matrix metalloproteinases and tissue factor *in vivo* and *in vitro*. *Circulation*, 103, 276–283, 2001.
46. Bea F, Blessing E, Bennett B, Levitz M, Wallace EP, and Rosenfeld ME, Simvastatin promotes atherosclerotic plaque stability in apoE-deficient mice independently of lipid lowering. *Arterioscl. Thromb. Vasc. Biol.*, 22, 1832–1837, 2002.
47. Mac Neill BD, Lowe HC, Takano M, Fuster V, and Jang IK, Intravascular modalities for detection of vulnerable plaque: current status. *Arterioscl. Thromb. Vasc. Biol.*, 23, 1333–1342, 2003.
48. Nissen SE, Pathobiology, not angiography, should guide management in acute coronary syndrome/non-ST-segment elevation myocardial infarction: the non-interventionist's perspective. *J. Am. Coll. Card.*, 41 (Suppl.), S103–S112, 2003.
49. Stefanadis C, Diamantopoulos L, Vlachopoulos C, et al., Thermal heterogeneity within human atherosclerotic coronary arteries detected *in vivo*: a new method of detection by application of a special thermography catheter. *Circulation*, 99, 1965–1971, 1999.

50. Madjid M, Naghavi M, Malik BA, Litovsky S, Willerson JT, and Casscells W, Thermal detection of vulnerable plaque. *Am. J. Card.*, 90, 36L-39L, 2002.

51. Moreno PR, Lodder RA, Purushothaman KR, Charash WE, O'Connor WN, and Muller JE, Detection of lipid pool, thin fibrous cap, and inflammatory cells in human aortic atherosclerotic plaques by near-infrared spectroscopy. *Circulation*, 105, 923–927, 2002.

52. Tearney GJ, Yabushita H, Houser SL, et al., Quantification of macrophage content in atherosclerotic plaques by optical coherence tomography. *Circulation*, 107, 113–119, 2002.

53. Weissleder R and Ntziachristos V, Shedding light onto live molecular targets. *Nature Medicine*, 9, 123–128, 2003.

54. Chen J, Tung CH, Mahmood U, et al., *In vivo* imaging of proteolytic activity in atherosclerosis. *Circulation*, 105, 2766–2771, 2002.

55. Bremer C, Tung CH, and Weissleder R, Molecular imaging of MMP expression and therapeutic MMP inhibition. *Acad Radiol*, 9 (Suppl.), S314–S315, 2002.

56. Rekhter M, How to evaluate plaque vulnerablity in animal models of atherosclerosis. *Cardiovasc. Res.*, 54, 36–41, 2002.

57. Badimon L, Atherosclerosis and thrombosis: lessons from animal models. *Thromb. Haemostasis*, 86, 356–365, 2001.

58. Fuster V, Ip JH, Badimon L, Badimon JJ, Stein B, and Chesebro JH, Importance of experimental models for the development of clinical trials on thromboatherosclerosis. *Circulation*, 83, IV15–IV25, 1991.

59. Shiomi M, Ito T, Hirouchi Y, and Enomoto M, Fibromuscular cap composition is important for the stability of established atherosclerotic plaques in mature WHHL rabbits treated with statins. *Atherosclerosis*, 157, 75–84, 2001.

60. Moons AHM, Levi M, and Peters RJG, Tissue factor and coronary artery disease. *Cardiovasc. Res.*, 53, 313–325, 2002.

61. Taubman MB, Fallon JT, Schecter AD, et al., Tissue factor in the pathogenesis of atherosclerosis. *Thromb. Haemostasis*, 78, 200–204, 1997.

62. Bennett MR, Apoptosis of vascular smooth muscle cells in vascular remodelling and atherosclerotic plaque rupture. *Cardiovasc. Res.*, 41, 361–368, 1999.

63. Galis ZS, Sukhova GK, Lark MW, and Libby P, Increased expression of matrix metalloproteinases and matrix degrading activity in vulnerable regions of human atherosclerotic plaques. *J. Clin. Invest.*, 94, 2493–2503, 1994.

64. Sukhova G, Shi GP, Simon DI, Chapman HA, and Libby P, Expression of the elastolytic cathepsins S and K in human atheroma and regulation of their production in smooth muscle cells. *J. Clin. Invest.*, 102, 576–583, 1998.

65. Constantinides P and Chakravarti RN, Rabbit arterial thrombosis production by systemic procedures. *Arch Pathol*, 72, 197–208, 1961.

66. Abela GS, Picon PD, Friedl SE, et al., Triggering of plaque disruption and arterial thrombosis in an atherosclerotic rabbit model. *Circulation*, 91, 776–784, 1995.

67. Nakamura M, Abe S, and Kinukawa N, Aortic medial necrosis with or without thrombosis in rabbits treated with Russell's viper venom and angiotensin II. *Atherosclerosis*, 128, 149–156, 1997.

68. Rekhter MD, Hicks GW, Brammer DW, et al., Animal model that mimics atherosclerotic plaque rupture. *Circ. Res.*, 83, 705–713, 1998.

69. Keelan PC, et al., A novel porcine model for *in vivo* detection of vulnerable plaque: deposition and localization of lipid-rich lesions in the coronary artery wall. *Circulation*, II-67, 2001, (abstr.)

70. Prescott MF, McBride CH, Hasler-Rapacz J, Von Linden J, and Rapacz J, Development of complex atherosclerotic lesions in pigs with inherited hyper-LDL cholesterolemia bearing mutant alleles for apolipoprotein B. *Am. J. Pathol.*, 139, 139–147, 1991.

71. Rapacz J, Hasler.-Rapacz J, Taylor KM, Checovich WJ, and Attie AD, Lipoprotein mutations in pigs are associated with elevated plasma cholesterol and atherosclerosis. *Science*, 234, 1573–1577, 1986.

72. Bennett MR, Breaking the plaque: evidence for plaque rupture in animal models of atherosclerosis. *Arterioscl. Thromb. Vasc. Biol.*, 22, 713–714, 2002.

73. Lowe HC, Jang IK, and Khachigian LM, Animal models of vulnerable plaque: clinical context and current status. *Thromb. Haemostasis*, 90, 774–780, 2003.

74. Reddick RL, Zhang SH, and Maeda N, Atherosclerosis in mice lacking apo E. Evaluation of lesional development and progression. *Arterioscl. Thromb.*, 14, 141–147, 1994.

75. Caligiuri G, Levy B, Pernow J, Thoren P, and Hansson GK, Myocardial infarction mediated by endothelin receptor signaling in hypercholesterolemic mice. *Proc. Natl. Acad. Sci. USA*, 96, 6920–6924, 1999.

76. Reddick RL, Zhang SH, and Maeda N, Aortic atherosclerotic plaque injury in apolipoprotein E deficient mice. *Atherosclerosis*, 140, 297–305, 1998.

77. Eitzman DT, Westrick RJ, Xu Z, Tyson J, and Ginsburg D, Plasminogen activator inhibitor-1 deficiency protects against atherosclerosis progression in the mouse carotid artery. *Arterioscl. Thromb. Vasc. Biol.*, 20, 846–852, 2000.

78. von der Thusen JH, van Vlijmen BJ, et al., Induction of atherosclerotic plaque rupture in apolipoprotein E–/– mice after adenovirus-mediated transfer of p53. *Circulation*, 105, 2064–2070, 2002.

79. Herrera VL, Makrides SC, Xie HX, et al., Spontaneous combined hyperlipidemia, coronary heart disease and decreased survival in Dahl salt-sensitive hypertensive rats transgenic for human cholesteryl ester transfer protein. *Nature Medicine*, 5, 1383–1389, 1999.

80. Seo HS, Lombardi DM, Polinsky P, et al., Peripheral vascular stenosis in apolipoprotein E-deficient mice. Potential roles of lipid deposition, medial atrophy, and adventitial inflammation. *Arterioscl. Thromb. Vasc. Biol.*, 17, 3593–3601, 1997.

81. Rosenfeld ME, Polinsky P, Virmani R, Kauser K, Rubanyi G, and Schwartz SM, Advanced atherosclerotic lesions in the innominate artery of the ApoE knockout mouse. *Arterioscl. Thromb. Vasc. Biol.*, 20, 2587–2592, 2000.

82. Getz GS, Mouse model of unstable atherosclerotic plaque? *Arterioscl. Thromb. Vasc. Biol.*, 20, 2503–2505, 2000.

83. Williams H, Johnson JL, Carson KGS, and Jackson CL, Characteristics of intact and ruptured atherosclerotic plaques in brachiocephalic arteries of apolipoprotein E knockout mice. *Arterioscl. Thromb. Vasc. Biol.*, 22, 788–792, 2002.

84. Calara F, Silvestre M, Casanada F, Napoli C, and Palinski W, Spontaneous plaque rupture and secondary thrombosis in apolipoprotein E-deficient and LDL receptor-deficient mice. *J. Pathol.*, 195, 257–263, 2001

85. Braun A, Trigatti BL, Post MJ, et al., Loss of SR-BI expression leads to the early onset of occlusive atherosclerotic coronary artery disease, spontaneous myocardial infarctions, severe cardiac dysfunction, and premature death in apolipoprotein E-deficient mice. *Circ. Res.*, 90, 270–276, 2002.

86. Kuhlencordt PJ, Chen J Han F, Astern J, and Huang PL, Genetic deficiency of inducible nitric oxide synthase reduces atherosclerosis and lowers plasma lipid peroxides in apolipoprotein E-knockout mice. *Circulation*, 103, 3099–3104, 2001.

87. Kuhlencordt PJ, Gyurko R, Han F, et al., Accelerated atherosclerosis, aortic aneurysm formation, and ischemic heart disease in apolipoprotein E/endothelial nitric oxide synthase double-knockout mice. *Circulation*, 104, 448–454, 2001.
88. Naghavi, M, Wyde P, Litovsky S, et al., Influenza infection exerts prominent inflammatory and thrombotic effects on the atherosclerotic plaques of apolipoprotein E-deficient mice. *Circulation*, 107, 762–768, 2001.
89. Westrick RJ, Bodary PF, Xu Z, Shen YC, Broze GJ, and Eitzman DT, Deficiency of tissue factor pathway inhibitor promotes atherosclerosis and thrombosis in mice. *Circulation*, 103, 3044–3046, 2001.
90. Caligiuri G, Rudling M, Ollivier V, et al., Interleukin-10 deficiency increases atherosclerosis, thrombosis, and low-density lipoproteins in apolipoprotein E knockout mice. *Mol. Med.*, 9, 10–17, 2003.
91. Dickson BC and Gotlieb AI, Towards understanding acute destabilization of vulnerable atherosclerotic plaques. *Cardiovasc. Pathol.*, 12, 237–248, 2003.
92. Libby P, Inflammation in atherosclerosis. *Nature*, 420, 868–874, 2002.
93. van der Wal AC, Becker AE, van der Loos CM, and Das PK, Site of intimal rupture or erosion of thrombosed coronary atherosclerotic plaques is characterized by an inflammatory process irrespective of the dominant plaque morphology. *Circulation*, 89, 36–44, 1994.
94. Tenaglia AN, Peters KG, Sketch MH Jr, and Annex BH, Neovascularization in atherectomy specimens from patients with unstable angina: implications for pathogenesis of unstable angina. *Am. Heart J.*, 135, 10–14, 1998.

4 Diagnosis of Vulnerable Plaques in the Cardiac Catheterization Laboratory

Johannes A. Schaar, Evelyn Regar,
Chourmouzios A. Arampatzis,
Arjen R.A. van der Ven, Cornelis J. Slager,
Frank J. Gijsen, Jolanda J. Wentzel,
Pim J. de Feyter, A.F.W. van der Steen,
and Patrick W. Serruys

CONTENTS

4.1 INTRODUCTION

Rupture of vulnerable plaques is the main cause of acute coronary syndrome and myocardial infarction. Identification of vulnerable plaque is, therefore, essential to enable the development of treatment modalities to stabilize such plaque. Because myocardial infarction and its consequences are so important, we must investigate options to identify areas that will be responsible for future events. A wide variety exists in the stability of coronary atherosclerotic plaques. A plaque may be stable for years but the abrupt disruption of its structure is the main cause of acute coronary syndrome.[1] The three forms of vulnerable plaques are thin cap fibroatheroma, erosion, and calcified nodules.

Thin cap fibroatheroma — Pathologic studies of plaque rupture with thrombosis suggest that prior to a thrombotic event, a plaque is an inflamed thin cap fibroatheroma (TCFA). TCFAs appear in 75% of all cases. The major components of the TCFA are: (i) an atheromatous core, (ii) a thin fibrous cap with macrophage and lymphocyte infiltration and decreased smooth muscle cell content, and (iii) expansive remodelling.

Erosion — Pathologic studies have shown that prior to an event, the endothelium was injured at the place where a thrombus formed. This endothelium consists of proteoglycan-rich endothelial cells. Erosion occurs in 30% of all cases.

Calcified nodules — Pathologic studies of plaques with thrombosis covering calcified nodules suggest that the plaque appeared heavily calcified and that calcified nodules projected into the lumens preceding 5% of all events.

The terms *vulnerable plaque*, *high-risk plaque*, and *thrombosis-prone plaque* can be used interchangeably. This chapter will discuss the current developments of imaging techniques that have the potential to detect vulnerable plaques. Since vulnerable plaques contain certain features that may be diagnosed by various specialized methods, an ideal technique would provide morphological, mechanical, and chemical information. To date, no single diagnostic modality providing such all-embracing assessment is available. The characteristics of vulnerable plaques have been described by numerous reviewers.[2,3] It is important to characterize the following features:

1. Size of the lipid core (40% of the entire plaque)
2. Thickness of the fibrous cap
3. Presence of inflammatory cells
4. Amount of remodeling and extent of plaque-free vessel wall
5. Three-dimensional morphology

4.2 ANGIOGRAPHY

Coronary angiography has become the "gold standard" for assessing the severity of obstructive lumenal narrowing. Furthermore, it serves as a decision-making tool for directing therapy such as percutaneous transluminal coronary angioplasty (PTCA) and coronary artery bypass graft (CABG). Coronary angiography can assess the lumen boundaries, but cannot reveal information about plaque burden, plaque delineation, and plaque components. The predictive power of occurrence of myocardial infarction is rather low because 70% of acute coronary occlusions are in areas that previously appeared angiographically normal, and only a minority occur at sites of severe stenosis.[4] Other studies have affirmed that the culprit lesion prior to a myocardial infarction involves in 48 to 78% of all cases a stenosis smaller than 50%.[5-7] Coronary angiograms also often fail to identify the culprit lesions of nontransmural myocardial infarctions.[8] The majority of ulcerated plaques are not large enough to be detected by angiography, but can be well assessed pathologically.[9]

We must consider that the predictive power of angiography is strongly dependent on the time interval between the angiogram and the myocardial infarction, because both time and interim therapy can influence atherosclerosis. In one study, the angiograms were performed between 1 and 77 mo preceding the events[4] and showed that atherosclerosis can be a rapidly progressive process. A recent study evaluated angiograms made 1 wk before acute myocardial infarction and indicated that signs of thrombosis and rupture were present in a majority of patients.[10] During the year after myocardial infarction, the presence of multiple complex plaques is associated with an increased incidence of recurrent acute coronary syndrome.[11]

Thus, patients with silent non-obstructive coronary atherosclerosis harbor vulnerable plaques associated with adverse clinical outcomes that cannot be detected by angiograms. If a disrupted ulcerated plaque is seen on angiography, the existence of additional rupture-prone plaques is to be expected. Angiography, therefore, has low discriminatory power for identifying vulnerable plaques but it does provide information about the entire coronary system and serves as a guide for invasive imaging techniques and therapy. In the future, noninvasive luminography and vessel wall assessments may become integral parts of daily diagnostic procedures.[12]

4.3 ANGIOSCOPY

Intracoronary angioscopy offers direct visualization of plaque surfaces and intraluminal structures like tears and thrombi. It allows assessment of the colors of plaques and thrombi[13] and displays a greater sensitivity than angiography in detecting such structures.[14] Angioscopic plaque rupture and thrombus have been shown to be associated with adverse clinical outcomes in patients with complex lesions.[15] Furthermore, yellow plaques seemed to show increased instability in a comparison of intravenous coronary ultrasound (IVUS) and angioscopy.[16] In patients with myocardial infarctions, all three coronary arteries were widely diseased and had multiple yellow plaques.[17]

In a 12-mo follow-up study of 157 patients with stable angina, acute coronary syndrome occurred more frequently in patients with yellow plaques than in those with white plaques. These results indicate that acute coronary syndromes occur more frequently in patients with yellow plaques, which can be imaged with angioscopy, but not with angiography.[18] However, angioscopy is difficult to perform and invasive, and only a limited part of the vessel tree can be investigated. Most importantly, to enable clear visualization of the vessel wall, the vessel must be occluded and the remaining blood flushed away with saline, thereby potentially inducing ischemia. Information regarding the degree of plaque extension into the vessel wall is not provided by angioscopy.

4.4 INTRAVENOUS CORONARY ULTRASOUND

IVUS provides real-time high-resolution images of vessel walls and lumens.[19] The size of IVUS catheters is between 2.9 and 3.5 French. Depending on the distance from the catheter, the axial resolution is about 150 microns, the lateral 300 microns. The images appear in real time at a frequency of up to 30 frames/sec. Features of the vessel can be detected based on the echogenicity and thickness of the material. Small structures can be visualized, but only those larger than 160 microns can be estimated accurately. The normal thickness of the medium is about 125 to 350 μm.

IVUS provides some insight into the composition of coronary plaques. In IVUS images, calcification is characterized by a bright echo signal with distal shadowing which hides plaque components and deeper vessel structures. In comparative studies of histology and IVUS, plaque calcification can be detected with a sensitivity of 86 to 97%.[20,21] The sensitivity for detecting microcalcification ranges around 60%.[22]

In IVUS images, lipid depositions are described as echolucent zones and can be detected with a sensitivity between 78 and 95% and specificity of 30%.[23,24] The sensitivity is dependent on the amount of lipid and can decrease if the echolucent area comprises less than a quarter of the plaque. Echolucent zones can also be caused by loose tissue and shadowing from calcium, which makes the interpretation of echolucent areas difficult. The sensitivity for differentiating fibrous and fatty tissue is 39 to 52%.[25]

The detection of vulnerable plaques by IVUS is mainly based on a series of case reports.[26,27] The main focus of these reports is the detection of already ruptured plaques. To evaluate the role of IVUS in detecting plaque rupture, a study of 144 patients with angina was performed. Ruptured plaques were characterized by cavities (echolucent areas within the plaques) and tears of the thin fibrous caps. They were identified in 31 patients of whom 23 (74%) presented with unstable angina. Plaque rupture was confirmed by injecting contrast medium and noting filling of the plaque cavities on IVUS. Of the patients without plaque rupture (n = 108), only 19 (18%) had unstable angina. The echolucent area (cavity)-to-total plaque area ratio was larger in the unstable group than in the stable group. The thickness of the fibrous cap in the unstable group was also found to be smaller than in the stable group.[28]

Two problems of these studies are the lacks of prospectivity and follow-up. Only Yamagishi et al. performed a prospective study with a follow-up period of about 2 yr. Large eccentric plaques containing echolucent zones revealed by IVUS were found to be at increased risk of instability even though the lumen area was preserved at the time of initial study.[29] It has been demonstrated, that plaques suspected to be vulnerable are associated with positive remodeling. Intravascular ultrasound assessment of vascular remodeling may help classify plaques with the highest probabilities of spontaneous rupture.[30]

A number of groups investigated the potential of ultrasound radio-frequency signal analysis for tissue characterization.[31–37] Many of these studies revealed the potential to identify calcified plaques, but although promising, none has yet produced a technique with sufficient spatial and parametric resolution to identify a lipid pool covered by a thin fibrous cap.

4.5 INTRAVASCULAR ELASTOGRAPHY AND PALPOGRAPHY

In 1991, a new ultrasound technique was introduced to measure the mechanical properties of tissue: elastography.[38] The underlying concept is that upon uniform loading, the local relative amount of deformation (strain) of a tissue is related to the local mechanical properties of that tissue. If we apply this concept to determine the local properties of arterial tissue, blood pressure acts as a stressor. At a given pressure difference, soft plaque components will deform more than hard components. Measurement of local plaque deformation in the radial direction can be obtained with ultrasound.

For intravascular purposes, a derivate of elastography called palpography may be a suitable tool.[39] In this approach, one strain value per angle is determined and plotted as a color-coded contour at the lumen vessel boundary. Since radial strain is obtained, the technique may have the potential to detect regions with elevated stress. Increased circumferential stress results in increased radial deformation of the plaque components. *In vitro* studies with histological confirmation have shown differences of strain normalized to pressure of fibrous, fibro-fatty, and fatty components of the plaques of coronary and femoral arteries.[40] The differences were evident mainly between fibrous and fatty tissue. The plaque types could not be differentiated by echo-intensity differences seen on IVUS echograms.

In an additional *in vitro* validation trial, postmortem coronary arteries were investigated with intravascular elastography and subsequently processed for histology. In histology, a vulnerable plaque was defined as consisting of a thin cap (<250 µm) with moderate to heavy macrophage infiltration and at least 40% atheroma. In elastography, a vulnerable plaque was defined as having a high strain region at the surface with adjacent low strain regions. Rotterdam Classification (ROC) analysis revealed a maximum predictive power for a strain value threshold of 1.26%. The area under the ROC curve was 0.85. The sensitivity was 88% and the specificity 89% for detecting thin cap fibroatheromas. Linear regression showed high correlation between the strain in the cap and the number of macrophages ($p < 0.006$) and an inverse relation between the number of smooth muscle cells and strain ($p < 0.0001$). Plaques declared vulnerable in elastography had thinner caps than non-vulnerable plaques ($p < 0.0001$).[41]

It is feasible to apply intravascular palpography during interventional catheterization procedures. In a recent study, data were acquired in patients (n = 12) during PTCA procedures with echo apparatus equipped with radiofrequency output. The systemic pressure was used to strain the tissue, and the strain was determined using cross-correlation analysis of sequential frames acquired at different pressures. A likelihood function was determined to obtain the frames with minimal motion of the catheter in the lumen since motion of the catheter impairs accuracy of strain estimation. Minimal motion was observed near the end of the passive filling phase. Reproducible strain estimates were obtained within one pressure cycle and over several pressure cycles. Validation of the results was limited to the information provided by the echogram. Significantly higher strain values were found in non-calcified plaques than in calcified plaques.[42]

Another *in vivo* validation study in atherosclerotic Yucatan pigs showed that fatty plaques had increased mean strain values. High-strain spots were also associated with the presence of macrophages, a further feature of vulnerable plaques.[43] Three-dimensional intravascular palpography detects strain patterns in human coronary arteries that are typical of deformable plaques.[44] The number of deformable plaques is correlated both with clinical presentation and levels of C-reactive protein.[45] The technique is highly reproducible.[46]

Palpography reveals information not revealed by IVUS. Differentiating hard and soft tissues may be important for the detection of a deformable plaque that is prone to rupture. Since palpography is based on clinically available IVUS catheters, the technique can be easily introduced into the catheterization laboratory. By acquiring data at the end of the filling phase, when catheter motion is minimal, the quality and reliability of the palpogram are increased. The clinical value of this technique is currently under investigation.

4.6 THERMOGRAPHY

Inflammation produces a temperature rise in affected tissues. Since atherosclerosis is accompanied by inflammation, one hypothesis suggests that a temperature rise can be measured at the surface of a plaque. Because a vulnerable plaque is a very active metabolic area, the hypothesis was extended to note that vulnerable plaques may exhibit even higher temperature rises.

Casscells et al. reported that carotid plaques taken from 48 patients during endarterectomies showed temperature heterogeneity.[47] The temperature difference noted in different areas was up to 2.2°C and correlated with cell density ($R^2 = -0.47$, p = 0.0001). A negative correlation between temperature difference and cap thickness ($R^2 = -0.34$, p = 0.0001) was also noted. The same group reported approximately the same *in vitro* findings in atherosclerotic rabbits.[48]

A correlation between temperature rise and macrophage infiltration has also been suggested in an *in vivo* rabbit trial.[49] Stefanadis et al. performed studies in humans. Patients with stable angina, unstable angina, and acute myocardial infarction were studied. The thermistor of the thermography catheter has a temperature accuracy of 0.05°C, a time constant of 300 msec, and a spatial resolution of 0.5 mm. The thermistor of the catheter was driven against the vessel wall by the force of blood flow, without the help of a mechanical device like a balloon. Temperature was constant within the arteries of the control subjects, whereas most atherosclerotic plaques showed higher temperatures compared with healthy vessel walls. Temperature differences between atherosclerotic plaque and healthy vessel wall increased progressively from stable angina to patients with acute myocardial infarction with a maximum difference of 1.5 ± 0.7°C.[50] Furthermore patients with high temperature gradients had significantly worse outcomes than patients with low gradients.[51] However, this data has yet to be confirmed prospectively in other centers and the influences of parameters such as coronary blood flow[52] and catheter design must be studied in the future.

4.7 OPTICAL COHERENCE TOMOGRAPHY

Optical coherence tomography (OCT) can provide images with ultrahigh resolution. The technique measures the intensity of back-reflected light in a similar way as IVUS measures acoustic waves.[53] It is an invasive technique with a catheter advanced over a 0.014-in. wire. With a Michelson interferometer, light is split into two signals. One signal is sent into the tissue and the other to a reference arm with a mirror. Both signals are reflected and cross-correlated by interfering light beams. To achieve cross-correlation at incremental penetration depths in the tissue, the mirror is dynamically translated. The intensity of the interfering signals at a certain mirror position represents back-scattering at a corresponding depth. High resolution images (resolution ranging from 4 to 20 μm) can be achieved[54] with a penetration depth up to 2 mm. Images can be acquired real time at 15 frames/sec.

Early attempts were made to validate OCT using histology. A lipid pool generates decreased signal areas and a fibrous plaque produces a homogenous signal-rich lesion.[55] *In vitro* comparison of OCT and IVUS demonstrated superior delineation by OCT of structural details like thin caps or tissue proliferations.[56]

The limitations of OCT are the low penetration depth that hinders studying large vessels and the light absorbance by blood that must be overcome by saline infusion or balloon occlusion with associated potential for ischemia. Special techniques like index matching may improve imaging through blood.[57]

4.8 RAMAN SPECTROSCOPY

Raman spectroscopy is a technique that can characterize chemical composition by utilizing the Raman effect[58] created when incident light (wave length 750 to 850 nm) excites molecules in a tissue sample that back-scatter the light while changing wavelength. The change in wavelength is the Raman effect.[59] The wavelength shift and the signal intensity are dependent on the chemical components of the tissue sample. Due to this unique feature, Raman spectroscopy can provide quantitative information about the molecular composition of a sample.[60] The spectra obtained from tissues require post-processing to differentiate plaque components.

Even in the presence of blood, Raman spectra have been shown to be obtainable *in vivo* from the aortic arches of sheep.[61] In a study using mice fed high fat–high cholesterol (HFC) diets for 0, 2, 4, or 6 months, Raman spectroscopy showed good correlation between cholesterol accumulation and total serum cholesterol exposure (R = approximately 0.87, $p < 0.001$). In female mice ($n = 10$) fed HFC diets with or without 0.01% atorvastatin, strong reductions in cholesterol accumulations (57%) and calcium salts (97%; $p < 0.01$) were demonstrated in the atorvastatin-treated group. Raman spectroscopy can, therefore, be used to quantitatively study the size and distribution of depositions of cholesterol and calcification.[62] Limitations of the technique are the limited penetration depth (1 to 1.5 mm), the long acquisition time, and the absorbance of the light by blood. Raman spectroscopy yields no geometrical information.

4.9 NEAR-INFRARED SPECTROSCOPY

Near-infrared (NIR) spectroscopy also provides information on the chemical components of coronary vessel walls. Molecular vibrational transitions measured in the NIR region (750 to 2500 nm) produce qualitative and quantitative results on plaque composition. NIR spectroscopy sensitivities and specificities for the histological features of plaque vulnerability were 90 and 93% for the lipid pools, 77 and 93% for the thin caps, and 84 and 89% for inflammatory cells.[63] A differentiation between vulnerable and non-vulnerable carotid plaques could be achieved *ex vivo*.[64] Future studies will address the question whether NIR spectroscopy is feasible *in vivo*. Problems like acquisition time, blood scattering, and influences of pH and temperature must be addressed.

4.10 MAGNETIC RESONANCE IMAGING

High-resolution magnetic resonance imaging (MRI) is a noninvasive modality for characterizing atherosclerotic plaques. Combining information from T1 and T2-weighted imaging can permit *in vitro* identification of atheromatous cores, collageneous caps, calcifications, media, adventitia, and perivascular fat.[65] In a small number of patients (n = 6) a matching between *in vivo* and *in vitro* measurements of carotid arteries was seen.[66] Yuan et al. determined the accuracy of *in vivo* MRI for measuring the cross-sectional maximum wall area of atherosclerotic carotid arteries in a group of 14 patients undergoing carotid endarterectomies. The authors showed a strong correlation between *in vivo* and *in vitro* measurements.[67] Although the results may not be perfect, it may be possible to identify carotid plaques at high risk for stroke using MRI.[68] Images of carotid arteries can be further improved using a coil placed close to the carotid artery at the surface of the neck.[69] An in-plane resolution of 0.4×0.4 mm and a slice thickness of 3 mm may allow assessment of fibrous cap thickness and integrity.[70]

Imaging of coronary arteries with MRI is more difficult than imaging carotid plaques since cardiac and respiratory motion, small plaque size, and the locations of the coronary arteries can cause acquisition problems. Nevertheless, high resolution MRI of the human coronary walls of angiographically normal and abnormal vessels has been shown to be feasible. In a study by Botnar et al., the coronary wall thickness and wall area were significantly enlarged in patients with coronary artery disease demonstrated by angiography.[71] Small plaque structures like fibrous caps cannot yet be assessed using current MRI techniques. Thinner slices and higher in-plane resolution are needed to better delineate coronary plaques.

4.11 ANGUS AND SHEAR STRESS

High-resolution reconstruction of three-dimensional (3D) coronary lumen and wall morphology is obtained by combining angiography and IVUS — a technique known as ANGUS.[72] Briefly, a biplane angiogram of a sheath-based IVUS catheter taken at end-diastole allows reconstruction of the 3D pull-back trajectory of the catheter.

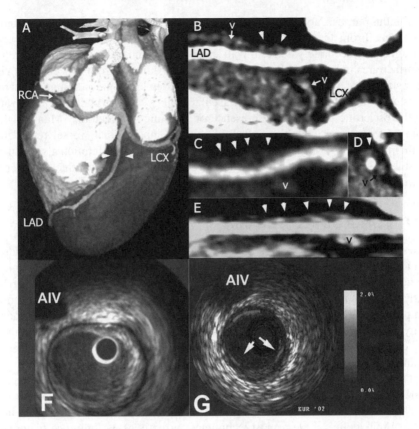

FIGURE 4.1 *(A color version of this figure follows page 112.)* Noninvasive coronary imaging, using a 16-slice spiral computed tomography scanner (Sensation 16, Siemens AG, Forchheim, Germany), suggested a nonobstructive lesion in the mid-LAD (A, arrowhead) confirmed with coronary angiography. The attenuation value of the plaque was measured as 80 Hounsfield units (HUs), suggesting a mixed plaque composition without calcification (C, D, arrowheads). The entire segment can be shown in a single plane by means of vessel tracking (E, arrowhead). The great cardiac vein can be differentiated from the plaque by the higher and homogeneous attenuation of the venous lumen (v). Palpography (G) delivers strain information about this plaque's surface. At right, a scale ranging from 0% (blue) to 2% (yellow) characterizes the strain pattern. The strain images are color-coded: blue indicates stiff (low strain) material and red indicates softer (higher strain) material. In the cross-section in the identical position with the IVUS image (F), an eccentric soft plaque is visible with shoulders of high strain (arrows) on both sides of the otherwise stable cap, while the strain at the left shoulder (left arrow) is 1.5% and on the right shoulder (right arrow) is 1.2%. Between 11 and 12 hr, the palpogram appears to show an area of high strain, but this is caused by the nearby cardiac vein (AIV).

Combining this path with lumen and wall information derived from IVUS images successively acquired during catheter pull-back at end-diastole accurately shows 3D lumen and wall reconstruction with resolution determined by IVUS. Filling the 3D lumen space with a high resolution 3D mesh allows calculation of the detailed blood velocity profile in the lumen.[73]

For this purpose, absolute flow and blood viscosity must be provided as boundary conditions. From the blood velocity profile, local wall shear stress on the endothelium can be accurately derived. Wall shear stress is the frictional force normalized to surface area induced by blood passing the wall. Although from a mechanical view, shear stress is of a very small magnitude compared to blood pressure-induced tensile stress, it has a profound influence on vascular biology[74] and explains the localization of atherosclerotic plaque in the presence of systemic risk factors.[75] Many of these biological processes including inflammation, thrombogenicity, vessel remodeling, intimal thickening or regression, and smooth muscle cell proliferation also influence the stability of vulnerable plaques. Therefore, the study of this parameter as derived by image-based modeling is of utmost importance.

4.12 CONCLUDING REMARKS

Assessment of atherosclerosis by imaging techniques is essential for *in vivo* identification of vulnerable plaques. Several invasive and noninvasive imaging techniques are currently in development. OCT has the advantage of high resolution; thermography measures metabolism; and NIR spectroscopy obtains information on chemical components. IVUS and IVUS-palpography are easy to perform and assess morphology and mechanical instability. Shear stress is an important mechanical parameter that deeply influences vascular biology. MRI and CT provide the advantages of noninvasive imaging.

Nevertheless all techniques are still under development and no single technique alone can yet identify a vulnerable plaque or predict its further development. This is related to fundamental methodological insufficiencies that may be resolved in the future. From a clinical view, most techniques currently assess only one feature of a vulnerable plaque. Thus, a combination of several modalities (see Figure 4.1)[76] will be of importance in the future to ensure high sensitivity and specificity in detecting vulnerable plaques.

REFERENCES

1. Libby P. Molecular bases of the acute coronary syndromes. *Circulation* 1995; 91: 2844–2850.
2. Falk E. Stable versus unstable atherosclerosis: clinical aspects. *Am Heart J* 1999, 1389: S421–S425.
3. Virmani R, Burke AP, Farb A, et al. Pathology of the unstable plaque. *Progr Cardiovasc Dis* 2002; 44: 349–356.
4. Little WC, Constantinescu M, Applegate RJ, et al. Can coronary angiography predict the site of a subsequent myocardial infarction in patients with mild-to-moderate coronary artery disease? *Circulation* 1988; 78: 1157–1166.
5. Nobuyoshi M, Tanaka M, Nosaka H, et al. Progression of coronary atherosclerosis: is coronary spasm related to progression? *J Am Coll Cardiol* 1991; 18: 904–910.
6. Ambrose JA, Tannenbaum MA, Alexopoulos D, et al. Angiographic progression of coronary artery disease and the development of myocardial infarction. *J Am Coll Cardiol* 1988; 12: 56–62.

7. Giroud D, Li JM, Urban P, et al. Relation of the site of acute myocardial infarction to the most severe coronary arterial stenosis at prior angiography. *Am J Cardiol* 1992; 69: 729–732.

8. Kerensky RA, Wade M, Deedwania P, et al. Revisiting the culprit lesion in non-Q-wave myocardial infarction: results from the VANQWISH trial angiographic core laboratory. *J Am Coll Cardiol* 2002; 39: 1456–1463.

9. Frink RJ. Chronic ulcerated plaques: new insights into the pathogenesis of acute coronary disease. *J Invasive Cardiol* 1994; 6: 173–185.

10. Ojio S, Takatsu H, Tanaka T, et al. Considerable time from the onset of plaque rupture and/or thrombi until the onset of acute myocardial infarction in humans: coronary angiographic findings within 1 week before the onset of infarction. *Circulation* 2000; 102: 2063–2069.

11. Goldstein JA, Demetriou D, Grines CL, et al. Multiple complex coronary plaques in patients with acute myocardial infarction. *New Engl J Med* 2000; 343: 915–922.

12. Kim WY, Danias PG, and Stuber M, Coronary magnetic resonance angiography for the detection of coronary stenoses. *New Engl J Med* 2001; 345: 1863–1869.

13. Mizuno K, Satomura K, Miyamoto A, et al. Angioscopic evaluation of coronary artery thrombi in acute coronary syndromes. *New Engl J Med* 1992; 326: 287–291.

14. Sherman CT, Litvack F, Grundfest W, et al. Coronary angioscopy in patients with unstable angina pectoris. *New Engl J Med* 1986; 315: 913–919.

15. Feld S, Ganim M, Carell ES, et al. Comparison of angioscopy, intravascular ultrasound imaging and quantitative coronary angiography in predicting clinical outcome after coronary intervention in high risk patients. *J Am Coll Cardiol* 1996; 28: 97–105.

16. Takano M, Mizuno K, Okamatsu K, et al. Mechanical and structural characteristics of vulnerable plaques: analysis by coronary angioscopy and intravascular ultrasound. *J Am Coll Cardiol* 2001; 38: 99–104.

17. Asakura M, Ueda Y, Yamaguchi O, et al. Extensive development of vulnerable plaques as a pan-coronary process in patients with myocardial infarction: an angioscopic study. *J Am Coll Cardiol* 2001; 37: 1284–1288.

18. Uchida Y, Nakamura F, Tomaru T, Morita T, Oshima T, Sasaki T, Morizuki S, and Hirose J. Prediction of acute coronary syndromes by percutaneous coronary angioscopy in patients with stable angina. *Am Heart J* 1995; 130: 195–203.

19. Bom N, Li W, van der Steen AF, Lancee CT, Cespedes EI, Slager CJ, and de Korte CL. Intravascular imaging. *Ultrasonics* 1998; 36: 625–628.

20. Di Mario C, The SH, Madretsma S, et al. Detection and characterization of vascular lesions by intravascular ultrasound: an *in vitro* study correlated with histology. *J Am Soc Echocardiogr* 1992; 5: 135–146.

21. Sechtem U, Arnold G, Keweloh T, et al. *In vitro* diagnosis of coronary plaque morphology with intravascular ultrasound: comparison with histopathologic findings. *Z Kardiol* 1993; 82: 618–627.

22. Friedrich GJ, Moes NY, Muhlberger VA, et al. Detection of intralesional calcium by intracoronary ultrasound depends on the histologic pattern. *Am Heart J* 1994; 128: 435–441.

23. Potkin BN, Bartorelli AL, Gessert JM, et al. Coronary artery imaging with intravascular high-frequency ultrasound. *Circulation* 1990; 81: 1575–1585.

24. Rasheed Q, Dhawale PJ, Anderson J et al. Intracoronary ultrasound-defined plaque composition: computer-aided plaque characterization and correlation with histologic samples obtained during directional coronary atherectomy. *Am Heart J* 1995; 129: 631–637.

64 High-Risk Atherosclerotic Plaques: Mechanisms, Imaging, Models, and Therapy

25. Hiro T, Leung CY, Russo RJ, et al. Variability of a three-layered appearance in intravascular ultrasound coronary images: a comparison of morphometric measurements with four intravascular ultrasound systems. *Am J Card Imaging* 1996; 10: 219–227.
26. Ge J, Haude M, Gorge G, et al. Silent healing of spontaneous plaque disruption demonstrated by intracoronary ultrasound. *Eur Heart J* 1995; 16: 1149–1151.
27. Jeremias A, Ge J, and Erbel R. New insight into plaque healing after plaque rupture with subsequent thrombus formation detected by intravascular ultrasound. *Heart* 1997; 77: 293.
28. Ge J, Chirillo F, Schwedtmann J, et al. Screening of ruptured plaques in patients with coronary artery disease by intravascular ultrasound. *Heart* 1999; 81: 621–627.
29. Yamagishi M, Terashima M, Awano K, et al. Morphology of vulnerable coronary plaque: insights from follow-up of patients examined by intravascular ultrasound before an acute coronary syndrome. *J Am Coll Cardiol* 2000; 35: 106–111.
30. von Birgelen C, Klinkhart W, Mintz GS, et al. Plaque distribution and vascular remodeling of ruptured and nonruptured coronary plaques in the same vessel: an intravascular ultrasound study *in vivo*. *J Am Coll Cardiol* 2001; 37: 1864–1870.
31. Nair A, Kuban BD, Obuchowski N, et al. Assessing spectral algorithms to predict atherosclerotic plaque composition with normalized and raw intravascular ultrasound data. *Ultrasound Med Biol* 2001; 10: 1319–1331.
32. Landini L, Sarnelli R, Picano E, et al. Evaluation of frequency dependence of backscatter coefficient in normal and atherosclerotic aortic walls. *Ultrasound Med Biol* 1986; 5: 397–401.
33. Wilson LS, Neale ML, Talhami HE et al. Preliminary results from attenuation-slope mapping of plaque using intravascular ultrasound. *Ultrasound Med Biol* 1994; 20: 529–542.
34. Jeremias A, Kolz ML, Ikonen TS, et al. Feasibility of *in vivo* intravascular ultrasound tissue characterization in the detection of early vascular transplant rejection. *Circulation* 1999; 100: 2127–2130.
35. Wickline SA, Miller JG, Recchia D, et al. Beyond intravascular imaging: quantitative ultrasonic tissue characterization of vascular pathology. *IEEE Ultrasonics Symposium* 1994; 3: 1589–1597.
36. Bridal SL, Beyssen B, Fornes P, Julia P, Berger G. Multiparametric attenuation and backscatter images for characterization of carotid plaque. *Ultrason Imaging* 2000; 22: 20–34.
37. Spencer T, Ramo MP, Salter DM et al. Characterisation of atherosclerotic plaque by spectral analysis of intravascular ultrasound: an *in vitro* methodology. *Ultrasound Med Biol* 1997; 23: 191–203.
38. Ophir J, Cespedes I, Ponnekanti H, et al. Elastography: a quantitative method for imaging the elasticity of biological tissues. *Ultrason Imaging* 1991; 13: 111–134.
39. Doyley MM, Mastik F, de Korte CL, et al. Advancing intravascular ultrasonic palpation toward clinical applications. *Ultrasound Med Biol* 2001; 27: 1471–1480.
40. de Korte CL, Pasterkamp G, van der Steen AF, et al. Characterization of plaque components with intravascular ultrasound elastography in human femoral and coronary arteries *in vitro*. *Circulation* 2000; 102: 617–623.
41. Schaar JA, de Korte CL, Mastik F et al. Characterizing vulnerable plaque features with intravascular elastography. *Circulation*. 2003; 108: 2636–2641.
42. de Korte CL, Carlier SG, Mastik F, et al. Morphological and mechanical information of coronary arteries obtained with intravascular elastography; feasibility study *in vivo*. *Eur Heart J* 2002; 23: 405–413.

43. de Korte CL, Sierevogel MJ, Mastik F, Strijder C, et al. Identification of athero-sclerotic plaque components with intravascular ultrasound elastography *in vivo*: a Yucatan pig study. *Circulation* 2002; 105: 1627–1630.

44. Schaar JA, Mastik F, de Korte CL, et al. Three-dimensional palpography: a new tool for detection of vulnerable plaque, a feasibility and reproducibility *in vitro*. *Eur Heart J* 2001; 22 (Suppl.) P2784.

45. Schaar JA, Mastik F, Regar E et al. Incidence of vulnerable plaques in humans: assessment with intravascular palpography. *Eur Heart J* 2003, 24 (Suppl.), P2210.

46. Schaar JA, Mastik F, Regar E et al. Reproducibility of three-dimensional palpography. *Eur Heart J* 2003, 24 (Suppl.), P2203.

47. Casscells W, Hathorn B, David M, et al. Thermal detection of cellular infiltrates in living atherosclerotic plaques: possible implications for plaque rupture and thrombo-sis. *Lancet* 1996; 347: 1447–1451.

48. Casscells W, David M, Bearman G et al. Thermography, in *The Vulnerable Athero-sclerotic Plaque*. V. Fuster (Ed.). Futura Publishing, 1999, p. 231–242.

49. Verheye S, De Meyer GR, Van Langenhove G et al. *In vivo* temperature heterogeneity of atherosclerotic plaques is determined by plaque composition. *Circulation* 2002; 105: 1596–1601.

50. Stefanadis C, Diamantopoulos L, Vlachopoulos C et al. Thermal heterogeneity within human atherosclerotic coronary arteries detected *in vivo*: A new method of detection by application of a special thermography catheter. *Circulation* 1999; 99: 1965–1971.

51. Stefanadis C, Toutouzas K, Tsiamis E, et al. Increased local temperature in human coronary atherosclerotic plaques: an independent predictor of clinical outcome in patients undergoing a percutaneous coronary intervention. *J Am Coll Cardiol* 2001; 37: 1277–1283.

52. Diamantopulos L, Liu X, De Scheerder I, et al. The effect of reduced blood-flow on the coronary wall temperature: are significant lesions suitable for intravascular ther-mography? *Eur Heart J* 2003: 1788–1795.

53. Huang D, Swanson EA, Lin CP, et al. Optical coherence tomography. *Science* 1991; 254: 1178–1181.

54. Boppart SA, Bouma BE, Pitris C, et al. *In vivo* cellular optical coherence tomography imaging. *Nat Med* 1998; 4: 861–865.

55. Jang IK, Bouma BE, Kang DH, et al. Visualization of coronary atherosclerotic plaques in patients using optical coherence tomography: comparison with intravascular ultra-sound. *J Am Coll Cardiol* 2002; 39: 604–609.

56. Brezinski ME, Tearney GJ, Weissman NJ, et al. Assessing atherosclerotic plaque morphology: comparison of optical coherence tomography and high frequency intra-vascular ultrasound. *Heart* 1997; 77: 397–403.

57. Brezinski M, Saunders K, Jesser C, et al. Index matching to improve optical coherence tomography imaging through blood. *Circulation* 2001; 103: 1999–2003.

58. Baraga JJ, Feld MS, Rava RP. *In situ* optical histochemistry of human artery using near-infrared Fourier transform Raman spectroscopy. *Proc Natl Acad Sci USA*. 1992; 89: 3473–3477.

59. Van de Poll SWE, Motz JT, Kramer JR. Prospects of laser spectroscopy to detect vulnerable plaque, in *Cardiovascular Plaque Rupture*. Brown, DL (Ed). Marcel Dekker, New York, 2002.

60. Hanlon EB, Manoharan R, Koo TW, et al. Prospects for *in vivo* Raman spectroscopy. *Phys Med Biol* 2000; 45: R1–R59.

61. Buschman HP, Marple ET, Wach ML, et al. *In vivo* determination of the molecular composition of artery wall by intravascular Raman spectroscopy. *Anal Chem* 2000; 72: 3771–3775.
62. van De Poll SW, Romer TJ, Volger OL, et al. Raman spectroscopic evaluation of the effects of diet and lipid-lowering therapy on atherosclerotic plaque development in mice. *Arterioscler Thromb Vasc Biol* 2001; 21: 1630–1635.
63. Moreno PR, Lodder RA, Purushothaman KR, et al. Detection of lipid pool, thin fibrous cap, and inflammatory cells in human aortic atherosclerotic plaques by near-infrared spectroscopy. *Circulation* 2002; 105: 923–927.
64. Wang J, Geng YJ, Guo B, et al. Near-infrared spectroscopic characterization of human advanced atherosclerotic plaques. *J Am Coll Cardiol* 2002; 39: 1305–1313.
65. Toussaint JF, Southern JF, Fuster V, et al. T2-weighted contrast for NMR characterization of human atherosclerosis. *Arterioscler Thromb Vasc Biol* 1995; 15: 1533–1542.
66. Toussaint JF, LaMuraglia GM, Southern JF, et al. Magnetic resonance images lipid, fibrous, calcified, hemorrhagic, and thrombotic components of human atherosclerosis *in vivo*. *Circulation* 1996; 94: 932–938.
67. Yuan C, Beach KW, Smith LH Jr, et al. Measurement of atherosclerotic carotid plaque size *in vivo* using high resolution magnetic resonance imaging. *Circulation* 1998; 98: 2666–2671.
68. Yuan C, Mitsumori LM, Beach KW, et al. Carotid atherosclerotic plaque: noninvasive MR characterization and identification of vulnerable lesions. *Radiology* 2001; 221: 285–299.
69. Hayes CE, Mathis CM, and Yuan C. Surface coil phased arrays for high-resolution imaging of the carotid arteries. *Thought* 1996; 6: 109–112.
70. Hatsukami TS, Ross R, Polissar NL, et al. Visualization of fibrous cap thickness and rupture in human atherosclerotic carotid plaque *in vivo* with high-resolution magnetic resonance imaging. *Circulation* 2000; 102: 959–964.
71. Botnar RM, Stuber M, Kissinger KV, et al. Noninvasive coronary vessel wall and plaque imaging with magnetic resonance imaging. *Circulation* 2000; 102: 2582–2587.
72. Slager, CJ, Wentzel JJ, Schuurbiers JCH et al., True 3-dimensional reconstruction of coronary arteries in patients by fusion of angiography and IVUS (ANGUS) and its quantitative validation. *Circulation*, 2000; 102: 511–516.
73. Thury A, Wentzel JJ, Schuurbiers JC, Ligthart JM, Krams R, de Feyter PJ, Serruys PW, and Slager CJ. Prominent role of tensile stress in propagation of a dissection after coronary stenting: computational fluid dynamic analysis on true 3D-reconstructed segment. *Circulation*. 2001; 104: E53–E54.
74. Malek AM, Alper, SL, and Izumo S. Hemodynamic shear stress and its role in atherosclerosis. *JAMA* 1999; 282: 2035–2042.
75. Asakura and T. and Karino T. Flow patterns and spatial distribution of atherosclerotic lesions in human coronary arteries. *Circ Res*, 1990; 66: 1045–1066.
76. Arampatzis CA, Ligthart JMR, Schaar JA et al. Detection of a vulnerable coronary plaque: a treatment dilemma. *Circulation* 2003; 108: E34–E35.

5 Imaging of High-Risk Atherosclerotic Plaque by Intravascular Ultrasound: Focal Assessment of Morphology and Vulnerability or Systemic Assessment of Disease Burden and Activity?

Paul Schoenhagen, Richard D. White, and Steven E. Nissen

CONTENTS

5.1 INTRODUCTION

Coronary artery disease (CAD) remains the leading cause of mortality in industrialized societies.[1-3] Most acute coronary events occur after sudden rupture or erosion of vulnerable plaques in the absence of prior significant luminal stenoses. Most of our knowledge about these high-risk lesions has been derived from postmortem studies in patients who died from coronary causes. Based on these studies, the interest has been focused on *focal* morphological characteristics including the necrotic cores, fibrous caps, and expansive remodeling. Animal models and clinical imaging studies have expanded these observations by demonstrating that plaque accumulation, vulnerability, and rupture are widespread and common processes that occur far more frequently than clinical syndromes. Our current understanding indicates that CAD is a diffuse disease process with a central role of inflammation. Acute coronary syndromes (ACSs) are the *focal* manifestations of this *systemic* disease process.[4-6]

The *in vivo* identification of focal, high-risk lesions before the occurrences of clinical events may have important implications for disease prevention. Using invasive and noninvasive imaging modalities, studies in patients presenting with ACS have retrospectively identified morphologic characteristics of the culprit lesion sites. Corresponding to histological studies, these include the necrotic cores, fibrous caps, plaque ruptures, and remodeling. The same characteristics have been prospectively observed in nonstenotic, asymptomatic lesions and have therefore been interpreted as evidence of vulnerability.

However, the observation that plaque vulnerability is a temporary, focal manifestation of a systemic disease process questions the paradigm of focal identification of high-risk lesions derived from postmortem studies. Alternatively, a quantitative assessment of disease burden and activity could identify individuals at high risk for future events. Several invasive and noninvasive imaging modalities are already used to assess coronary plaque burden, and our knowledge about the relationship to biochemical markers of disease activity is constantly growing. Future studies will be necessary to evaluate the relationships of plaque burdens, biochemical markers, and clinical events.[7-9]

In this chapter, we will review the role of atherosclerosis imaging for the detection of high-risk lesions. Based on our experience with intravascular ultrasound (IVUS) and multidetector computed tomography (MDCT), we will discuss the potential impact for understanding CAD in research settings, disease prevention, and novel focal and systemic treatment approaches.

5.2 FOCAL ASSESSMENT OF LESION MORPHOLOGY AND VULNERABILITY: A PARADIGM DERIVED FROM POSTMORTEM STUDIES

Most of the early knowledge about vulnerable plaques was derived from histological postmortem studies in patients who died related to cardiac causes.[10-13] In these patients, the culprit lesion sites were typically characterized by large, often eccentric, necrotic cores separated from the lumens by thin fibrous caps. Because of the expansion of vessel diameter at the lesion site, a process described as expansive or positive arterial remodeling,[14-17] the lumen was often relatively maintained. However, expansive remodeling appeared to be associated with plaque vulnerability.[18-20]

A consistent characteristic of vulnerable plaques is a prominent inflammatory response.[21-24] In early atherosclerotic lesions, macrophages accumulate at a plaque site and, by incorporating cholesterol, become so-called foam cells. This cell accumulation develops into the necrotic cores of more advanced lesions. Macrophages are also found in the shoulder regions of fibrous caps at the borders of necrotic core areas, where mechanical stress and inflammation add to instability.[25-27] The accumulation and activation of macrophages and other inflammatory cells induce the secretion of enzymes including the matrix metalloproteinases (MMPs). Enzymatic weakening of the connective tissue framework (extracellular matrix) of the fibrous cap is the pathophysiologic process underlying arterial remodeling and plaque rupture.[28,29]

Similar to these postmortem observations, initial *in vivo* imaging studies have focused on culprit lesions identified by angiography in patients presenting with acute coronary events. Angiography is a *planar* imaging modality. By projecting a silhouette of the lumen, angiography allows exact assessment of luminal dimension for the identification of stenosis severity. Angiographic studies demonstrated that certain high-risk plaque characteristics are reflected by the shapes of the luminal plaque borders.[30] However, angiography does not allow assessment of the plaques. The development of intravascular ultrasound (IVUS), a *tomographic* imaging modality, allowed direct assessment of vessel walls and further descriptions of plaque morphology in patients with stable and unstable presentations.[31-34] Several groups used IVUS to examine differences between stable and unstable coronary plaques in symptomatic patients.

Reproducing the above-described findings of postmortem studies, echolucent appearance and expansive (positive) remodeling by intravascular ultrasound have been associated with the clinical presentation of unstable angina.[35-40] Our group studied 85 patients with unstable and 46 patients with stable coronary syndromes using IVUS. Expansive (positive) remodeling and plaque echolucency were significantly more frequent in unstable than in stable lesions, while constrictive (negative) remodeling was more frequent in stable lesions.[39] In further work we demonstrated that increased MMP3 is found more frequently in expansive remodeled lesions.[41]

Most of the postmortem and early imaging observations *retrospectively* described anatomical and ultrastructural characteristics of highly stenotic lesions that had already caused clinical symptoms. However, plaque vulnerability is a *prospective* definition of a plaque at risk of rupturing in the future. It has been inferred that the characteristics present in symptomatic lesions are identical to those of vulnerable lesions before rupture. However, the lesions exhibit important differences.

Angiographic studies have consistently demonstrated that patients who eventually develop myocardial infarctions typically only demonstrate mild stenosis at future culprit lesion sites in the months before the events.[42-47] The proof that high-risk characteristics identified in already ruptured lesions represent those of vulnerable lesions could only come from prospective, serial examinations. This has become feasible with *in vivo* imaging modalities but the current data are very limited.

Using IVUS, Yamagishi et al. prospectively examined whether the identification of these morphologic features in mild to moderately stenotic plaques would be associated with acute coronary syndromes during follow-up.[48] The authors examined 114 atherosclerotic coronary sites without significant stenosis by angiography (<50% diameter stenosis) in 106 patients. The lesions consisted of 22 concentric and 92 eccentric plaques with plaque area averaging 59 ± 12%. During a 2-year follow-up, 12 patients had acute coronary events related to previously examined coronary sites at an average of 4.0 ± 3.4 months after the initial IVUS study.

The preexisting plaques related to the subsequent acute events demonstrated an eccentric pattern and the mean percent plaque area was greater than in the patients without acute events. However, no statistically significant difference in lumen area existed between two patient groups. Among the 12 future culprit sites, 10 contained echolucent zones, likely representing a lipid-rich, necrotic core at baseline. In contrast, of the 90 sites without acute events, echolucent zones were seen at only 4 sites. These results suggest that imaging equivalents of necrotic cores could in fact identify lesions at increased risk for future instability. The study also confirms prospectively that despite significant plaque accumulation, lumen area is preserved at the time of initial study secondary to expansive remodeling of the vessel wall.

Recent technical developments in ultrasound equipment, utilizing several characteristics of the digitized ultrasound signal with radiofrequency analysis and elastography, allow advanced tissue characterization.[49–53] Alternatively, light waves are used in optical coherence tomography, to more precisely characterize the compositions of atherosclerotic plaques.[54,55] Yet another approach is the focal assessment of temperature differences with sensitive intravascular thermography catheters, presumably reflecting focal inflammatory changes of vulnerable lesions.[56,57]

These results must be confirmed in larger studies using serial imaging and advanced imaging modalities. This will be possible in several ongoing large progression–regression studies using serial IVUS examinations 1 or 2 years apart, testing different pharmacological treatment strategies. These studies should include several focal arterial segments with minimal disease that show progression and changes in morphology.

However, despite the critical importance of identifying focal morphological characteristic of vulnerable plaques, the clinical application of results may be limited. Increasing evidence indicates that the paradigm of identifying and treating individual culprit lesions (vulnerable plaques) based on experience with angiography and postmortem studies may not be adequate for the understanding and modification of coronary atherosclerosis in vulnerable patients because of its diffuse, systemic nature as described below.[8,9]

5.3   EVIDENCE OF A MULTIFOCAL, SYSTEMIC DISEASE PROCESS: IMPACT ON EXISTING DIAGNOSTIC AND THERAPEUTIC PARADIGMS

Recent histological studies suggest that episodes of plaque destabilization and rupture are common and most frequently not associated with clinical symptoms.[58–61] Presumably, after episodes of rupture, the local balance between thrombosis and spontaneous thrombolysis prevents occlusion in most vessel segments. The nonocclusive clot formation is then followed by a "healing" process characterized by fibrosis. It is now accepted that this sequence of events represents the most frequent mode of lesion progression. On the other hand, studies in patients at the times of acute coronary events suggest that multiple ruptured plaques can be found distant from the "culprit" lesion throughout the coronary tree.[5,62]

Presumably, such patients have underlying milieus conducive to the development of multifocal plaque ulcerations.[62–64] This systemic vulnerability at the time of acute coronary syndromes is associated with evidence of systemic inflammation and may explain the high propensity for recurrent events. Plaque vulnerability therefore describes a temporary, systemic biochemical stage of plaque activation with increased risk of rupture. These results have been confirmed *in vivo*. Angiographic studies in patients presenting with ACS have demonstrated lesions with character-istics of plaque rupture at multiple sites other than the culprit lesions.[65-67] The findings of these additional lesions may correspond to the documented accelerated rates of atherosclerotic disease progression and repeat coronary events in the months after acute coronary events.[68–71]

Recent IVUS studies also demonstrated the presence of diffuse destabilization throughout the coronary tree.[72–75] Rioufol et al.[72] examined all three coronary arteries with IVUS in 24 patients 1 to 2 weeks after acute coronary syndromes. Plaque rupture, arterial remodeling, lesion eccentricity, and plaque calcifications were ana-lyzed. A total of 72 epicardial coronary arteries were explored and 50 distinct plaque ruptures were detected (mean = 2.08 per patient; range = 0 to 6). Nine cases of plaque rupture in nine patients (37.5%) were clearly identified at the culprit lesions; 41 cases of plaque rupture were located in arteries other than the culprit artery.

Culprit lesions with or without plaque ruptures exhibited the same morphologic criteria by angiography and IVUS, including similar minimum luminal diameter, plaque burden, and remodeling ratio. At least one plaque rupture somewhere other than on the culprit lesion was found in 79% of the patients; at least one rupture diagnosed in an artery other than the culprit artery was present in 70.8% of the patients, and 12.5% showed ruptures (at least one) in all three arteries. Ruptured plaques distant from the culprit lesions demonstrated lower echogenicity and less calcification than ruptured culprit lesions, suggesting a less chronic atherosclerotic disease process.

Asakura et al.[74] took a similar approach using coronary angioscopy. Over the 4 wk following myocardial infarction, angioscopic examinations of 73 coronary arteries revealed yellow (vulnerable) plaques at 90% of the culprit lesions and also diffusely (3.2 ± 1.7 per artery) in all three coronary arteries. Intracoronary thrombi were frequently found at the culprit lesion sites, but only exceptionally on additional lesions. The fact that angioscopy assesses lesion surface rather than rupture[76] likely explains the lower number of distinct ruptures found by IVUS compared with the higher frequency of yellow plaques revealed by angioscopy. The higher sensitivity of angioscopy also explains the remarkably high rate (60%) of yellow plaque found in stable coronary subjects in whom IVUS estimated the incidence of plaque rupture at 5 to 20%,[75,77] a percentage close to findings in postmortem studies.

Our group took a different approach by comparing morphology and frequency of ulcerated additional plaques proximal to the culprit lesions in patients with acute

MI and stable clinical presentation.[75] The high-risk patient group who had high anticipated frequencies of vulnerable lesions was enrolled from the CADILLAC study — a prospective multicenter study of stenting or balloon angioplasty during acute evolving MI.[78] A low-risk control group with a low anticipated frequency of vulnerable lesions included patients with stable clinical presentations undergoing elective stenting.

A total of 197 patients constituted the study population; 105 with acute evolving MIs and 92 patients with stable presentation. IVUS imaging was performed in the segment proximal to the culprit lesion. The presence of additional focal atherosclerotic lesions with or without plaque ulceration was examined. Plaque ulceration was defined as a cavity in a vessel wall with disruption of the intima and flow observed within the plaque cavity. Lumen and external elastic membrane (EEM) areas were traced manually using the intimal leading edge boundary and the leading edge of the adventitia, respectively. The plaque area was calculated as the difference between lumen and EEM area. Plaque morphology was classified according to commonly used definitions as recommended by American College of Cardiology/American Heart Association (ACC/AHA) guidelines into echolucent plaques, echodense plaques, calcified plaques, and mixed plaques.[33,34]

In the overall group of 197 patients, a total of 106 atherosclerotic lesions proximal to the treated culprit lesion were identified (54%). Proximal focal lesions were identified in 50% of patients presenting with acute MIs and 59% in patients of the stable group (p = 0.2). Considering the two cohorts, a total of 12 ulcerated lesions were identified within the 106 identified proximal lesions (11%) and they were unequally distributed. Ten ulcerated plaques were found in the proximal vessel segments of the acute MI group and only two ulcerations were found in the stable group.

The prevalence of ulceration was significantly higher in the acute infarct group compared to the stable group (19% versus 4%; p = 0.014). After adjusting for age and smoking, a multivariable logistic regression model showed that the prevalence of ulceration in the acute MI group remained statistically higher than in the stable group (p = 0.04; odds ratio = 5.6; 95% confidence interval [CI] = 1.1 to 28.4%). Other than the higher frequency of ulceration, additional plaques distant from the culprit lesion in patients with acute myocardial infarction were undistinguishable from plaques in patients with stable presentations. In particular, the frequency of plaque echolucency was not significantly different.

While confirming the systemic nature of plaque vulnerability, the finding that characteristics previously associated with vulnerability at culprit lesion sites such as echolucency and eccentricity were present with similar frequency at nonculprit lesions in both the stable and unstable groups was striking. These studies demonstrate the limitations of identifying morphological characteristics of focal vulnerable plaques *in vivo*:

1. The inability to distinguish additional, nonruptured plaques in patients with acute MI and stable presentation may reflect the fact that the temporal, biochemical changes associated with plaque vulnerability are below the detection threshold of *in vivo* imaging.

2. The simultaneous presence of multiple plaque ruptures demonstrates that the successful identification of a focal vulnerable lesion does not completely describe the overall disease process.
3. The presence of imaging characteristics of rupture and vulnerability remote from the episodes of rupture[58–61] provides further evidence that the morphologic findings at focal lesion sites are not sufficient to describe systemic disease activity.

Based on these findings, it is attractive to hypothesize that the paradigm of morphologic changes of individual focal vulnerable plaques based on autopsy studies of patients with fatal coronary events[79] is not completely applicable to *in vivo* imaging of nonfatal events. The *in vivo* identification of vulnerability may require an assessment of plaque morphology and plaque burden with imaging modalities integrated with systemic markers of disease activity (e.g., serum markers of inflammation).[62,80–85] These findings have already initiated a paradigm shift in our approach to coronary atherosclerosis as described below.

5.4 SYSTEMIC ASSESSMENT OF CORONARY ATHEROSCLEROTIC DISEASE BURDEN AND ACTIVITY: AN EMERGING NEW PARADIGM

Based on the above description of the multifocal nature of coronary artery disease (CAD), an assessment of risk may require knowledge about plaque burden and disease activity. Accurate and reproducible methods for the detection and quantification of subclinical coronary atherosclerosis and disease activity could identify high-risk patients and allow serial monitoring during various therapeutic interventions. Several invasive and noninvasive imaging methods are already used to follow plaque burden in atherosclerosis progression–regression studies.

The tomographic orientation of IVUS images enables visualization of the full thickness of vessel walls and, therefore, measurements of lumens *and* atheromas. For these measurements, the leading edge of the intima and the external elastic membrane (EEM) are traced by manual or automated planimetry. From these two measurements, the atheroma area is calculated as EEM area minus lumen area. Maximum and minimum plaque thicknesses are defined as the longest and shortest distances between the lumen and EEM leading edges, respectively.

In quantitative, volumetric, coronary IVUS studies, consecutive plaque area measurements are integrated along a vessel segment between two fiduciary points. Typically, a long target segment (>40 mm) with moderate disease (angiographic stenoses <50%) is chosen. The ultrasound catheter is placed distal to a fiduciary point such as a coronary branch and subsequently a motorized pull-back is performed at constant speed of usually at 0.5 mm/sec. Beginning at the distal fiduciary point, frames at 1-mm distance are selected and EEM and lumen areas are planimetered (Figure 5.1). In serial studies, patients return for repeat IVUS examinations after follow-up periods of 12 to 24 mo and the same methodology is repeated. This

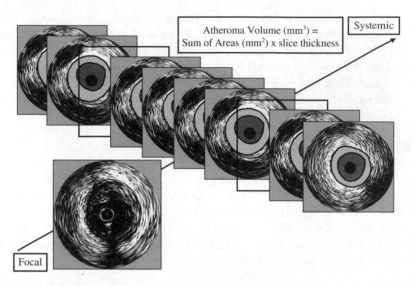

$$\text{Atheroma Volume (mm}^3\text{)} = \text{Sum of Areas (mm}^2\text{) x slice thickness}$$

Systemic

Focal

FIGURE 5.1 *(A color version of this figure follows page 112.)* An optimal atherosclerosis imaging modality would combine noninvasiveness, high resolution, and the capability of assessing the overall disease process. As shown for the examples of histology, IVUS, and MDCT, each existing modality can be placed into this context in order to reveal its strengths and weaknesses.

methodology allows the assessment of the percent change in atheroma volume with considerable statistical power to detect small changes.[86]

Serial intravascular ultrasound studies in native coronary arteries have described an attenuated increase in plaque volume and changes in plaque morphology during lipid-lowering treatment.[86–91] In an early study, the progression of plaque burden was examined during 3-year treatment with pravastatin or diet in mildly diseased vessels.[87] Follow-up plaque area increased by 41% in the control group and decreased by 7% in the treatment group. In another study examining the effects of low density lipoprotein (LDL) apharesis, plaque regression was found in the treatment group.[88]

Schartl et al. described plaque volume and plaque morphology in a serial IVUS study during lipid-lowering treatment.[89] One hundred-thirty-one patients were randomized to treatment with atorvastatin or "usual care" that could include statin therapy. After 12 mo, mean LDL cholesterol (LDL-C) was reduced from 155 to 86 mg/dL in the atorvastatin group and from 166 to 140 mg/dL in the usual care group. Mean absolute plaque volume showed an insignificant smaller increase in the atorvastatin group compared with the usual care group (1.2 ± 30.4 mm^3 versus 9.6 ± 28.1 mm^3; p = 0.19). Echogenicity increased to a larger extent in the atorvastatin group than in the usual care group.

Several other large IVUS regression–progression studies using volumetric analysis of plaque burden have recently been finalized or are close to completion. These include the Reversal of Atherosclerosis with Aggressive Lipid Lowering (REVERSAL) trial comparing two lipid-lowering regimens and the Norvasc for Regression of Manifest Atherosclerotic Lesions (NORMALISE) trial comparing amlodipine, enalapril, and placebo.

In the recently reported REVERSAL trial,[90] IVUS was performed in patients with LDL-C levels of 125 to 210 mg/dL. Subjects were randomized to 80 mg atorvastatin or 40 mg pravastatin for 18 mo. At study completion, a repeat IVUS examination was performed under identical conditions and analyzed in a blinded core laboratory. At 34 centers in the United States, 655 patients were randomized and 502 completed the protocol.

The baseline LDL-C (mean = 150.2 mg/dL) was reduced to 110 mg/dL with pravastatin versus 79 mg/dL with atorvastatin (p = <0.0001). C-reactive protein (CRP) levels decreased 5.2% with pravastatin and 36.4% with atorvastatin (p = <0.0001). The primary endpoint (percent change in atheroma volume) showed progression in the pravastatin-treated cohort (+2.7%; p = 0.001 compared to baseline). In contrast, atheroma volume decreased slightly in the atorvastatin group (–0.4%), indicating absence of progression (p = 0.98 compared to baseline). Comparing the two groups, the progression rate was significantly lower in the atorvastatin cohort (p = 0.024). The lower progression rate in the atorvastatin arm was independent of baseline LDL-C levels. These results show that intensive treatment using 80 mg of atorvastatin can arrest progression of coronary atherosclerosis.

The smaller Milano trial in patients presenting with acute coronary syndromes[91] assessed the effect of an intravenous recombinant apo A-I Milano/phospholipid complex (ETC-216), a variant of apolipoprotein A-I, on atheroma burdens in patients with acute coronary syndromes (ACSs). In this double blind, randomized, placebo-controlled multicenter study, 123 patients consented, 57 were randomly assigned, and 47 completed the protocol. In a ratio of 1:2:2, patients received five weekly infusions of placebo or ETC-216 at 15 mg/kg or 45 mg/kg.

Intravascular ultrasound was performed within 2 wk following ACS and repeated after five weekly treatments. The primary efficacy parameter was the change in percent atheroma volume (follow-up minus baseline) in the combined ETC-216 cohort. The mean (standard deviation or SD) percent atheroma volume decreased by –1.06% (3.17%) in the combined ETC-216 group (median = –0.81%; 95% CI = –0.34 to –1.53%; p = 0.02 compared with baseline). In the placebo group, mean (SD) percent atheroma volume increased by 0.14% (3.09%; median = 0.03%; p = 0.97 compared with baseline). The absolute reduction in atheroma volume in the combined treatment groups was –14.1 mm³ or a 4.2% decrease from baseline (p = <0.001).

Although promising, these results require confirmation in larger clinical trials with morbidity and mortality endpoints. Eventually, for the application in clinical settings of disease prevention, assessments with noninvasive modalities will be required. Several imaging modalities including cardiovascular computed tomography (CT) are currently under study for that purpose. The effect of pharmacological intervention on (calcified) coronary plaque burden has been observed in CT "calcium scoring" studies.[92,93] More recently, the differentiation of calcified and noncalcified plaques has become possible noninvasively with contrast-enhanced MDCT.[94–96]

Our group compared IVUS and MDCT findings in 14 patients.[95] An IVUS pullback through segments of the left coronary artery with <50% angiographic diameter stenosis was performed. Based on a review of the angiographic and IVUS images, individual mildly stenotic coronary segments were identified in the left main trunk, left anterior descending, and left circumflex coronary arteries using characteristic landmarks. In each segment, the site with maximum plaque area and a proximal normal reference site were identified. Lumen and external elastic membrane (EEM) areas were manually traced. Presence of plaque was defined as a maximal intimal thickness >0.5 mm. Plaque morphology was classified visually as calcified or non-calcified. Plaque distribution in cross-sectional images was defined as symmetric or asymmetric.

The remodeling responses of the segments were described by a remodeling ratio (RR) defined as EEM area at the lesion site divided by EEM area at the proximal reference site. The presence and absence of expansive (positive) remodeling were defined as RR >1.05 and RR 1.05, respectively. Subsequently, a contrast-enhanced MDCT acquisition was performed and segments corresponding to the IVUS analysis were identified.

The presence of plaque, plaque composition (calcified versus noncalcified), plaque distribution, and remodeling were described. The semiquantitative assessment of the remodeling response was based on the size of the outer vessel contour on longitudinal images. Expansive (positive) remodeling was considered when the outer contour of the most diseased site was larger than that of a normal proximal reference site. For each MDCT plaque characteristic, a level of confidence was assigned on a scale: 0% indicated absolute confidence that the characteristic was absent and 100% indicated absolute confidence of its presence. Agreement between MDCT readers for the different characteristics was described based on two-alternative (yes or no) forced-choice answers.

The accuracy of MDCT in comparison with IVUS for distinguishing the different parameters was measured by the area under the ROC curve (AUC) using percent-confidence levels supplied by each reader for each segment. Forty-six segments were identified based on angiography and IVUS. MDCT analysis could be performed for 80.4% of segments. Analysis of the remaining nine segments was not possible secondary to degradation by motion artifacts (n = 3) or due to distal location (n = 6). IVUS demonstrated plaque in 27 of the 37 MDCT-analyzable segments. MDCT readers 1 and 2 agreed in their assessments of the absence of presence of plaque in 31 of 37 segments (84%); calcified or noncalcified plaque in 22 of 24 segments (92%); symmetric or asymmetric plaque distribution in 15 of 24 segments (63%); and remodeling or absence of remodeling in 17 of 27 segments (63%). The results for the accuracy of MDCT based on percent-confidence ratings demonstrated high accuracy for all characteristics studied when compared with IVUS. Other studies demonstrated the potential value of further plaque characterization based on Houns-field unit values.[94]

These results demonstrate that advances in temporal and spatial resolution of MDCT will allow the noninvasive detection of atherosclerotic plaque. Future studies need to address the reliability of disease quantification before these modalities can be applied to research and clinical settings similar to IVUS. Corresponding results have been described with other noninvasive modalities including B-mode ultrasound and MRI.[97-102]

While detailed analysis of morphological plaque composition and detection of the inflammatory changes central to unstable lesions are beyond the resolution of

MDCT and other noninvasive imaging modalities,[7] these modalities allow assessment of overall plaque burden similar to IVUS. Although the prognostic role of plaque burden in disease destabilization is not completely understood, it is an attractive hypothesis that systemic triggers cause more instability when acting upon a lager plaque mass, therefore increasing the statistical chance of a clinical event. Therefore, the assessment of plaque burden may be an important component in the assessment of plaque vulnerability if combined with markers of disease activity. Future studies comparing imaging criteria of individual lesions and diffuse plaque burden with systemic markers of vulnerability are necessary to define the clinical role of atherosclerosis imaging.

5.5 CONCLUDING REMARKS: IMAGING OF VULNERABLE PLAQUES: NEED FOR PROSPECTIVE TRIALS

Sudden complications related to the destabilization of vulnerable plaques initiate most acute coronary syndromes. Early detection of such high-risk lesions with imaging modalities could lead to innovative preventive strategies.[103] However, it has become obvious that most vulnerable lesions never lead to clinical symptoms and that plaque destabilization is a systemic process. Based on this evolving understanding of CAD and the pathophysiology of ACS, the assessment of future risk will require us to identify and quantify plaque and disease activity. Several invasive and noninvasive imaging modalities are already used to assess coronary plaque burden (Figure 5.2). Fusion of anatomic and functional image information (e.g., positron

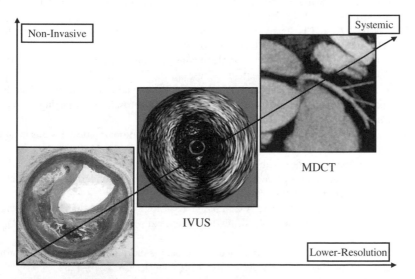

FIGURE 5.2 *(A color version of this figure follows page 112.)* Because atherosclerotic plaque accumulation and vulnerability are systemic disease processes, a comprehensive assessment of the risk for the development of acute coronary syndromes may require both the assessment of focal lesion characteristics (vulnerable plaque) and the systemic plaque burden (vulnerable patient). An IVUS pull-back through a vessel segment can provide information about plaque morphology and plaque burden.

emission tomography and computerized tomography) may allow simultaneous insights into disease burden and activity. In addition, our knowledge about the relationship between plaque burden and biochemical markers of disease activity is constantly growing.[104]

However, because plaque vulnerability is a prospective definition, only serial prospective studies will allow identification of focal or systemic characteristics of high-risk lesions. This will require multicenter trials evaluating the relationship of plaque burden, biochemical markers, and clinical events.[8]

REFERENCES

1. American Heart Association. *2002 Heart and Stroke Statistical Update*. Dallas, TX, 2001.
2. The Euro Heart Survey of Acute Coronary Syndromes (Euro Heart Survey ACS). *Eur Heart J* 2002; 23: 1190–1201.
3. Sekikawa, A. et al. Coronary heart disease mortality among men aged 35–44 years by prefecture in Japan in 1995–1999 compared with that among white men aged 35–44 by state in the United States in 1995–1998: vital statistics data in recent birth cohort. *Jpn Circ J* 2001; 65: 887–892.
4. Ross, R. The pathogenesis of atherosclerosis: a perspective for the 1990s. *Nature* 1993; 362: 801–809.
5. Libby, P. Current concepts of the pathogenesis of the acute coronary syndromes. *Circulation* 2001; 104: 365–372.
6. Davies, M.J. Stability and instability: two faces of coronary atherosclerosis. *Circulation* 1996; 94: 2013–2020.
7. Fayad, Z.A. and Fuster, V. Clinical imaging of the high-risk or vulnerable atherosclerotic plaque. *Circ Res* 2001; 89: 305–316.
8. Naghavi, M. et al. From vulnerable plaque to vulnerable patient: a call for new definitions and risk assessment strategies, part I. *Circulation* 2003; 108: 1664–1672.
9. Tuzcu, E.M. and Schoenhagen, P. Acute coronary syndromes, plaque vulnerability, and carotid artery disease: the changing role of atherosclerosis imaging. *J Am Coll Cardiol* 2003; 42: 1033–1036.
10. Davies, M.J. and Thomas, A. Thrombosis and acute coronary artery lesions in sudden cardiac ischemic death. *New Engl J Med* 1984; 310: 1137–1140.
11. Falk, E. Plaque rupture with severe pre-existing stenosis precipitating coronary thrombosis: characteristics of coronary atherosclerotic plaques underlying fatal occlusive thrombi. *Br Heart J* 1983; 50: 127–134.
12. Davies, M.J. and Thomas, A.C. Plaque fissuring: the cause of acute myocardial infarction, sudden ischemic death and crescendo angina. *Br Heart J* 1985; 53: 363–373.
13. Burke, A.P. et al. Coronary risk factors and plaque morphology in men with coronary disease who died suddenly. *New Engl J Med* 1997; 336: 1276–1282.
14. Glagov, S. et al. Compensatory enlargement of human atherosclerotic coronary arteries. *New Engl J Med* 1987; 316: 1371–1375.
15. Gibbons, G.H. and Dzau, V.J. The emerging concept of vascular remodeling. *New Engl J Med* 1994; 330: 1431–1438.

16. Schoenhagen, P. et al. Arterial remodeling and coronary artery disease: the concept of "dilated" versus "obstructive" coronary atherosclerosis. *J Am Coll Cardiol* 2001; 38: 297–306.
17. Ward, M.R. et al. Arterial remodeling: mechanisms and clinical implications. *Circulation* 2000; 102: 1186–1191.
18. Pasterkamp, G. et al. Relation of arterial geometry to luminal narrowing and histologic markers for plaque vulnerability: the remodeling paradox. *J Am Coll Cardiol* 1998; 32: 655–662.
19. Varnava, A.M., Mills, P.G., and Davies, M.J. Relationship between coronary artery remodeling and plaque vulnerability. *Circulation* 2002; 105: 939–943.
20. Burke, A.P. et al. Morphological predictors of arterial remodeling in coronary atherosclerosis. *Circulation* 2002; 105: 297–303.
21. Pasterkamp, G. et al. Inflammation of the atherosclerotic cap and shoulder of the plaque is a common and locally observed feature in unruptured plaques of femoral and coronary arteries. *Arterioscler Thromb Vasc Biol* 1999; 19: 54–58.
22. Moreno, P.R. et al. Macrophage infiltration in acute coronary syndromes: implications for plaque rupture. *Circulation* 1994; 90: 775–778.
23. Moreno, P.R. et al. Macrophages, smooth muscle cells and tissue factor in unstable angina. *Circulation* 1996; 94: 3090–3097.
24. Shah, P.K. et al. Human monocyte-derived macrophages induce collagen breakdown in fibrous caps of atherosclerotic plaques. *Circulation* 1995; 92: 1565–1569.
25. Loree, H.M. et al. Effects of fibrous cap thickness on peak circumferential stress in model atherosclerotic vessels. *Circ Res* 1992; 71: 850–858.
26. Cheng, G.C. et al. Distribution of circumferential stress in ruptured and stable atherosclerotic lesions. *Circulation* 1993; 87: 1179–1187.
27. Lee, R.T. et al. Circumferential stress and matrix metalloproteinase 1 in human coronary atherosclerosis. *Arterioscler Thromb Vasc Biol* 1996; 16: 1070–1073.
28. Galis, Z.S. et al. Increased expression of matrix metalloproteinases and matrix degrading activity in vulnerable regions of human atherosclerotic plaques. *J Clin Invest* 1994; 94: 2493–2503.
29. Sukhova, G.K. et al. Expression of the elastolytic cathepsins S and K in human atheroma and regulation of their production in smooth muscle cells. *J Clin Invest* 1998; 102: 576–583.
30. Ambrose, J.A. et al. Angiographic evolution of coronary artery morphology in unstable angina. *J Am Coll Cardiol* 1986; 7: 472–478.
31. Nissen, S.E. et al. Intravascular ultrasound assessment of lumen size and wall morphology in normal subjects and patients with coronary artery disease. *Circulation* 1991; 84: 1087–1099.
32. Nissen, S.E. and Yock, P. Intravascular ultrasound: novel pathophysiological insights and current clinical applications. *Circulation* 2001; 103: 604–616.
33. Mintz, G.S. et al. American College of Cardiology Clinical Expert Consensus document on standards for acquisition, measurement and reporting of intravascular ultrasound studies (IVUS): a report of the American College of Cardiology Task Force on Clinical Expert Consensus Documents. *J Am Coll Cardiol* 2001; 37: 1478–1492.
34. Di Mario, C. et al. Clinical application and image interpretation in intracoronary ultrasound: Study Group on Intracoronary Imaging of the Working Group of Coronary Circulation and of the Subgroup on Intravascular Ultrasound of the Working Group of Echocardiography of the European Society of Cardiology. *Eur Heart J*, 1998; 19: 207–229.

35. Gussenhoven, E.J. et al. Arterial wall characteristics determined by intravascular ultrasound imaging: an *in vitro* study. *J Am Coll Cardiol* 1989; 14: 947–952.

36. Hodgson, J.Mc.B. et al. Intracoronary ultrasound imaging: Correlation of plaque morphology with angiography, clinical syndrome and procedural results in patients undergoing coronary angioplasty. *J Am Coll Cardiol* 1993; 21: 35–44.

37. Fukuda, D. et al. Lesion characteristics of acute myocardial infarction: an investigation with intravascular ultrasound. Heart. 2001; 85: 402–406.

38. Smits, P.C. et al. Angioscopic complex lesions are predominantly compensatory enlarged: an angioscopic and intracoronary ultrasound study. *Cardiovasc Res* 1999; 41: 458–464.

39. Schoenhagen, P. et al. Extent and direction of arterial remodeling in stable and unstable coronary syndromes. *Circulation* 2000; 101: 598–603.

40. Nakamura, M. et al. Impact of coronary artery remodeling on clinical presentation of coronary artery disease: an intravascular ultrasound study. *J Am Coll Cardiol.* 2001; 37: 63–69.

41. Schoenhagen, P. et al. Relation of matrix-metalloproteinase 3 found in coronary lesion samples retrieved by directional coronary atherectomy to intravascular ultrasound observations on coronary remodeling. *Am J Cardiol* 2002; 89: 1354–1359.

42. Ambrose, J.A. et al. Angiographic progression of coronary artery disease and the development of myocardial infarction. *J Am Coll Cardiol* 1988; 12: 56–62.

43. Giroud, D. et al. Relation of the site of acute myocardial infarction to the most severe coronary arterial stenosis prior to angiography. *Am J Cardiol* 1992; 69: 729–732.

44. Little, W.C. et al. Can coronary angiography predict the site of a subsequent myocardial infarction in patients with mild-to-moderate coronary artery disease? *Circulation* 1988; 78: 1157–1166.

45. Hackett, D., Davies, G., and Maseri, A. Pre-existing coronary stenoses in patients with first myocardial infarction are not necessarily severe. *Eur Heart J* 1988; 9: 1317–1323.

46. Ambrose, J.A. et al. Coronary angiographic morphology in myocardial infarction: a link between the pathogenesis of unstable angina and myocardial infarction. *J Am Coll Cardiol* 1985; 6: 1233–1238.

47. Ojio, S. et al. Considerable time from the onset of plaque rupture and/or thrombi until the onset of acute myocardial infarction in humans: coronary angiographic findings within 1 week before the onset of infarction. *Circulation* 2000; 102: 2063–2069.

48. Yamagishi, M. et al. Morphology of vulnerable coronary plaque: insights from follow-up of patients examined by intravascular ultrasound before and acute coronary syndrome. *J Am Coll Cardiol* 2000; 35: 106–111.

49. Nair, A. et al. Coronary plaque classification with intravascular ultrasound radiofrequency data analysis. *Circulation* 2002; 106: 2200–2206.

50. Kawasaki, M. et al. Noninvasive quantitative tissue characterization and two-dimensional color-coded map of human atherosclerotic lesions using ultrasound integrated backscatter: comparison between histology and integrated backscatter images. *J Am Coll Cardiol* 2001; 38: 486–492.

51. Takiuchi, et al. Quantitative ultrasonic tissue characterization can identify high-risk atherosclerotic alteration in human carotid arteries. *Circulation* 2000; 102: 766–770.

52. Stahr, P.M. et al. Discrimination of early/intermediate and advanced/complicated coronary plaque types by radiofrequency intravascular ultrasound analysis. *Am J Cardiol* 2002; 90: 19–23.

53. de Korte, C.L. et al. Characterization of plaque components with intravascular ultra-sound elastography in human femoral and coronary arteries *in vitro*. *Circulation* 2000; 102: 617–623.

54. Guillermo, J.T. et al. Quantification of macrophage content in atherosclerotic plaques by optical coherence tomography. *Circulation* 2003; 107: 113–119.

55. Yabushita, H. et al. Characterization of Human Atherosclerosis by Optical Coherence Tomography. *Circulation* 2002; 106: 1640–1645.

56. Casscells, W. et al. Thermal detection of cellular infiltrates in living atherosclerotic plaques: possible implications for plaque rupture and thrombosis. *Lancet* 1996; 347: 1447–1451.

57. Stefanadis, C. et al. Thermal heterogeneity within human atherosclerotic coronary arteries detected *in vivo*: A new method of detection by application of a special thermography catheter. *Circulation* 1999; 99: 1965–1971.

58. Frink, R.J. Chronic ulcerated plaques: new insights into the pathogenesis of acute coronary disease. *J Invasive Cardiol* 1994; 6: 173–185.

59. Williams, H. et al. Characteristics of intact and ruptured atherosclerotic plaques in brachiocephalic arteries of apolipoprotein E knockout mice. *Arterioscler Thromb Vasc Biol* 2002; 22: 788–792.

60. Burke, A.P. et al. Healed plaque ruptures and sudden coronary death: Evidence that subclinical rupture has a role in plaque progression. *Circulation* 2001; 103: 934–940.

61. Mann, J. and Davies, M.J. Mechanisms of progression in native coronary artery disease: role of healed plaque disruption. *Heart* 1999; 82: 265–268.

62. Buffon, A. et al. Widespread coronary inflammation in unstable angina. *New Engl J Med* 2002; 347: 5–12.

63. Mazzone, A. et al. Increased expression of neutrophil and monocyte adhesion mole-cules in unstable coronary artery disease. *Circulation* 1993; 88: 358–363.

64. Biasucci, L.M. et al. Intracellular neutrophil myeloperoxidase is reduced in unstable angina and acute myocardial infarction, but its reduction is not related to ischemia. *J Am Coll Cardiol* 1996; 27: 611–616.

65. Goldstein, J.A. et al. Multiple complex coronary plaques in patients with acute myo-cardial infarction. *New Engl J Med* 2000; 343: 915–922.

66. Serruys, P.W.J.C. et al. Fluvastatin for prevention of cardiac events following suc-cessful first percutaneous coronary intervention. *JAMA*, 2002, 287, 3215–3222.

67. Zairis, M.N. et al. C-reactive protein and multiple complex coronary artery plaques in patients with primary unstable angina. *Atherosclerosis* 2002; 164: 355–359.

68. Chen, L. et al. Angiographic stenosis progression and coronary events in patients with "stabilized" unstable angina. *Circulation* 1995; 91: 2319–2324.

69. Chen, L. et al. Differential progression of complex culprit stenoses in patients with stable and unstable angina pectoris. *J Am Coll Cardiol* 1996; 28: 597–603.

70. Kaski, J.C. et al. Coronary stenosis progression differs in patients with stable angina pectoris with and without a previous history of unstable angina *Eur Heart J* 1996; 17: 1488–1494.

71. Guazzi, M.D. et al. Evidence of multifocal activity of coronary disease in patients with acute myocardial infarction. *Circulation* 1997; 96: 1145–1151.

72. Rioufol, G. et al. Multiple atherosclerotic plaque rupture in acute coronary syndrome: a three-vessel intravascular ultrasound study. *Circulation* 2002; 106: 804–808.

73. Maehara, A. et al. Morphologic and angiographic features of coronary plaque rupture detected by intravascular ultrasound. *J Am Coll Cardiol* 2002; 40: 904–910.

74. Asakura, M. et al. Extensive development of vulnerable plaques as a pan-coronary process in patients with myocardial infarction: an angioscopic study. *J Am Coll Cardiol.* 2001; 37: 1284–1288.
75. Schoenhagen, P. et al. Coronary plaque morphology and frequency of ulceration distant from culprit lesions in patients with unstable and stable presentation. *Arterioscler Thromb Vasc Biol* 2003; 23: 1895–1900.
76. Takano, M. et al. Mechanical and structural characteristics of vulnerable plaques: analysis by coronary angioscopy and intravascular ultrasound. *J Am Coll Cardiol* 2001; 38: 99–104.
77. Ge, J. et al. Screening of ruptured plaques in patients with coronary artery disease by intravascular ultrasound. *Heart* 1999; 81: 621–627.
78. Stone, G.W. et al. Controlled Abciximab and Device Investigation to Lower Late Angioplasty Complications (CADILLAC) Investigators: comparison of angioplasty with stenting, with or without abciximab, in acute myocardial infarction. *New Engl J Med.* 2002, 346: 957–966.
79. Muller, J.E., Tofler, G.H., and Stone, P.H. Circadian variation and triggers of onset of acute cardiovascular disease. *Circulation* 1989; 79: 733–743.
80. Ridker, P.M. et al. Inflammation, aspirin, and the risk of cardiovascular disease in apparently healthy men. *New Engl J Med* 1997; 336: 973–979.
81. Ridker, P.M. et al. Comparison of C-reactive protein and low-density lipoprotein cholesterol levels in the prediction of first cardiovascular events. *New Engl J Med* 2002; 347: 1557–1565.
82. Zhang, R. et al. Association between myeloperoxidase levels and risk of coronary artery disease. *JAMA* 2001; 286: 2136–2142.
83. Koenig, W. et al. C-reactive protein, a sensitive marker of inflammation, predicts future risk of coronary heart disease in initially healthy middle-aged men. *Circulation* 1999; 99: 237–242.
84. Blake, G.J. et al. Soluble CD40 ligand levels indicate lipid accumulation in carotid atheroma: an *in vivo* study with high-resolution MRI. *Arterioscler Thromb Vasc Biol* 2003; 23: E11–E14.
85. Lutgens, E. et al. Transforming growth factor-beta mediates balance between inflammation and fibrosis during plaque progression. *Arterioscler Thromb Vasc Biol* 2002; 22: 975–982.
86. Schoenhagen, P. and Nissen, S.E. Coronary atherosclerotic disease burden: an emerging endpoint in progression/regression studies using intravascular ultrasound. *Curr Drug Targets Cardiovasc Haematol Disord* 2003; 3: 218–226.
87. Takagi, T. et al. Intravascular ultrasound analysis of reduction in progression of coronary narrowing by treatment with pravastatin. *Am J Cardiol* 1997, 79, 1673–1676.
88. Matsuzaki, M. et al. Intravascular ultrasound evaluation of coronary plaque regression by low density lipoprotein apheresis in familial hypercholesterolemia. *J Am Coll Cardiol* 2002, 40, 220–227.
89. Schartl, M. et al. Use of intravascular ultrasound to compare effects of different strategies of lipid-lowering therapy on plaque volume and composition in patients with coronary artery disease. *Circulation* 2001; 104: 387–392.
90. Nissen, S.E. et al. for the REVERSAL Investigators. Effect of intensive compared with moderate lipid-lowering therapy on progression of coronary atherosclerosis: a randomized controlled trial. *JAMA* 2004; 291: 1071–1080.
91. Nissen, S.E. et al. Effect of recombinant ApoA-I Milano on coronary atherosclerosis in patients with acute coronary syndromes: a randomized controlled trial. *JAMA* 2003; 290: 2292–2300.

92. Callister, T.Q. et al. Effect of HMG-CoA reductase inhibitors on coronary artery disease by electron-beam computed tomography. *New Engl J Med* 1998; 339: 1972–1978.

93. Achenbach, S. et al. Influence of lipid-lowering therapy on the progression of coronary artery calcification. *Circulation* 2002; 106: 1077–1082.

94. Schroeder, S. et al. Noninvasive detection and evaluation of atherosclerotic coronary plaques with multislice computed tomography. *J Am Coll Cardiol* 2001; 37: 1430–1435.

95. Schoenhagen, P. et al. Noninvasive assessment of plaque morphology and remodeling in mildly stenotic coronary segments: comparison of 16-slice computed tomography and intravascular ultrasound. *Cor Artery Dis* 2003; 14: 459–462.

96. Achenbach, S. et al. Detection of calcified and noncalcified coronary atherosclerotic plaque by contrast-enhanced, submillimeter multidetector spiral computed tomography: a segment-based comparison with intravascular ultrasound. *Circulation* 2004; 109: 14–17.

97. Fayad, Z.A. et al. Computed tomography and magnetic resonance imaging for noninvasive coronary angiography and plaque imaging: current and potential future concepts. *Circulation* 2002; 106: 2026–2034.

98. Zhao, X.Q. et al. Effects of prolonged intensive lipid-lowering therapy on the characteristics of carotid atherosclerotic plaques *in vivo* by MRI. *Arterioscler Thromb Vasc Biol* 2001, 21, 1623–1629.

99. Kim, W.Y. et al. Three-dimensional black-blood cardiac magnetic resonance coronary vessel wall imaging detects positive arterial remodeling in patients with nonsignificant coronary artery disease. *Circulation* 2002; 106: 296–299.

100. de Groot, E. et al. B-mode ultrasound assessment of pravastatin treatment effect on carotid and femoral artery walls and its correlation with coronary arteriographic findings: a report of the Regression Growth Evaluation Statin Study (REGRESS). *J Am Coll Cardiol* 1998; 31: 1561–1567.

101. Taylor, A.J. et al. ARBITER: Arterial Biology for the Investigation of the Treatment Effects of Reducing Cholesterol: a randomized trial comparing the effects of atorvastatin and pravastatin on carotid intima medial thickness. *Circulation* 2002; 106: 2055–2060.

102. Corti, R. et al. Effects of lipid-lowering by simvastatin on human atherosclerotic lesions: a longitudinal study by high-resolution, noninvasive magnetic resonance imaging. *Circulation* 2001; 104: 249–252.

103. Bonow, R.O. Primary Prevention of Cardiovascular Disease. A Call to Action. *Circulation* 2002, 106, 3140–3141.

104. Brennan, M.L. et al. Prognostic value of myeloperoxidase in patients with chest pain. *New Engl J Med* 2003; 349: 1595–1604.

6 Optical Coherence Tomography for Detection of Vulnerable Plaque

Fabian Moselewski, Stephan Achenbach, and Ik-Kyung Jang

CONTENTS

6.1 INTRODUCTION

Optical coherence tomography (OCT) is a high resolution, cross-sectional imaging technique. It is based on the analysis of the back-scatter of infrared light and provides a spatial resolution in the micrometer range. Developed in the early 1990s, it is a relatively new technique, but rapid technological development has made it possible to apply this new imaging modality to intracoronary imaging of atherosclerotic plaques. The feasibility and safety of OCT for *in vivo* coronary plaque characterization has been established. The unique capability of this high resolution imaging modality can serve as a powerful tool to detect vulnerable plaques and also evaluate therapeutic interventions including pharmacologic, genetic, and local therapies.

In this chapter, we will introduce the technical background of OCT as a high resolution imaging tool and will provide an overview of experimental and clinical data concerning its feasibility for characterizing atherosclerotic plaques in coronary arteries. Advantages and disadvantages of atherosclerotic plaque imaging by OCT and the potential clinical role for the detection and characterization of coronary lesions will be described.

6.2 PATHOPHYSIOLOGY OF PLAQUE DISRUPTION AND RATIONALE FOR HIGH RESOLUTION IMAGING

Disruption of atherosclerotic plaque with subsequent thrombosis is the main cause of acute coronary syndromes including unstable angina, myocardial infarction, and sudden cardiac death.[1,2] Atherosclerotic plaques that are prone to rupture are frequently referred to as "vulnerable" or "high risk" plaques,[3–6] representing a subgroup of coronary atherosclerotic lesions with a high likelihood of causing acute coronary events. While *vulnerable plaque* is a prospective definition,[7] postmortem pathologic studies have identified certain morphologic features that predispose plaques to rupture.[8,9]

Plaques that exhibit these features are frequently referred to as high risk plaques.[10–13] These features include (1) large lipid-rich cores, (2) thin fibrous caps, and (3) focal accumulations of inflammation cells e.g., macrophages, in the fibrous cap region. While the large size of a lipid core[13] may make it amenable to clinical imaging methods (intracoronary ultrasound and possibly magnetic resonance imaging [MRI] and computed tomography [CT]), the dimensions of a fibrous cap (less than 65 μm in high risk plaques) and the presence and density of macrophage infiltration are beyond the resolution of intracoronary ultrasound, MRI, and CT. OCT has a spatial resolution high enough to detect and differentiate all these components. Thus, OCT may play a central role in the development and evaluation of strategies for treating high risk plaques.

6.3 TECHNICAL PRINCIPLES OF OPTICAL COHERENCE TOMOGRAPHY

Optical coherence tomography is a cross-sectional imaging technique based on the analysis of the back-scatter of light. It was first described by Huang and Swanson in 1991.[14] Initially, the method was used primarily to image the peripapillary area of the retina — a transparent tissue. Subsequently, its applications were expanded to nontransparent tissues. Similarly to ultrasound, OCT analyzes the signal that is back-scattered after sending energy with wave characteristics into the tissue to be evaluated.[15] However, while ultrasound uses acoustic waves, OCT uses electromagnetic waves (typically, infrared light at a wavelength of 1300 nm).

Because infrared light travels much faster than ultrasound, OCT uses low coherence interferometry for the calculation of the acquired data distance. A laser source generates coherent infrared light pulses; a reference and sample arm reflect

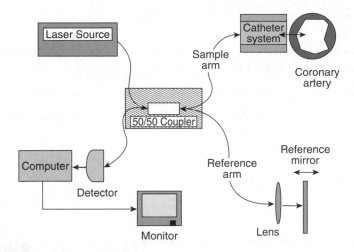

FIGURE 6.1 OCT system. The signals of sample and reference arm are unified in the OCT system. Interference may occur and can be displayed on a monitor or saved digitally. (From Jang, I.K. et al. *J Am Coll Cardiol*, 2002. 39: 604–609. With permission.)

the back-scattered light to the system; and both arms are recombined almost simultaneously. In order to measure distances within the scattered light of the sample arm, the length of the reference arm is changed. Depending on the structural delay and attenuation within the sample arm, interference will occur (Figure 6.1). OCT measures the intensity of interference as output. Results are displayed in grey scale and saved digitally. Depending on the wavelength, a spatial resolution of 4 to 16 μm can be achieved. The typical penetration depth in nontransparent tissue is about 2 to 3 mm. The acquisition time of one image is about 200 msec, permitting high resolution imaging without motion artifacts.

Because the bandwidth is inversely proportional to the coherence length of the light source and the coherence length is directly related to the axial resolution, the broader the bandwidth, the higher the resolution. For a typical bandwidth of 75 nm (full width at half maximum), OCT has been shown to achieve an axial resolution between 4 and 16 μm. The transversal resolution depends on the size of the focal spot. Thus, a small aperture focusing the source to a small spot relates to high transversal resolution (typically 10 μm). Light penetration in tissue depends on absorption and scattering (according to index mismatch) of the light within the tissue. Therefore, near-infrared light with a wavelength in the range of 1300 nm is applied.

Infrared light is characterized by substantially lower scattering and absorption than light in the visible range. On the other hand, infrared light has a wavelength short enough to avoid induction of vibrational transitions in water. The image acquisition time of one image is currently limited by the time needed for the modulation of the reference arm length. Currently, a sampling rate of four to eight frames per second with an acquisition time of 200 msec per image is typically achieved. Technical characteristics of OCT in comparison to intravascular ultrasound (IVUS) are illustrated in Table 6.1.

TABLE 6.1

Comparison of Technical Features of Optical Coherence Tomography and Intravascular Ultrasound

Technical Feature	Optical Coherence Tomography	Intravascular Ultrasound
Light source	Infrared light (1300 nm)	Ultrasound (40 MHz)
Acquisition time	200 msec	250 msec
Spatial resolution	4 to 16 μm	130 μm
Penetration depth	2 to 3 mm	5 mm
Position of transducer	In system	In catheter
Main limitation	Blood cells significantly scatter signal	Resolution

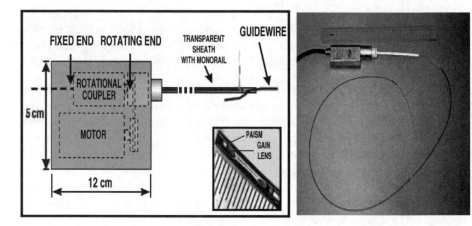

FIGURE 6.2 Intracoronary OCT catheter. The modified intravascular ultrasound catheter contains a rotating core with a single optical fiber. The light beam is reflected perpendicularly toward the vessel wall by a prism attached to the tip of the optical fiber. (From Tearney, G.J., et al. *Circulation*, 2003. 107: 113–119. With permission.)

Commercially available IVUS catheters were modified for intracoronary OCT imaging for our studies. The intracoronary OCT catheter contains a rotating core that carries a single optical fiber. The end of the outer sheath is transparent and a prism attached to the tip of the optical fiber reflects the light beam in a 90 angle toward the vessel wall (Figure 6.2).

In most *in vivo* studies, a 3.0-French catheter was employed. Images are acquired at four frames per second. Because blood reflects the optical signal and would cause significant artifacts, images of the vessel lumen and surrounding vessel wall can only be acquired in the absence of red blood cells. The saline flush technique has shown to be an adequate method to resolve this issue.[15]

After injection of 8 to 10 cc of saline solution through the guiding catheter, clear image acquisition is possible for approximately 2 sec.[16] The necessity for repeated saline flushes is a limitation of OCT and currently restricts its use to relatively short predefined segments of the coronary arteries. Our current and recent research efforts are focused on that issue. Index matching is an alternative to decrease the index and thus the grade of optical reflection between plasma and red blood cells.[17]

6.4 CHARACTERIZATION OF ATHEROSCLEROTIC PLAQUE

Initially, OCT was primarily applied to transparent tissues at the peripapillary area of the retina. It was used for diagnosis of retina–macula related diseases such as glaucoma, where high resolution imaging of microstructures is warranted. Expanding the technique to nontransparent tissues, OCT was investigated in the field of dermatology[18,19] for noninvasive detection of skin abnormalities such as skin cancer and psoriasis. It is feasible for the detection of different layers of tissues in gastroenterology for the diagnosis of Barrett esophagus.

6.4.1 *Ex Vivo* Validation

In 2002, our group established the OCT criteria for different plaque components[20] (see Table 6.2). A total of 357 postmortem atherosclerotic segments from 90 cadavers were investigated. By validating imaging results to histology, sensitivity and specificity of 75% and 97.5%, respectively, were found for fibrous plaques. Characterization of fibrocalcified plaque was possible with sensitivity and specificity of 96% and 97%, respectively. Sensitivity and specificity for the detection of lipid-rich plaque were 90% and 92%. The interobserver agreement regarding the initial histological diagnosis was high (Cohen's $= 0.83$)

Fibrous Plaque (American Heart Association, Stary Type IV lesion[21]) — In OCT, fibrous plaques are characterized by homogeneous, highly back-scattering, signal-rich regions with or without small signal-poor regions (see Figure 6.3).

Fibrocalcific plaque (American Heart Association, Stary Type Vb lesion[21]) — Plaque calcification regions typically appear as sharply bordered, signal-poor regions in OCT images (see Figure 6.4). Calcified plaques thus demonstrate such sharply delineated calcified regions surrounded by fibrous tissue.

Lipid-rich plaque (American Heart Association, Stary Type Va lesion[21]) — Lipid-rich regions within atherosclerotic plaques show diffusely bordered, signal-poor regions, and will usually show thin, homogenous overlying bands of tissue (see Figure 6.5). This signal-rich band corresponds to the fibrous cap. The signals within lipid-rich regions are similar to those of calcium, but the lack of a sharply delineated border permits distinction of lipid-rich lesions from plaque calcification.

6.4.2 Fibrous Cap Imaging

The thickness of a fibrous cap may provide important information related to the vulnerability of a coronary plaque.[22–24] The fibrous cap that covers a necrotic plaque core predominantly consists of extracellular collagen-rich matrix and smooth muscle cells.[10] Often, the thinnest portion of the overlaying cap is the shoulder region[25]

TABLE 6.2
OCT Image Features of Arterial Vessel Wall Structure by Histopathologic Finding[15,34,41]

Histologic Structure	Intravascular Ultrasound Finding	Optical Coherence Tomography Finding
Intimal hyperplasia	Not appropriately detectable	Signal-rich layer nearest lumen
Media	Less echogenic than intima	Signal-poor middle layer
Adventitia	Signal-rich outer layer	Signal-rich, heterogeneous outer layer (fairly detectable)
Internal elastic lamina (IEL)	Cannot always be distinguished clearly	Signal-rich band between intima and media
External elastic lamina (EEL)	Not detectable	Signal-rich band between media and adventitia
Atheroma	Area between EEM and luminal border	Loss of layered appearance, narrowing of lumen between outer side of IEL and inner side of EEL
Fibrous plaque	Intermediate echogenicity between echolucent atheroma and highly echogenic calcific lesions	Homogeneous, signal-rich region
Macrocalcification	Bright echoes with characteristic "acoustic shadow"	Large, heterogeneous, sharply delineated
Lipid pool	Not detectable	Large, homogeneous, poorly delineated, signal-poor (echolucent) region
Fibrous cap	Not detectable	Signal-rich band overlying signal-poor region

Source: Modified after Jang, I.K. et al., *J. Am. Coll. Cardiol.*, 39, 604, 2002.

where peak circumferential stress is highest. Using the high resolution of OCT and its high contrast between fibrous and lipid-rich tissue, visualization of the fibrous cap and measurement of its dimensions are possible (see Figure 6.5).[16,20,26]

6.4.3 MACROPHAGE DETECTION IN VULNERABLE PLAQUES

Activated macrophages weaken fibrous caps and thus lead to higher vulnerability and aptness to disrupt. OCT has been shown to be able to detect and quantify the number of macrophages in atherosclerotic plaques in an *ex vivo* study.[27] Twenty-six lipid-rich cadaveric atherosclerotic coronary artery plaques were investigated. OCT imaging was performed within 72 hr postmortem. The obtained results were compared to immunohistologic stains of the corresponding plaque segment. We used an OCT system with a light source of 1310 nm and an axial resolution of ~10 µm. The transverse resolution was 25 µm. Since the average size of a macrophage is

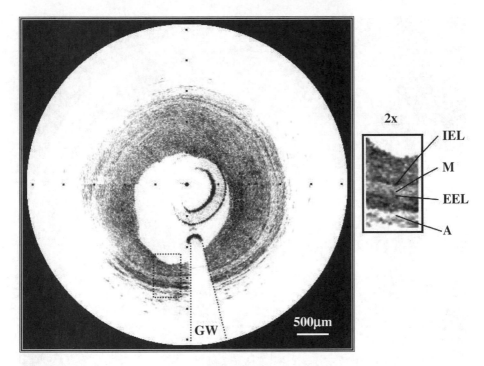

FIGURE 6.3 Fibrous coronary artery plaque imaged by OCT. The plaque tissue shows high signal due to intense back-scatter. The internal elastic lamina (IEL), tunica media (M), and external elastic lamina (EEL) are clearly visualized. The internal part of the adventitia (A) is also depicted. GW = guide wire artifact.

between 20 and 50 μm, it was assumed that OCT imaging might be appropriate to detect cell characteristics of the fibrous cap region.

During postprocessing of the obtained images, a region of interest was set and the background level and speckle noise of the OCT images were subtracted. Raw and logarithmic-based OCT imaging was compared quantitatively to immunohistologic results. For the raw OCT data, a correlation of 84% (p = <0.0001) was found between OCT signal intensity and macrophage content as determined by histology. When using a threshold of macrophage content of 10% of the area,[28] the sensitivity and specificity of OCT to detect plaque rich in macrophages reached 100% (see Figure 6.6).

6.5 ANIMAL EXPERIMENT

Using a swine model, we investigated the ability of OCT to image *in vivo* coronary arteries.[29] Normal coronary arteries, intimal dissections, and stents were visualized with OCT and compared to IVUS. Significant advantages of OCT were identified: all layers of the vessel wall, including the intima were detected with OCT whereas IVUS could not provide any detailed structural information.

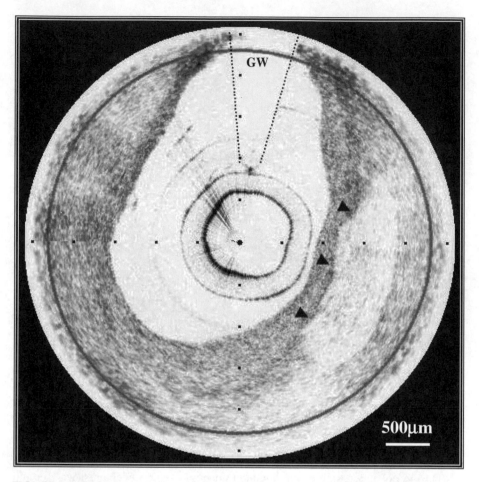

FIGURE 6.4 OCT image of a fibrocalcific plaque. It illustrates a region of low signal intensity within the internal elastic lamina (IEL) sharply bounded by a signal-richer fibrous area. GW = guide wire artifact.

Layered structures including intimal defects, disruption of the media wall, dissections, and the microanatomic relationships between stents and the vessel walls were clearly detected by OCT. The mechanical properties of the OCT catheter were found to be almost identical to those of the IVUS catheter. In this preclinical experiment, we showed that *in vivo* identification of clinically relevant coronary artery morphology with high resolution and contrast by OCT is feasible.

6.6 *IN VIVO* VALIDATION

We performed the first *in vivo* application of OCT for visualization of coronary atherosclerotic plaques in patients.[16] In 10 patients undergoing percutaneous coronary intervention, 17 mild to moderate coronary artery lesions were investigated.

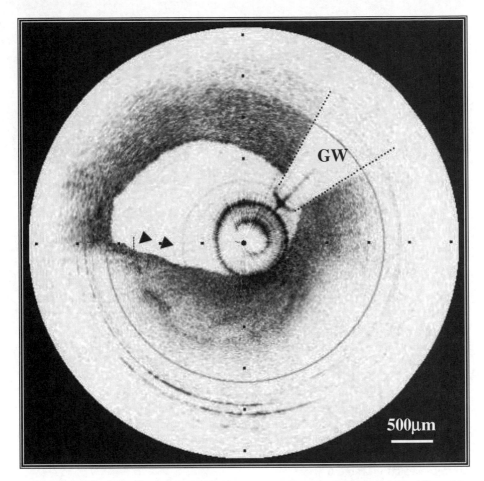

FIGURE 6.5 OCT image of a lipid-rich, high risk plaque. The lipid pool covered by a thin fibrous cap can be clearly seen. GW = guide wire artifact.

IVUS and OCT images of the same lesion were compared for detection of various vessel wall components.

OCT imaging was performed during repeated 8- to 10-cc saline flushes of the coronary lumen. Each flush generated a 2-sec image acquisition time. Axial resolution of the used OCT system was 13 ± 3 μm; the axial IVUS resolution was 98 ± 19 μm. The acquired penetration depth of OCT was 1.25 mm (5 mm for IVUS). On average, the additional time required for OCT was 10 min per procedure. The overall safety of the OCT procedure was excellent. All enrolled patients tolerated the procedure without any complaints or complications.

OCT was able to detect all vessel wall structures identified by IVUS. All calcifications detected by IVUS were also seen by OCT; OCT provided higher contrast between calcifications and surrounding tissues. The characteristic acoustic shadow of calcification in IVUS prevented exact assessments of the sizes and depths of coronary calcifications, while no shadowing was apparent with OCT.

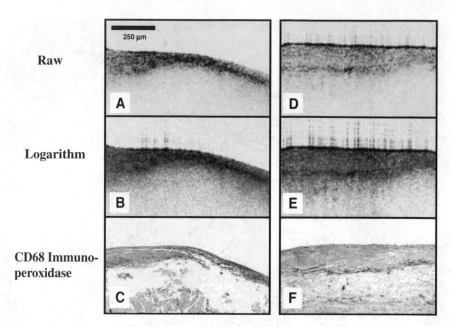

FIGURE 6.6 Corresponding OCT images (A,B,D,E) and histology (C,F) of an atherosclerotic plaque with lipid-rich pool and thin fibrous cap (CD68 immunoperoxidase, original magnification ×100).

All echolucent regions noted with IVUS were also detected with OCT. In addition, OCT depicted two echolucent areas, most probably corresponding to lipid pools. Intravascular ultrasound could demonstrate intimal hyperplasia in three segments while OCT was able to detect eight additional sites of intimal hyperplasia due to its higher resolution. IVUS and OCT findings for corresponding image pairs are represented in Table 6.3.

In summary, this study demonstrated that OCT imaging can be performed reliably and safely *in vivo*. In comparison to intravascular ultrasound, OCT may provide significant additional information concerning plaque morphology, composition, and vulnerability.

6.7 *IN VIVO* EVALUATION OF INTRACORONARY STENTS

Both IVUS and OCT provide the opportunity to assess the outcome of coronary stenting. Although IVUS has been shown to permit evaluation of stent expansion apposition,[30] additional detailed information about the stent and surrounding tissue cannot be obtained by IVUS and artifacts caused by the metal struts of a stent frequently impair image quality.

Our group demonstrated that OCT is able to assess the postinterventional status of lesions and stents with extremely high resolution.[31] In 43 imaged stents, the ability of OCT to demonstrate vessel dissection, tissue prolapse, stent apposition, and stent

TABLE 6.3
IVUS and OCT Findings for Corresponding Image Pairs

Feature	Identified by both OCT and IVUS	Identified by OCT alone
Intimal hyperplasia	3 (3 patients)	8 (7 patients)
Internal elastic lamina	Not evaluated	11 (8 patients)
External elastic lamina	Not evaluated	10 (7 patients)
Plaque (both types)	17 (10 patients)	0
Fibrous Plaque	13 (10 patients)	0
Calcific plaque	4 (4 patients)	0
Echolucent region	2 (2 patients)	2 (2 patients)

Note: All features of vessel wall structure identified by the IVUS reader were seen in the corresponding OCT image (middle column). Additional findings by OCT not identified by the IVUS reader cited in the right column. N = 17.

Source: Modified after Jang, I.K. et al., *J. Am. Coll. Cardiol.*, 39, 604, 2002.

asymmetry was investigated. Because we lacked a better "gold standard," IVUS was used as a reference tool. OCT was performed without any complications and a significant difference from the information provided by IVUS was found. Dissections were identified in eight cases by OCT, while IVUS showed only two dissections. In 29 cases, tissue prolapse was recognized by OCT, while IVUS demonstrated only 12 cases (see Figure 6.7). Incomplete stent deployment was found in seven stents with OCT and in three stents with IVUS. Given the substantially higher resolution of OCT, these results are not astonishing. The study shows the feasibility of OCT imaging in stents, but clinical benefit remains questionable, especially since recent studies found only marginal benefits of IVUS-guided stenting.[32,33]

6.8 LIMITATIONS OF OCT

Intravascular OCT provides visualization of plaque components with a resolution similar to histology and is able to identify characteristics of vulnerable or high risk plaques *in vivo*. However, in spite of the impressive image quality, OCT reveals no physiologic information about plaques.

A major limitation of OCT comes from the intrinsic property of optical imaging. Blood produces significant attenuation of emitted infrared light. During all *in vivo* OCT measurements performed, the interfering blood was displaced by a saline flush which permitted subsequent imaging for about 2 sec. The short duration of clear visualization makes imaging of an entire vessel difficult. Current developments and studies are addressing that limitation. Index matching — a technique of administering agents to the blood to decrease the scattering effects of red blood cells — constitutes an attractive approach and may significantly increase the penetration of OCT.[17] Other possible solutions include proximal or distal balloon occlusion of a

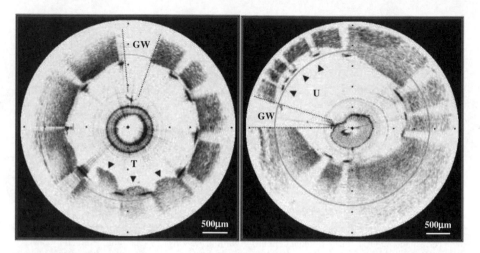

FIGURE 6.7 Optical coherence tomography image of an intracoronary stent. Tissue prolapse (T) and an underdeployed part of the stent (U) can be detected. GW = guide wire artifact.

vessel or a continuous saline flush via a separate catheter. The next generation of the OCT system now under development may allow scanning of long vessel segments.

The limited penetration depth constitutes another major limitation of CT since it frequently precludes visualization and measurement of the complete plaque and does not allow for evaluation of the remodeling process. Reliable detection of morphologic structures is only possible within a radius of approximately 2 to 3 mm.

6.9   CONCLUDING REMARKS

OCT can provide detailed information about the characteristics of coronary athero-sclerotic lesions including lipid pools, thin fibrous caps, and presence of macro-phages and may be useful for the detection of vulnerable plaque. The value of OCT relative to other intracoronary imaging techniques aimed to determine plaque sta-bility and vulnerability must still be determined.

Competing methods that provide complementary physiologic and structural information include thermography, Raman spectroscopy, infrared spectroscopy, and angioscopy.[34–40] Recently, IVUS has been combined with virtual histology and pal-pography–elastography and revealed promising results. The comparison of the var-ious diagnostic modalities with their ability to detect different components of vul-nerable plaques is shown in Table 6.4. Combining these imaging tools to obtain both physiologic and structural information will thus enhance diagnostic yields. In sum-mary, OCT is a novel imaging modality with a histology level resolution that has proven capable of characterizing coronary plaques *in vivo*.

TABLE 6.4
Comparison of Noninvasive and Invasive Imaging Modalities for Detection of Individual Characteristics of Vulnerable Plaque

Imaging Modality	Resolution	Penetration	Fibrous Cap	Lipid Core	Inflammation	Calcium	Thrombus	Current Status
IVUS	100 μm	Good	+	++	–	+++	+	CS/CA
Angioscopy	UK	Poor	+	++	–	–	+++	CS/CA*
OCT	10 μm	Poor	+++	+++	+	+++	+	CS
Thermography	0.5 mm	Poor	–	–	+++	–	–	CS
Spectroscopy	NA	Poor	+	++	++	++	–	PCS
Intravascular MRI	160 μm	Good	+	++	++	++	+	PCS

Note: NA = not applicable; CS = clinical studies; CA = clinically approved for commercial use; CA* = clinically approved for commercial use in Japan; PCS = preclinical studies; UK = unknown; +++ = sensitivity > 90%; + = sensitivity 80–90%; ++ = sensitivity 50–80%; – = sensitivity <50%.

Source: From MacNeill, B., Lowe, H.C., Takano, M., Fuster, V., and Jang, I.K., *Arterioscler. Thromb. Vasc. Biol.*, 23, 1333–1342, 2003. With permission.

REFERENCES

1. Dalager-Pedersen, S., H.B. Ravn, and E. Falk, Atherosclerosis and acute coronary events. *Am J Cardiol*, 1998. 82: 37T–40T.
2. Schroeder, A.P. and E. Falk, Pathophysiology and inflammatory aspects of plaque rupture. *Cardiol Clin*, 1996. 14: 211–220.
3. Muller, J.E. et al. Triggers, acute risk factors and vulnerable plaques: the lexicon of a new frontier. *J Am Coll Cardiol*, 1994. 23: 809–813.
4. Muller, J.E. and B. Mangel, Circadian variation and triggers of cardiovascular disease. *Cardiology*, 1994. 85 (Suppl. 2): 3–10.
5. Muller, J.E., G.H. Tofler, and P.H. Stone, Circadian variation and triggers of onset of acute cardiovascular disease. *Circulation*, 1989. 79: 733–743.
6. Kondo, N.I. and J.E. Muller, Triggering of acute myocardial infarction. *J Cardiovasc Risk*, 1995. 2: 499–504.
7. Nagavi M et al. From vulnerable plaque to vulnerable patient: a call for new definitions and risk assessment strategies. *Circulation*, 2003, in press.
8. Virmani, R. et al. Lessons from sudden coronary death: a comprehensive morphological classification scheme for atherosclerotic lesions. *Arterioscler Thromb Vasc Biol*, 2000. 20: 1262–1275.
9. Davies, M.J. and A.C. Thomas, Plaque fissuring — the cause of acute myocardial infarction, sudden ischaemic death, and crescendo angina. *Br Heart J*, 1985. 53: 363–373.
10. Falk, E., P.K. Shah, and V. Fuster, Coronary plaque disruption. *Circulation*, 1995. 92: 657–671.
11. Davies, M.J., Detecting vulnerable coronary plaques. *Lancet*, 1996. 347: 1422–1423.
12. Lee, R.T. and P. Libby. The unstable atheroma. *Arterioscler Thromb Vasc Biol*, 1997. 17: 1859–1867.
13. Can atherosclerosis imaging techniques improve the detection of patients at risk for ischemic heart disease? Proceedings of 34th Bethesda Conference, October 7, 2002. *J Am Coll Cardiol*, 2003. 41: 1856–1917.
14. Huang, D., et al. Optical coherence tomography. *Science*, 1991. 254: 1178–1181.
15. Fujimoto, J.G., et al. High resolution *in vivo* intra-arterial imaging with optical coherence tomography. *Heart*, 1999. 82: 128–133.
16. Jang, I.K. et al. Visualization of coronary atherosclerotic plaques in patients using optical coherence tomography: comparison with intravascular ultrasound. *J Am Coll Cardiol*, 2002. 39: 604–609.
17. Brezinski, M. et al. Index matching to improve optical coherence tomography imaging through blood. *Circulation*, 2001. 103: 1999–2003.
18. Welzel, J., M. Bruhns, and H.H. Wolff, Optical coherence tomography in contact dermatitis and psoriasis. *Arch Dermatol Res*, 2003.
19. Welzel, J., et al. Optical coherence tomography of the human skin. *J Am Acad Dermatol*, 1997. 37: 958–963.
20. Yabushita, H. et al. Characterization of human atherosclerosis by optical coherence tomography. *Circulation*, 2002. 106: 1640–1645.
21. Stary, H.C. et al. A definition of advanced types of atherosclerotic lesions and a histological classification of atherosclerosis: report from the Committee on Vascular Lesions of the Council on Arteriosclerosis, American Heart Association. *Circulation*, 1995. 92: 1355–1374.
22. Kristensen, S.D., H.B. Ravn, and E. Falk, Insights into the pathophysiology of unstable coronary artery disease. *Am J Cardiol*, 1997. 80: 5E–9E.

23. Pasterkamp, G. et al. Techniques characterizing the coronary atherosclerotic plaque: influence on clinical decision making? *J Am Coll Cardiol*, 2000. 36: 13–21.

24. Zhou, J. et al. Plaque pathology and coronary thrombosis in the pathogenesis of acute coronary syndromes. *Scand J Clin Lab Invest Suppl*, 1999. 230: 3–11.

25. Fuster, V., Lewis A. Conner Memorial Lecture: mechanisms leading to myocardial infarction: insights from studies of vascular biology. *Circulation*, 1994. 90: 2126–2146.

26. MacNeill, B.D., M. Hayase, and I.K. Jang, The comparison between optical coherence tomography and intravascular ultrasound. *Minerva Cardioangiol*, 2002. 50: 497–506.

27. Tearney, G.J., et al. Quantification of macrophage content in atherosclerotic plaques by optical coherence tomography. *Circulation*, 2003. 107: 113–119.

28. Moreno, P.R., et al. Macrophage infiltration in acute coronary syndromes: implications for plaque rupture. *Circulation*, 1994. 90: 775–778.

29. Tearney, G.J. et al. Porcine coronary imaging *in vivo* by optical coherence tomography. *Acta Cardiol,* 2000. 55: 233–237.

30. Colombo, A. et al. Intracoronary stenting without anticoagulation accomplished with intravascular ultrasound guidance. *Circulation*, 1995. 91: 1676–1688.

31. Bouma, B.E. et al. Evaluation of intracoronary stenting by intravascular optical coherence tomography. *Heart*, 2003. 89: 317–320.

32. Mudra, H. et al. Randomized comparison of coronary stent implantation under ultrasound or angiographic guidance to reduce stent restenosis (OPTICUS Study). *Circulation*, 2001. 104: 1343–1349.

33. Schiele, F. et al. Impact of intravascular ultrasound guidance in stent deployment on 6-month restenosis rate: a multicenter, randomized study comparing two strategies — with and without intravascular ultrasound guidance. RESIST Study Group on Restenosis after IVUS-guided stenting. *J Am Coll Cardiol*, 1998. 32: 320–328.

34. Stefanadis, C. et al. Thermal heterogeneity within human atherosclerotic coronary arteries detected *in vivo*: a new method of detection by application of a special thermography catheter. *Circulation*, 1999. 99: 1965–1971.

35. Verheye, S. et al. *In vivo* temperature heterogeneity of atherosclerotic plaques is determined by plaque composition. *Circulation*, 2002. 105: 1596–1601.

36. Brennan, J.F., III et al. Determination of human coronary artery composition by Raman spectroscopy. *Circulation*, 1997. 96: 99–105.

37. Romer, T.J. et al. Histopathology of human coronary atherosclerosis by quantifying its chemical composition with Raman spectroscopy. *Circulation*, 1998. 97: 878–885.

38. Moreno, P.R. et al. Detection of lipid pool, thin fibrous cap, and inflammatory cells in human aortic atherosclerotic plaques by near-infrared spectroscopy. *Circulation*, 2002. 105: 923–927.

39. Arakawa, K. et al. Angioscopic coronary macromorphology after thrombolysis in acute myocardial infarction. *Am J Cardiol*, 1997. 79: 197–202.

40. Ueda, Y. et al. The healing process of infarct-related plaques: insights from 18 months of serial angioscopic follow-up. *J Am Coll Cardiol*, 2001. 38: 1916–1922.

41. Brezinski, M.E. et al. Optical coherence tomography for optical biopsy: properties and demonstration of vascular pathology. *Circulation*, 1996. 93: 1206–1213.

7 Magnetic Resonance Imaging of High-Risk Plaque

Stephen G. Worthley and Juan J. Badimon

CONTENTS

7.1   INTRODUCTION

What is clear from reviewing the pathogenetic mechanisms behind atherosclerosis and the acute coronary syndromes is that we are extremely limited in our ability to accurately identify patients at risk for acute coronary events.[1] The current armamentarium of clinically available diagnostic investigations, both noninvasive and invasive, can only provide us with data related to the stenotic severity of a coronary artery. The noninvasive testing can determine stress-induced (exercise or pharmacologic) ischemic changes in electrical repolarization, wall motion, and myocardial radioactive tracer uptake. The invasive test of coronary angiography, although the

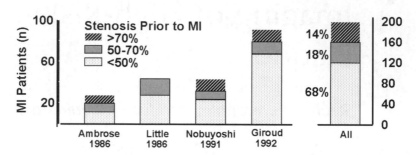

FIGURE 7.1 Meta-analysis of studies showing the association of stenosis severity and associated risk of coronary occlusion and myocardial infarction (MI). (Modified from Falk, E. et al., *Circulation*, 92, 657, 1995. With permission.)

current "gold standard" for the detection of coronary atherosclerotic disease, provides no data about the composition of an atherosclerotic lesion.[2,3]

However, the vast majority of acute coronary events involve noncritically stenosed atherosclerotic lesions[4] that would be undetected by currently available stress testing and imaging techniques (Figure 7.1). Thus, given the critical role that atherosclerotic lesion composition has been shown to play in the risk of plaque rupture, subsequent thrombogenicity, and an ensuing acute coronary event, new detection techniques must be investigated for purposes of documenting atherosclerotic lesion composition.[5] The imaging of such vulnerable plaques should provide information about composition and degree of encroachment on the vessel lumen by the atherosclerotic plaque. The ideal imaging modality should be safe, noninvasive, accurate, and reproducible, thus allowing longitudinal studies in the same patient.[6]

Magnetic resonance imaging (MRI) is a unique technology that allows the noninvasive visualization of cardiovascular anatomy.[7] Of all imaging modalities currently available in all fields, MRI provides the greatest intrinsic contrast between soft tissue structures. Thus, it is a powerful tool for defining pathoanatomical processes of the visceral organs, including the heart and vascular structures. Furthermore, the absence of ionizing radiation and the free choice of tomographic planes enhance the potential of this technique for the future. However, MRI does have limitations, including relatively long imaging time, relative isolation of the patient from medical care during image acquisition, and contraindication in patients with certain metallic implants (e.g., permanent pacemakers). Imaging time and quality are rapidly improving with technological advances in the field, and the information that MRI can provide in the cardiovascular field is rapidly growing.

MRI has the potential to provide information about cardiac anatomy, function (myocardial and valvular), perfusion, and metabolism. Application to the coronary arteries suggests that MRI may supply information about coronary angiography, flow velocity, and even the characterization of atherosclerotic lesions within coronary artery walls. Because of the excellent soft tissue contrast provided by MRI

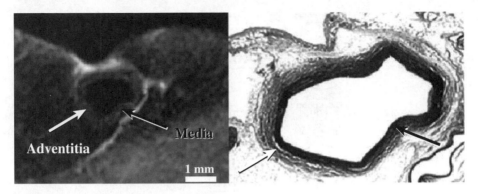

FIGURE 7.2 MR image (T2W) of the right coronary artery showing no obvious athero-sclerotic plaque but defining the media (high signal, white) with a black arrow from the dense adventitia (low signal, black) with a white arrow. The corresponding histopathology section confirms the accurate identification of the vessel wall. Surrounding the vessel wall is another high signal structure on the T2W image representing connective tissue. (Modified from Worthley, S.G. et al., *Atherosclerosis*, 150, 321, 2000. With permission.)

techniques, the ability of MRI to differentiate between these plaque components has been investigated recently.[8–12] Experimental data have shown that MRI is effective in identifying both normal vessel wall components (Figure 7.2) and atherosclerotic plaques.[8,11]

In this chapter, we will review some of the underlying pathobiology of athero-sclerosis and discuss the basics of MRI with respect to the concept of atherosclerosis imaging, bringing us to the current status of atherosclerosis imaging with MR.

7.2 PATHOGENESIS OF ATHEROTHROMBOSIS

The clinical manifestations of atherosclerosis remain the leading causes of death and morbidity in western society. Thrombosis of a disrupted atherosclerotic plaque appears to be a crucial event for a patient who experiences a clinical complication of atherosclerosis. However, such plaque disruption and subsequent thrombosis may lead to one of two scenarios (1) nonocclusive luminal thrombosis leading to silent, rapid plaque growth or (2) occlusive (transiently or permanently) luminal thrombosis associated with unstable angina pectoris, acute myocardial infarction, or sudden cardiac death (Figure 7.3).

Plaques containing large atheromatous cores are more prone to disruption, and indeed three-quarters of such plaques are responsible for the atherothrombotic com-plications leading to acute coronary syndromes.[13,14] Most other cases are associated with plaque thrombosis atop a macrophage-rich intimal erosion in a more fibrotic plaque, often in association with a severe arterial stenosis.[13,14] However, it is worth-while to explore these concepts more thoroughly, including factors for both plaque disruption and subsequent thrombosis.

Plaque disruption is a central feature of atherothrombotic syndromes and the risk that it will occur relates to intrinsic properties (vulnerability) and extrinsic factors

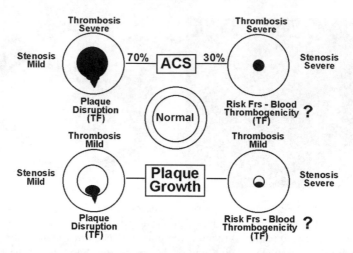

FIGURE 7.3 Various outcomes resulting from thrombotic complications of atherosclerotic disease. Plaque disruption and subsequent thrombosis are associated with 70% of the acute coronary syndromes; the remaining 30% seem to be caused by a severe stenosis triggering thrombosis. ACS = acute coronary syndrome. Question marks refer to the potential effect of a newly reported systemic pool of tissue factor (TF).(From Worthley, S.G. et al. *Mt Sinai J Med*, 68, 167–181, 2001. With permission.)

(triggers) of the plaque. Atherosclerotic plaque disruption tends to occur at sites where the fibrous cap is thinnest and most heavily infiltrated with macrophage-derived foam cells (i.e., its weakest point). This tends to be at the shoulder region of an eccentric lesion (the juncture between the normal vessel wall and the athero-sclerotic plaque).[14] Factors shown to be associated with risk of rupture of the fibrous cap are:

1. Size of the atheromatous core
2. Thickness, collagen content, and smooth muscle cell content of the fibrous cap
3. Inflammation within the fibrous cap
4. Cap fatigue

It is true that the composition of most atherosclerotic lesions is mainly fibrotic, but significant atheromatous cores exist in the majority of so-called culprit lesions for acute coronary syndromes as we described earlier.[4] A number of studies have confirmed the association between size of the atheromatous core and risk for sub-sequent plaque rupture. One study found that in aortic plaque, an atheromatous core of >40% of the plaque content was at a particularly high risk of disruption and subsequent thrombosis.[15] This concept helps explain the postulated mechanism by which lipid lowering is felt to reduce clinical events. Based on numerous animal studies, lipid lowering therapy is believed to decrease the lipid content of a plaque (i.e., decrease the size of the lipid-rich core) resulting in a more fibrotic and stable plaque.[16-18]

Fibrous caps vary widely in their thickness and composition but they tend to be thinnest at the shoulder regions of the plaques.[14] Collagen, in particular type 1 collagen, is a critical determinant of fibrous cap strength and in disrupted aortic plaques, smooth muscle cells (sources of collagen in the caps) and the collagen content are decreased.[15,19] One mechanism postulated for the reduction of smooth muscle cells in the fibrous cap is apoptosis, although it is uncertain whether apoptosis is the only mechanism responsible.[19]

Evidence of active inflammation (with immunohistochemical staining of pathological samples) within the fibrous caps at sites of disruption is strong, and studies have shown macrophage infiltration at the disrupted shoulder regions of fibrous caps.[13] An important mechanism appears to be the production of matrix-degrading enzymes including the matrix metalloproteinases (MMPs) that play an important role in atherogenesis also. Activated macrophages within the fibrous cap produce a variety of MMPs and *in vitro* studies have confirmed the ability of these enzymes to degrade fibrous caps.[20] Although many of these enzymes have been implicated, only gelatinase B (MMP-9) has been associated with rupture-prone areas in human atherectomy specimens.[21] T cells are also present in increased numbers at these rupture-prone sites and are able to stimulate macrophages to produce MMP-9.[22]

7.3 MAGNETIC RESONANCE IMAGING

Magnetic resonance can provide information about cardiac anatomy, function (myocardial and valvular), perfusion, and metabolism. Application to coronary arteries suggests that MRI may supply information about coronary angiography, flow velocity, and even the characterization of atherosclerotic lesions within coronary artery walls.[7] Although we are still a long way from "one-stop shopping" with cardiac MR imaging, the field is exciting and will surely play a significant role in cardiovascular imaging in the future.

7.3.1 MRI BASICS

Hydrogen (^{1}H) is the simplest and most abundant element in the human body and thus most MR studies assess hydrogen nuclei (protons) in water. By subjecting an object or patient to a strong local magnetic field, usually 1.5 T, these protons or spins are relatively aligned. They are excited by a radiofrequency pulse and subsequently detected with receiver coils. The detected signals are influenced by the relaxation times (T1 and T2), proton density, motion and flow, molecular diffusion, magnetization transfer, and changes in susceptibility. Three additional magnetic (gradient) fields are applied during MRI: one to select the slice and two to encode spatial information. The timing of the excitation pulses and the successive magnetic field gradients determine the image contrast.

7.3.2 TECHNICAL CONSIDERATIONS

An MR image is encoded into its constituent spatial frequency components. In order to generate an image of a specific spatial resolution and image field of view (FOV), data for a minimal set of spatial frequencies or k-space lines must be sampled so that the spatial frequency distribution of the object can be determined. With a single k-space line sampled after a single radiofrequency excitation pulse, the number of k-space lines in an image directly determines the total image acquisition time.

Current MRI techniques have evolved to a highly specialized degree and the processes involved are extremely complex. However, the concept of MRI is worth exploring on a simplistic level. One basic of MRI is that a person placed within an external magnetic field will become partially magnetized although the magnetization is orders of magnitude less than the strength of the external magnetic field. Much of this effect is associated with hydrogen ions (protons) within the body, the largest source of which is water. A physical principle of changing magnetic fields is that they emit radiofrequency waves, and the collection of radiofrequency information can be translated into the MR image to be analyzed.

The characteristics of these radiofrequency waves are determined by many factors including the parameters of MRI techniques and, importantly, the various tissues investigated. The technique allows accurate differentiation of the soft tissue components of the body. Two main imaging sequences or techniques known as spin echo sequences and gradient echo sequences form the basis for much of the MRI performed today.

7.3.2.1 Spin Echo Sequences

Spin echo imaging can provide excellent discrimination of various components of the heart and has flexible contrast characteristics, depending on the programmed parameters of the imaging sequence (T1-weighted = T1W, proton density-weighted = PDW, T2-weighted = T2W). With this technique, blood within the vascular compartment appears black (so-called black blood imaging; see Figure 7.4). Due to the often longer imaging times, this imaging sequence has traditionally been used for the imaging of static phenomena including myocardial wall thickness, cardiac chamber volumes, intracardiac thrombi and more recently, atherosclerotic plaques.

The conventional single-phase, multiple-slice ECG-gated spin echo (SE) is the most common imaging sequence traditionally used for cardiac MRI. The SE technique generates images where the blood signals appear dark (black blood images) because of the requirement that any spins excited by the initial 90° radiofrequency pulse dephase and are rephased by the subsequent 180° radiofrequency pulse. Flowing spins (such as blood) transiting through the imaged slice are affected by one but not both radiofrequency pulses. Hence, the spins flowing through the slice will not refocus and return a signal, i.e., they appear dark in the image. However, slow-flowing blood will not appear dark in SE images, as it may remain within the imaged slice and thus "see" both the 90° and 180° radiofrequency pulses. Saturation radiofrequency pulses are usually placed above and below the image planes to ensure that the blood signal is dark.

The repetition time (TR) is equal to the R–R interval and the minimum echo time (TE) is selected for T1-weighted images. For T2-weighted images, TR is equal to two or more R–R intervals and a TE of 80 to 100 msec. In each R–R interval, data at different spatial locations are acquired with the same k-space encoding value.

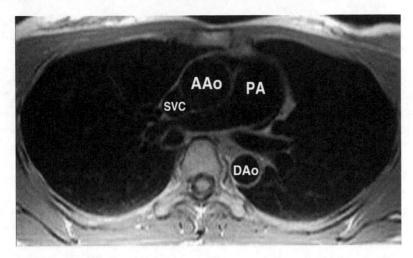

FIGURE 7.4 So-called black blood image (spin echo-based sequence) taken through the chest wall (axial slice). Suppression of the signal from the blood pool was obtained using a double inversion recovery sequence described in the text. AAo = ascending aorta. PA = pulmonary artery. DAo = descending aorta. SVC = superior vena cava.

Images at the different spatial locations are then at a different temporal phase of the cardiac cycle. Since only one k-space is acquired per cardiac trigger, a typical scan with 128 k-spaces in the phase encoding direction will take 128 heart beats to complete for a T1-weighted image or 256 heart beats for a T2-weighted image with TR equal to 2 R–R. Typically the SE images are acquired with two signal averages and, therefore, the imaging time is usually 6 to 8 min for a T1-weighted acquisition or 12 to 18 min for a T2-weighted acquisition, depending on heart rate. The quality of T2-weighted images is lower than that of T1-weighted images because of lower signal-to-noise ratio due to the long TE and longer acquisition time.

The long scan times make gated SE images extremely sensitive to respiratory motion and dependent on consistent ECG gating. In order to minimize the image artifacts from respiratory motion, respiratory view ordering (respiratory compensation) can be used,[23] but it further extends the total scan time (10 to 20 min) and is sometimes ineffective.

In gated SE, data for each scan location are acquired at a fixed delay from the cardiac R wave. With variation in the cardiac rhythm (approximately 5%), the heart may be at different phase of the cardiac cycle even though the cardiac delay time may be the same.[24] As normal variation of the cardiac cycle usually results in changes during diastole, gated SE images acquired at the end of a cardiac cycle often exhibit blurring or ghosting artifacts. However, the contrast between the heart, epicardial fat, and ventricular cavities is relatively good. T1-weighted images are useful for anatomical evaluations, whereas the utility of T2-weighted imaging includes visualizing soft tissue T2 contrast and characterizing cardiac or paracardiac masses, intramyocardial tumors, and vegetations.

Conventional SE with its acquisition of a single line of k-space data per slice excitation is susceptible to respiratory artifacts, but this can be overcome by using techniques that provide shorter imaging times. By encoding for multiple k-space lines after a single 90° radiofrequency excitation pulse via a train of refocusing 180° radiofrequency pulses, the fast spin echo (FSE or turbo spin echo) sequence provides shorter imaging with reduced respiratory motion artifacts. The number of echoes acquired after the 90° excitation is named echo train length (ETL) or turbo factor. With an ETL of 8, the scan time for a T2-weighted sequence (TR = 2 R–R) is reduced to 32 heart beats for a 128-phase encoding image.

In order to ensure that a signal from blood is adequately suppressed, a double inversion recovery magnetization preparation pulse (velocity-selective inversion) is used.[25] This is quickly followed by a slice-selective inversion pulse that restores the magnetization within the imaged slice. An inversion time (TI = ~600 msec) is selected to null the signal from blood when the 90° radiofrequency excitation pulse is applied. In order to minimize image blurring artifacts from T2 decay in a long echo train, the acquisition is segmented over several heart beats and the spacing between each echo (echo spacing or ESP) is minimized. With an ETL of 32, a gated T2-weighted FSE image can be acquired in 16 heart beats for 256 k-space lines. This allows fast data acquisition during suspended respiration and provides artifact-free images of cardiovascular anatomy. One of the disadvantages of the current double inversion recovery FSE sequence is that images are acquired a single slice at a time, in order not to affect the effectiveness of the inversion pulses used to null signals from blood. A recent extension of the FSE sequence is the single or segmented shot HASTE (half Fourier turbo spin echo) technique.[26] Image acquisition can be achieved in the time required for a single heart beat.

7.3.2.2 Gradient Echo Sequences

Gradient echo imaging is especially useful for vascular lumen angiography. Flowing blood appears white (so-called bright blood imaging; see Figure 7.5). This form of imaging sequence may be acquired rapidly, allowing cardiac cycle (cine) imaging of the heart and thus the assessment of myocardial function. The advent of extremely rapid image acquisition (10 to 15 images per second) with this technique allows for real-time imaging and with further improvements in the resolution and image quality, the potential for performing interventional vascular procedures with MR real-time imaging exists.

This technique of imaging is less able to provide varying tissue contrast compared with spin echo imaging and images are mainly T1-weighted. The technique is characterized by short sequence repetition times (TRs), flip angles less than 90°, and substantially greater signal intensity of the ventricular blood pool compared to that of the myocardium. The latter effect is due to an in-flow refreshment phenomenon whereby fresh unsaturated blood continues to course through the imaged slice and experience fewer radiofrequency pulses than myocardial tissue that remains in the imaged slice throughout the data acquisition period. Consequently, the ventricular blood pool returns a much higher signal than the saturated spins of myocardial tissue, providing contrast between the ventricular cavity and the endocardium.

Short TR-gated gradient echo pulse sequences are used to generate cine images at multiple time frames of the cardiac cycle. Conventional cine pulse sequences

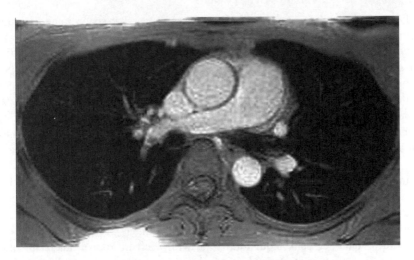

FIGURE 7.5 Bright blood imaging (gradient echo-based image) of the same patient and at the exact location shown in Figure 7.4.

run asynchronously to the cardiac cycle with the spatial frequency (phase) encoding value updated on detection of the R wave trigger. Each radiofrequency excitation pulse is applied at the same spatial location and repeated at intervals of TR in the cardiac cycle. Since the sequence runs asynchronously, the radiofrequency excitation pulses may occur at varying time delays from the R wave from one cardiac cycle to the next. On detection of the next cardiac R wave, the k-space encoding value is updated and the acquired temporal data from the previous R–R interval is resorted and interpolated into evenly distributed time frames within each cardiac cycle. This method of gating is also known as retrospective gating because data from the current R–R interval is resorted only after the next R wave trigger is detected.

As noted earlier, conventional gradient echo cine pulse sequences acquire only one k-space encoding view per heart beat. The total image acquisition time is then of the order of 128 heart beats. As this time is beyond the ability of a patient to maintain an effective breath-hold, conventional cine scans suffer respiratory motion artifacts and require some form of respiratory gating or an intelligent k-space acquisition view reordering to maintain an artifact-free image. These gating and reordering measures, however, are only marginally effective and cannot substitute for a breath-held acquisition.

Faster cardiac magnetic resonance (CMR) techniques have dramatically shortened image acquisition times to as little as 10 to 15 heart beats, making breath holding a feasible option to reduce respiratory motion artifacts. Faster scan times have been achieved by segmenting k-spaces and acquiring multiple k-space lines per R–R interval.[27] The scan time is speeded up by a factor equal to that of the number of k-space lines acquired per image per R–R interval. In this manner, a typical cine acquisition with a matrix size of 128 pixels in the phase encoding direction can be completed in as few as 16 heart beats, with 8 k-space lines per segment (or views per segment). The k-space is divided into several segments, with each k-space line in a segment acquired in a single R–R interval.

Due to the need to rapidly acquire data for several k-space lines in order to minimize motion-blurring artifacts, segmented k-space techniques are almost exclusively used with fast gradient echo pulse sequences that have very short TR times. Fast gradient-recalled echo acquisitions can also be radiofrequency-phase spoiled for better myocardium–blood pool contrast. However, shorter TR times require smaller flip angles and as a consequence, image signal-to-noise ratio is lower than in conventional gradient echo cine acquisitions. Multiple phases of the cardiac cycle can be visualized by repeated acquisition of the same k-space segment within an R–R interval and assigning the data acquired at different time points in the cardiac cycle to different temporal phases.

In segmented k-space scans, the total scan time is inversely proportional to the number of views per segment. The large the number of views acquired per segment, the shorter the scan time. However, the reduction in scan time is obtained at the expense of reducing the temporal resolution of the image. Significant motion of the heart during data segment acquisition time will result in loss of spatial resolution from cardiac motion-related blurring. Minimizing artifacts from cardiac motion by decreasing the number of views per segment would conversely lead to an increase in the total scan time, reducing the ability of a patient to hold his breath and reintroducing respiratory-related motion artifacts.

Fortunately, the minimum temporal resolution needed to sample the cardiac motion, especially during systole, is about 40 msec. With fast gradient echo pulse sequences, TR can be reduced to about 5 to 8 msec, permitting the collection of at least five to eight k-space lines per segment. Similar to the conventional cine acquisition, a higher effective temporal resolution can be obtained by a simple interpolation or nearest neighbor view-sharing process.[28]

Each temporal phase image represents the cardiac motion at specific delays from the cardiac R wave trigger averaged over the acquisition time per segment. The true image temporal resolution is unchanged but the effective temporal resolution is now doubled. View sharing can thus increase the number of phases reconstructed without affecting the manner in which the k-space data is acquired.

In addition to the acquisition of images at the same spatial location at different time points in the cine, a single-phase multislice acquisition can also be performed. A segmented k-space gradient–echo multiplanar acquisition would then acquire images at different spatial locations, each at a different phase of the cardiac cycle. Although the image quality is somewhat limited, a wide range of pathology can be detected from these images. Major structures such as the aorta, main pulmonary arteries, liver, spleen, and spine may be viewed. Another application of this technique is the imaging of uncooperative or sedated patients for whom breath-holding is not possible.

With imaging of so-called gradient–echo sequences, the MR signal is usually discarded (spoiling) so as to prevent cross-contamination of signals from different excitations. However, with the increased speed of gradient switching in more recent MRI units, this residual MR signal can be preserved and placed into a steady state by very rapid sequential excitation pulses. Such sequences are also known as steady state free precession images and are becoming extensively utilized in cardiovascular imaging (Figure 7.6). Various venders use terms such as true Fast Imaging with Steady-State Precession (FISP), balanced Fast Field Echo (FFE),

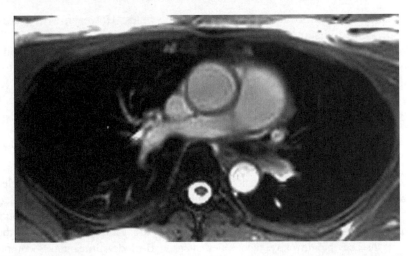

FIGURE 7.6 Steady-state free precession imaging performed in the same patient and at the exact location shown in Figure 7.4 and Figure 7.5. Note the high intrinsic signal generated by the blood pool.

and Fast Imaging Employing Steady-State Acquisition (FIESTA) to describe such sequences. The sequences produce a high signal intensity related to the ratio of the T2:T1 of the object imaged. The technique is, however, sensitive to off-resonance artifacts due to in-field inhomogeneities. Thus, metallic objects such as sternal wires remaining after cardiac surgery and prosthetic cardiac valves with metallic components are associated with obvious artifacts.

7.3.3 PATIENT SAFETY

MRI is generally well tolerated, although patients with musculoskeletal ailments (including chronic back pain) are less able to tolerate long imaging times. Claustrophobia prevents imaging in 2 to 10% of patients, although patient education, reassurance by staff, and sedation can assist in reducing this. Patient safety involves potential adverse events that can occur from placement within a strong magnetic field.

Patients with metallic implants such as mechanical heart valves (except for a prior version of the Starr–Edwards valve) and sternal wires resulting from thoracotomies and hip prostheses can safely undergo MRI studies. Such materials are not ferromagnetic and thus present no hazard to the patient. They will however, lead to artifacts with signal losses on images in the region of the metallic device. Endovascular metallic implants such as arterial stents and intravascular coils are unlikely to dislodge even if imaged within a few days after implantation. However, waiting more than 6 weeks after implantation before undergoing MRI is often recommended. As with all metallic devices, these endovascular implants will allow MRI signal loss in the regions of the objects.[29]

Permanent pacemakers and implanted cardioverter defibrillators are considered absolute contraindications to MRI due to the risk of pacemaker failure or rapid rhythm induction due to the oscillating magnetic fields. However, MRI has been safely performed in some patients with pacemakers.

External metallic objects such as intravenous drip stands and oxygen cylinders can act as potentially lethal projectiles if brought inside an MRI room due to the strong magnetic field present. Special MRI ECG leads and pulse oximetry leads must be used because any metallic components within these devices can heat within a magnetic field and thus burn a patient.

7.4   MRI OF ATHEROSCLEROSIS

When imaging atherosclerotic lesions, two important features need to be clearly differentiated: the degree of lumen obstruction and the composition of the plaque. Several invasive imaging techniques such as angiography, intravascular ultrasound,[30] angioscopy,[31] and optical coherence tomography[32] are available to assess atherosclerotic disease. Noninvasive techniques such as B-mode ultrasound,[33] computed tomography,[34] magnetic resonance,[35] and nuclear imaging techniques such as scintigraphy[36] and positron emission tomography[37] are also available. Most of these techniques are very useful in identifying luminal diameter and stenosis or wall thickness and some techniques provide assessments of relative risk for a future cardiovascular event. However, most fail to characterize completely the composition of atherosclerotic lesions and are therefore unable to assess accurately vulnerable plaques.[38]

High resolution MR has emerged as the potential leading noninvasive *in vivo* imaging modality for atherosclerotic plaque characterization. MR differentiates plaque components on the basis of biophysical and biochemical parameters such as chemical composition and concentration, water content, physical state, molecular motion, and diffusion. The ability to obtain images of the atherosclerotic vessels is dependent on the amount of available signal, contrast, and the lack of noise.

MR images can be "weighted" to T1, T2, or proton density values through manipulation of the MR parameters (i.e., repetition time and echo time). In a T1-weighted (T1W) image, tissues with low T1 values will be displayed as hyperintense picture elements or pixels (high signal intensity). Conversely, high T1 values will be displayed as hypointense pixels (low signal intensity). In a T2-weighted (T2W) image, tissues with high T2 values will be portrayed as hyperintense pixels, and those with low T2 values as hypointense pixels. Thus, T1W and T2W images for the same anatomy can appear quite different because an MR image is not a photograph; it is a computerized map of radio signals emitted by the human body. Finally, in a proton density–weighted (PDW) image, the differences in contrast are proportional to the density of water and fat protons within the tissue. A PDW image is also referred to as an intermediate-weighted image because the contrast in the image is a combination of mild T1 and T2 contrasts.

Plaque imaging requires the acquisition of high spatial resolution (<1 mm) and contrast resolution, due to the small size of the vessels under consideration, the adjacent lumen, and the size of each plaque structure. *In vivo* MR plaque imaging and characterization have been performed utilizing a multicontrast approach as previously validated.[11,12,39] The stabilization of an atherosclerotic plaque can be achieved by a multifactorial approach.[40] First, modifications of diet and lifestyle

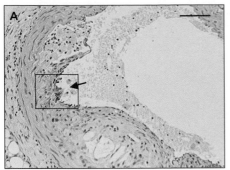
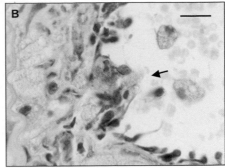

COLOR FIGURE 3.1 Acute plaque rupture: Apo E knockout mouse, brachiocephalic artery. Cleaved caspase-3 expression in a ruptured atherosclerotic lesion within a brachiocephalic artery of an 8-week-old, high-fat fed Apo E knockout mouse. Brown color in both panels indicates cleaved caspase-3 positive cells (apoptotic). Arrows indicate site of plaque rupture. Right panel shows detail of insert in left panel. Scale bars equal 100 μm (A) and 20 μm (B).

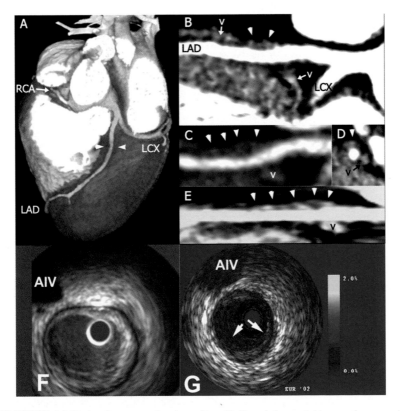

COLOR FIGURE 4.1 Noninvasive coronary imaging, using a 16-slice spiral computed tomography scanner (Sensation 16, Siemens AG, Forchheim, Germany), suggested a nonobstructive lesion in the mid-LAD (A, arrowhead) confirmed with coronary angiography. The attenuation value of the plaque was measured as 80 Hounsfield units (HUs), suggesting a mixed plaque composition without calcification (C, D, arrowheads). The entire segment can be shown in a single plane by means of vessel tracking (E, arrowhead). The great cardiac vein can be differentiated from the plaque by the higher and homogeneous attenuation of the venous lumen (v). Palpography (G) delivers strain information about this plaque's surface. At right, a scale ranging from 0% (blue) to 2% (yellow) characterizes the strain pattern. The strain images are color-coded: blue indicates stiff (low strain) material and red indicates softer (higher strain) material. In the cross-section in the identical position with the IVUS image (F), an eccentric soft plaque is visible with shoulders of high strain (arrows) on both sides of the otherwise stable cap, while the strain at the left shoulder (left arrow) is 1.5% and on the right shoulder (right arrow) is 1.2%. Between 11 and 12 hr, the palpogram appears to show an area of high strain, but this is caused by the nearby cardiac vein (AIV).

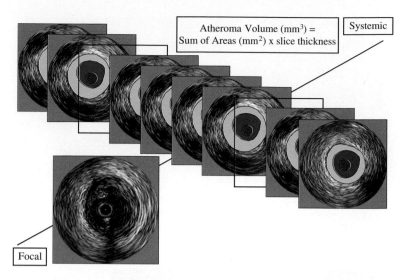

COLOR FIGURE 5.1 An optimal atherosclerosis imaging modality would combine noninvasiveness, high resolution, and the capability of assessing the overall disease process. As shown for the examples of histology, IVUS, and MDCT, each existing modality can be placed into this context in order to reveal its strengths and weaknesses.

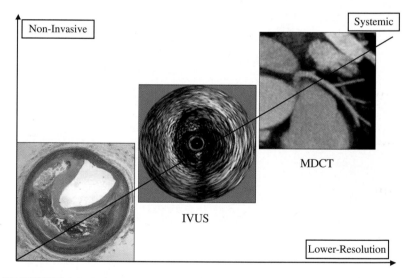

COLOR FIGURE 5.2 Because atherosclerotic plaque accumulation and vulnerability are systemic disease processes, a comprehensive assessment of the risk for the development of acute coronary syndromes may require both the assessment of focal lesion characteristics (vulnerable plaque) and the systemic plaque burden (vulnerable patient). An IVUS pull-back through a vessel segment can provide information about plaque morphology and plaque burden.

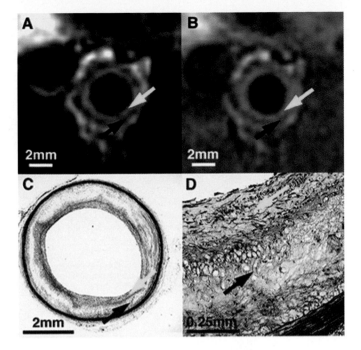

COLOR FIGURE 7.8 Differentiation of lipidic area (black arrow) from fibrotic area (yellow arrow) of abdominal aortic lesions with *in vivo* T2W image (A) and PDW (B) images. The greater contrast between fibrotic and lipidic components of the atherosclerotic plaque with T2W imaging is evident. C is a corresponding histopathological section stained with a combined Masson's elastin stain. D is a magnification of C showing lipid-laden foam cells and the fibrotic cap. (From Helft, G. et al., *J Am Coll Cardiol*, 37, 1149, 2001. With permission.)

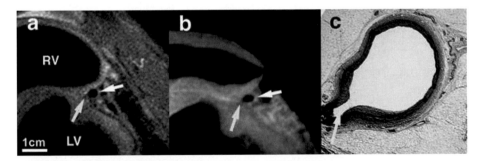

COLOR FIGURE 7.12 MRI of a noninjured coronary arterial segment (LAD). Images a and b are PDW fat-suppressed images from the same position as evidenced by the appearance of the left ventricular contours and the origin of the first septal perforator artery (yellow arrow). The thin vessel wall of the noninjured LAD (white arrow) is readily discerned from the surrounding epicardial fat. The comparable appearances of the two images demonstrate the ability of motion suppression: the *in vivo* image (a) has the same appearance as the *ex vivo* image (b). The corresponding histopathology section (c) confirms the thinness of the vessel wall. The presence of the first septal perforator from the histopathology section aids co-registration with the MR images. (From Worthley, S.G. et al., *Circulation*, 101, 2956, 2000. With permission.)

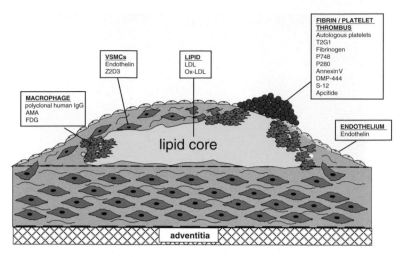

COLOR FIGURE 8.3 Ruptured atherosclerotic plaque with surface thrombus formation. The text boxes represent substrates labelled with radiotracer molecules related to their targets within the plaque. Further explanation is provided in text. AMA = aminomalonic acid. FDG = fluorodeoxyglucose. LDL = low-density lipoprotein. Ox-LDL = oxidized low-density lipoprotein.

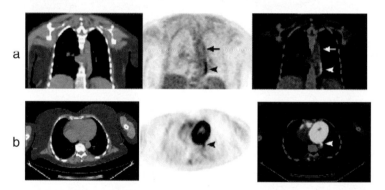

COLOR FIGURE 8.4 (a) Coronal CT (left), PET (middle), and fused PET/CT (right) images. FDG uptake is seen in the middle and lower descending aorta (arrow and arrowhead). (b) Transaxial CT (left), PET (middle), and fused PET/CT (right) images. [18F]FDG uptake is clearly demonstrated in the aortic wall (arrowhead). (Modified from Tatsumi M. et al., *Radiology*, 229, 831, 2003. With permission.)

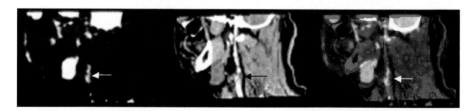

COLOR FIGURE 8.5 Sagittal images of carotid artery in patient with transient ischemic attack showing FDG accumulation (white arrow) on the [18F]FDG-PET image (left panel), carotid artery stenosis (black arrow) on the CT angiogram (middle panel), and co-localization of [18F]FDG uptake and carotid artery stenosis (white arrow) on the fused image (right panel)

produce tremendous benefits in reducing coronary risk.[41] In addition, several pharmacotherapeutic approaches have been established with the ultimate goal of reducing cardiovascular morbidity and mortality. Among them, statins have clearly demonstrated clinical benefit, in part through plaque stabilization.[42–45] In addition to their hypolipidemic effect, it has long been postulated that statins reduce the lipid contents of lesions, thus decreasing their vulnerability.[2,46] Statins may also work by reducing plaque inflammation and matrix metalloproteinase activity, thereby decreasing the risk of plaque rupture and reducing plaque thrombogenicity.[47]

7.4.1 EX VIVO MRI PLAQUE STUDIES

Early work on applying MR techniques to characterizing plaque focused on lipid assessment with nuclear MR spectroscopy and chemical shift imaging.[48–50] These techniques suffer from poor signal-to-noise (SNR) ratio because the concentration of lipid present in the plaque is very low in comparison with water. Therefore, it has been difficult to extend these methods to *in vivo* settings. Current studies have focused on MRIs of water protons and are more applicable to clinical settings.[9,51]

7.4.2 MR MULTICONTRAST PLAQUE IMAGING

After an *ex vivo* study, Herfkens et al. performed the first *in vivo* patient imaging study of aortic atherosclerosis.[52,53] Only anatomic or morphological features such as wall thickening and luminal narrowing were assessed. Improvements in MR techniques (faster imaging and detection coils) conducive to high resolution and contrast imaging permitted studies of the different plaque components using multicontrast MR generated by T1, T2, and PDW imaging.[8,9] Atherosclerotic plaque characterization by MR is based on the signal intensities and morphological appearance of the plaque on T1W, PDW, and T2W images as previously validated (Figure 7.7).[9,51]

The plaque fibrous tissues consisting mainly of extracellular matrix elaborated by smooth muscle cells are associated with a short T1. The origin of the T1 shortening (increased signal intensity on T1W images) is specific to protein–water interactions.[54] The plaque lipids consist primarily of unesterified cholesterol and cholesteryl esters and are associated with a short T2.[10]

The short T2 (decreased signal intensity of T2W images) of the lipid components is in part due to the micellar structures of lipoproteins, their denaturation by oxidation, or the exchange between cholesteryl esters and water molecules (both from fatty chains and from the cholesterol ring), with a further interchange between free and bound water.[10]

Perivascular fat, mainly composed of triglycerides, appears different from atherosclerotic plaque lipids on MRI.[55] The plaque-calcified regions consist primarily of calcium hydroxylapatite and are associated with low signal intensities on MRI because of their low proton density and diffusion-mediated susceptibility effects.[56] The MR appearance and evolution of thrombi or hemorrhages have been investigated in the central nervous system,[57] pelvis,[58] and aorta.[59] These studies showed that the different MR signal intensities of hemorrhages depend on the structure of hemoglobin and its oxidation state.[57]

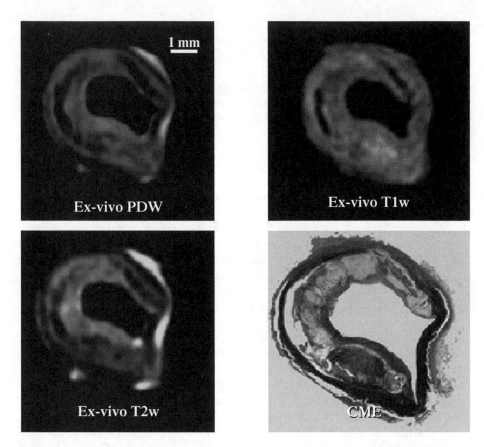

FIGURE 7.7 Series of three different MR imaging sequences of the same abdominal aortic section and the corresponding histopathology section, highlighting the various signal intensities for each atherosclerotic plaque component with the different MR imaging sequences. (Modified from Worthley, S.G. et al., *Atherosclerosis*, 150, 321, 2000. With permission.)

Additional studies in the context of arterial thrombus and atherosclerosis are necessary. *Ex vivo* studies in which atherosclerotic specimens were analyzed via MR and histopathological examination have been performed.[9,51] Cross-sections were matched between the multicontrast MR images and histopathology. The overall sensitivity and specificity for each component were very high. Calcifications, fibrous tissues, lipid cores, and thrombi were readily identified. Diffusion imaging that probes the motions of water molecules facilitated thrombus detection.[60]

7.4.3 *In Vivo* MRI Experimental Studies

MR has been used to study plaques in several animal models. Skinner et al. induced aortic plaques in rabbits through a combination of atherogenic diet and double-balloon denudation and found *in vivo* aortic plaque progression.[61] In a similar rabbit model, the ability of MRI to quantify lipid-rich and fibrous components of lesions and follow their progression or regression in response to dietary modification has

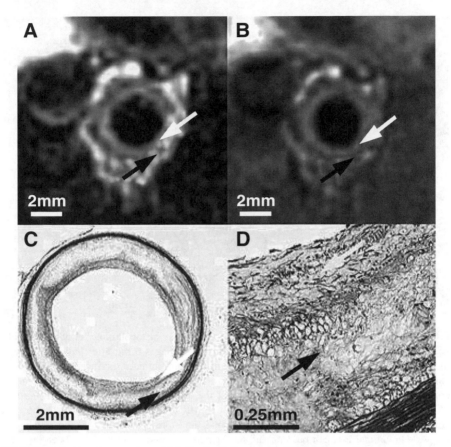

FIGURE 7.8 *(A color version of this figure follows page 112.)* Differentiation of lipidic area (dark arrow) from fibrotic area (white arrow) of abdominal aortic lesions with *in vivo* T2W image (A) and PDW (B) images. The greater contrast between fibrotic and lipidic components of the atherosclerotic plaque with T2W imaging is evident. C is a corresponding histopathological section stained with a combined Masson's elastin stain. D is a magnification of C showing lipid-laden foam cells and the fibrotic cap. (From Helft, G. et al., *J Am Coll Cardiol*, 37, 1149, 2001. With permission.)

been shown (Figure 7.8).[62,63] Fast-spin echo multicontrast sequences with in-plane resolution of 0.35 mm and slice thickness of 3 mm were obtained. Furthermore, aortic MR atherosclerotic imaging can be used as a tool for documentation of arterial remodeling in a rabbit model (Figure 7.0).[64]

Using conventional MR systems (i.e., 1.5 T), an in-plane spatial resolution 350 microns can be achieved with a high SNR and contrast-to-noise ratio for *in vivo* vessel wall imaging. To study smaller structures such as the abdominal aortas of mice (1 mm in luminal diameter), it is necessary to increase the SNR by using high magnetic field scanners equipped with small radiofrequency coils and strong magnetic field gradients. In transgenic apolipoprotein E knockout mice, MR microscopy (MRM) with a spatial resolution of 50 to 100 microns in-plane and a slice thickness of 500 microns, an excellent agreement between MRM and histological findings for

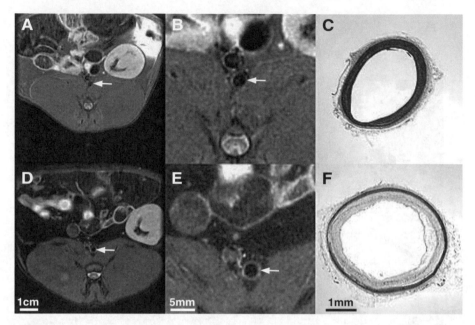

FIGURE 7.9 A through C: MR images and corresponding histopathology of atherosclerotic aortas at baseline (3 mo of age). D through F: aortic images 6 mo after balloon injury (9 mo of age). The aortic images, although from different animals sacrificed as part of the validation subgroup, were selected at approximately the same level in the abdomen for comparability as evidenced by the presence of the left kidney (right of image) at baseline (A) and 6 mo after balloon injury (D). Magnified MR images in A and D clearly show the very thin aortic wall at baseline (B, arrow) and the more thickened wall 6 mo later (E, arrow). No luminal loss can be seen and the increase in vessel wall area has been outward. Corresponding histopathology sections from A–B and D–E (C and F, respectively) confirm the MRI findings. The atherosclerotic burden is greater 6 mo after the balloon injury, but the lumen is preserved. Scale bars in D, E and F also apply to A, B, and C, respectively). (From Worthley, S.G. et al., *Circulation*, 101, 586, 2000. With permission.)

aortic plaque size, shape, and characteristics has been shown.[65] Therefore, high-resolution MRI and MRM may allow convenient and noninvasive quantitative assessment of serial changes in atherosclerosis in different animal models of disease progression and regression.

Another option is to utilize intravascular MR receive coils to enhance SNR and thus increase resolution.[7] To date, reports of atherosclerotic imaging with an intravascular MR coil have noted the requirement to use occlusive balloons to stabilize the coils[66,67] or they were performed postmortem.[68] However, one study reports the utility of a novel IV MR coil that affords a high SNR at the level of the artery wall without occluding the artery lumen in Watanabe heritable hyperlipidemic (WHHL) rabbits (Figure 7.10).[69] However, further work is needed to explore the utility of such coils for the purposes of atherosclerotic imaging in humans.

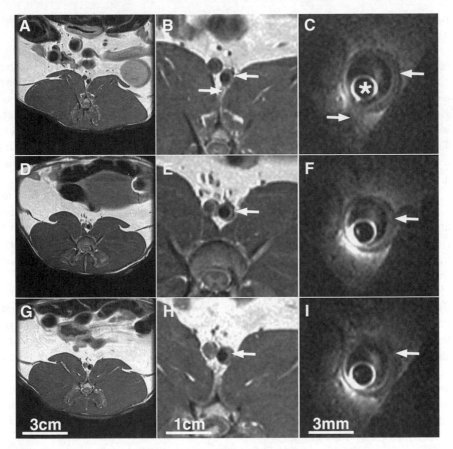

FIGURE 7.10 A, D, and G: Surface coil MR images (T2W) from three animals showing atherosclerotic aortae at the origins of their first spinal arteries. The images are magnified to better show the atherosclerotic aortae in the adjacent panels (B, E, and H). The corresponding IV MR coil images are adjacent to the magnified surface coil images, as confirmed by the origin of the first spinal artery (arrows, C, F, and I). Panel C shows the high signal ring structure within the artery lumen representing the IV MR coil (asterisk) and the minimal obstruction to the aortic lumen caused by the IV coil. Excellent flow suppression can be noted in all images by the homogeneous dark appearance of the lumen. Fat suppression has not been used; the periaortic fat appears bright. Eccentric atherosclerotic plaque can be appreciated on the external phased-array coil MR images (white arrows) in several aortic sites (B, E, and H). (From Worthley, S.G. et al., *Arterioscler Thromb Vasc Biol*, 23, 346, 2003. With permission.)

7.4.4 *IN VIVO* MRI STUDIES ON HUMAN CAROTID ARTERY PLAQUE

MRI has been used for the study of atherosclerotic plaque in human carotid,[11,12] aortic,[70] and peripheral arterial disease.[71] *In vivo* images of advanced lesions in carotid arteries were obtained from patients referred for endarterectomies. The superficial location and relative absence of motion of carotid arteries present less of a technical challenge for imaging than do the coronary arteries or aorta.

Some of the MR studies of carotid arterial plaques included imaging and characterization of normal and pathological arterial walls,[11] quantification of plaque size,[72] and detection of fibrous cap "integrity."[73] Typically the images are acquired with resolution of 0.4 to 0.5 mm using a carotid phased-array coil. Most of the *in vivo* MR plaque imaging and characterization involved a multicontrast approach with high resolution black blood spin echo- and fast spin echo-based MR sequences. The signal from the blood flow is rendered black by the use of preparatory pulses (e.g., radiofrequency spatial saturation or inversion recovery pulses) to better visualize the adjacent vessel wall.

Hatsukami et al. introduced the use of bright blood imaging (i.e., three-dimensional fast time-of-flight imaging) for the visualization of the fibrous cap thickness and morphological integrity.[73] This sequence provides enhancement of the signal from flowing blood and a mixture of T1 and proton density contrast weighting that highlights the fibrous cap. MR angiography (MRA) and high resolution black blood imaging of the vessel wall can be combined.

Comparison studies of MRA and contrast angiography have shown good sensitivity and specificity in the aorta and in the carotid, renal, and other peripheral vessels.[74] MRA demonstrates the severity of stenotic lesions and their spatial distribution, whereas the high resolution black blood wall characterization technique may show the compositions of the plaques and may facilitate risk stratification and selection of the treatment modality. Improvements in spatial resolution (250 microns) are now possible with the design of new phased-array coils tailored for carotid imaging[75] and new imaging sequences such as long echo train fast-spin echo imaging with "velocity-selective" flow suppression or double-inversion recovery preparatory pulses (black blood imaging).

7.4.5 *In Vivo* MRI Studies on Human Aortic Plaque

In vivo black blood MR atherosclerotic plaque characterization of the human aorta has been reported.[70,76] The principal challenges associated with MRI of the thoracic aorta are obtaining sufficient sensitivity for submillimeter imaging and exclusion of artifacts caused by respiratory motion and blood flow. Summers et al. used MRI to show that the wall thickness of the ascending aorta is increased in patients with homozygous familial hypercholesterolemia.[76] However, conventional T1W spin echo images were obtained and no plaque composition analysis was performed.

Fayad et al. assessed thoracic aorta plaque composition and size using T1W, T2W, and PDW images.[70] The acquired images had a resolution of 0.8×0.8 mm in plane with a slice thickness of 5 mm using a torso phased-array coil. Rapid high resolution imaging was performed with a fast spin echo sequence in conjunction with velocity-selective flow suppression preparatory pulses. Matched cross-sectional aortic imaging with MR and TEE showed a good correlation for plaque composition and mean maximum plaque thickness. A recent study using MR in asymptomatic subjects from the Framingham Heart Study demonstrated that aortic plaque burden (i.e., plaque volume:aortic volume) increased significantly with age and was higher

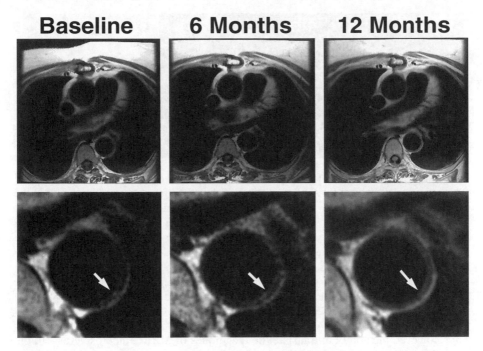

FIGURE 7.11 Serial T2-weighted images of the same patient. Note adequate matching of the images with a similar pattern of coronary vessels (top). In detail of the descending aorta (bottom), arrows indicate maximal atherosclerotic plaque size. Despite the subtle visual changes in atherosclerotic burden evident in these images, the reproducibility of this MRI technique allowed the detection of a significant reduction in atherosclerotic burden. (Modified from Corti R. et al., *Circulation*, 104, 249, 2001. With permission.)

in the abdominal aorta compared with the thoracic aorta.[77] Results ascertained that long-term measures of risk factors and Framingham Heart Study coronary risk score were strongly associated with asymptomatic aortic atherosclerosis as detected by MR.[77]

Using these techniques for aortic and carotid plaque imaging, Corti et al. showed that MRI could be used to monitor changes in atherosclerotic lesions at these sites in response to statin therapy, showing that much of the plaque regression was associated with a reduction in the outer vessel wall area, with minimal change in the lumen areas of the vessels (Figure 7.11).[39]

7.4.6 *IN VIVO* MRI STUDIES ON CORONARY ARTERY PLAQUE

As extensively reviewed earlier, the ability to accurately define the components of a complex coronary atherosclerotic lesion (fibrous cap, lipid core, calcium, hemorrhage) would potentially allow risk stratification of patients for future acute coronary syndromes. Given the excellent soft tissue contrast provided by MR imaging techniques, the ability of MR to differentiate these plaque components could potentially lead to the assessment of plaque vulnerability in the coronary artery system.

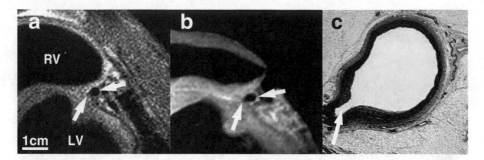

FIGURE 7.12 *(A color version of this figure follows page 112.)* MRI of a noninjured coronary arterial segment (LAD). Images a and b are PDW fat-suppressed images from the same position as evidenced by the appearance of the left ventricular contours and the origin of the first septal perforator artery (yellow arrow). The thin vessel wall of the noninjured LAD (white arrow) is readily discerned from the surrounding epicardial fat. The comparable appearances of the two images demonstrate the ability of motion suppression: the *in vivo* image (a) has the same appearance as the *ex vivo* image (b). The corresponding histopathology section (c) confirms the thinness of the vessel wall. The presence of the first septal perforator from the histopathology section aids co-registration with the MR images. (From Worthley, S.G. et al., *Circulation*, 101, 2956, 2000. With permission.)

However, the ability to translate the techniques of MRI of atherosclerosis in the aorta and carotid systems described above to coronary arteries *in vivo* has the same limitations that initially faced MR coronary angiography, namely, motion (cardiac and respiratory), small vessel size, and tortuosity of the vessels. In order to visualize the components of coronary atherosclerotic lesions, submillimeter resolution will be required. The first description of the feasibility of performing high resolution black blood atherosclerotic imaging *in vivo* was in a porcine model.[8] This study by Worthley et al. confirmed the ability of high resolution MRI with breath-holding techniques and cardiac gating to overcome motion artifacts (Figure 7.12)[78] and showed excellent agreement of MRI and histopathology of coronary artery lesions (Figure 7.13).[8]

These techniques have been translated to humans, using both the breath-hold sequences cited in the initial porcine experiments[35] and also using respiratory navigator techniques[79] described earlier (Figure 7.14). These techniques still lack the resolution to accurately quantify the various components of complex atherosclerotic lesions in the coronary arteries of patients. Thus, despite the incredible potential for MR characterization of coronary atherosclerotic lesions, its feasibility has yet to been shown. However, the future is very exciting with the advent of advances in MRI technology including coil design, high field imaging, and novel sequence development.

7.5 TARGETED MRI

Targeted MR contrast agents that characterize thrombus are under development. Fibrin can be identified by lipid-encapsulated perfluorocarbon paramagnetic nano-

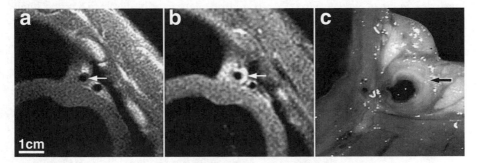

FIGURE 7.13 MRI and gross pathology of an injured LAD artery. The magnified images transverse to the LAD artery after balloon injury are taken without (a) and with (b) fat suppression. Suppression of the perivascular fat allows a clearer definition of the outer vessel wall. A good agreement between MR images and the corresponding gross pathological specimen (c) can be seen, as indicated by the eccentric coronary plaque that is mainly fibrocellular (white arrows in a and b; black arrow in c). (From Worthley, S.G. et al., *Circulation*, 101, 2956, 2000. With permission.)

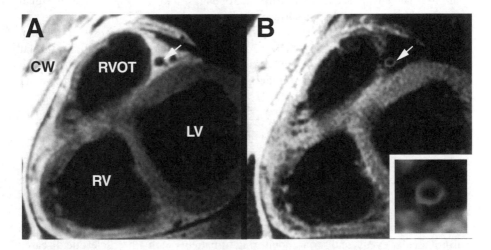

FIGURE 7.14 *In vivo* cross-sectional black blood MR images of lumen (A) and wall (B) of proximal LAD from normal subject (see arrow). Lumen image was obtained without fat saturation; wall image was obtained with fat saturation to better delineate coronary artery wall. Blood flow in coronary artery lumen was suppressed with velocity-selective inversion preparatory pulses. Images show normal circular lumen surrounded by uniform thin coronary wall. Average wall thickness of LAD measures 0.8 mm. B, Inset: magnified view of LAD. Some imaging parameters were TR = 2 R–R intervals, TE = 40 msec, 24 × 18-cm FOV, 3-mm slice thickness, 384 × 384 acquisition matrix, NSA 1, 32 echo train length, 125-kHz data sampling. LV = left ventricle. RV = right ventricle. RVOT = right ventricular outflow tract. CW = chest wall. (From Fayad, Z.A. et al., *Circulation*, 102, 506, 2000. With permission.)

particles *in vitro*[80] and *in vivo*.[81] Activated platelets may be targeted via the inter-action of an ultrasmall superparamagnetic iron oxide–arginine–glycine–aspartic acid (RGD) peptide construct with the IIb/III receptor.[82] Some preliminary work has also looked at the uptake of ultrasmall superparamagnetic nanoparticles of iron oxide (USPIOs) that have unique magnetic properties and appear to be taken up by fresh nonendothelialized thrombi.[83] However, thrombus imaging using USPIOs has some limitations including the lack of a shortening of T2* and an effect that was not present at all thrombus ages.[83] Thus, more work is required to determine whether this technique has merit for the purpose of thrombus imaging.

Another MRI contrast agent for detecting apoptotic cells based on the first C2 domain of the protein is synaptotagmin I.[84] This protein, like annexin V, binds to the phosphatidylserine that redistributes from the inner to the outer leaflet of the plasma membrane as an early event in the apoptotic program. The combination of MRI and a targeted contrast agent for apoptosis may prove useful in the understand-ing and detection of apoptosis in atherosclerosis.

MRI of the location and distribution of macrophages may be facilitated by the use of superparamagnetic nanoparticles of iron oxide (SPIOs) because these particles are avidly taken up by macrophages.[85] Injection of SPIOs into hyperlipidemic rabbits was associated with accumulation in macrophages, and the appearance of signal voids studded on the luminal surface of the aorta was noted when imaging was performed. In two studies performed on this model, the signal voids were present when imaging was performed 2 hr[86] or 5 days[87] after injection of the SPIOs. Similar appearances were observed in the aortas and intrapelvic arteries of humans who were given SPIO for oncological imaging.[88] This type of specific cellular targeting approach warrants further investigation.

7.6 CONCLUDING REMARKS

MRI is a powerful tool in the field of atherosclerosis and thrombosis research because it provides insights into crucial structural processes via a noninvasive and safe technology. However, the potential role that MRI may play in the clinical manage-ment of patients with or at risk of atherothrombotic events is yet to be determined and will require further study. However, the potential to predict risk for future cardiovascular events and serial monitoring of patients with atherosclerotic diseases using MRI appears great.

REFERENCES

1. Worthley SG, Helft G, Zaman AG, Fuster V, and Badimon JJ. Atherosclerosis and the vulnerable plaque — pathogenesis, part I. *Aust NZ J Med* 2000; 30: 600–607.
2. Fuster V and Badimon JJ. Regression or stabilization of atherosclerosis means regression or stabilization of what we don't see in the arteriogram. *Eur Heart J* 1995; 16 (Suppl.): E:6–E12.

3. Topol EJ and Nissen SE. Our preoccupation with coronary luminology: the dissociation between clinical and angiographic findings in ischemic heart disease. *Circulation* 1995; 92: 2333–2342.
4. Falk E, Shah PK, and Fuster V. Coronary plaque disruption. *Circulation* 1995; 92:
   657–671.
5. Fuster V, Fayad ZA, and Badimon JJ. Acute coronary syndromes: biology. *Lancet*
   1999; 353 (Suppl. 2): S115–119.
6. Celermajer DS. Noninvasive detection of atherosclerosis. *New Engl J Med* 1998;
   339: 2014–2015.
7. Worthley SG, Helft G, Zaman AG, Fuster V, and Badimon JJ. Atherosclerosis and
   the vulnerable plaque — imaging, part II. *Aust NZ J Med* 2000; 30: 704–710.
8. Worthley SG, Helft G, Fuster V, Fayad ZA, Rodriguez OJ, Zaman AG, Fallon JT,
   and Badimon JJ. Noninvasive *in vivo* magnetic resonance imaging of experimental
   coronary artery lesions in a porcine model. *Circulation* 2000; 101: 2956–2961.
9. Worthley SG, Helft G, Fuster V, Fayad ZA, Fallon JT, Osende JI, Roque M, Shinnar
   M, Zaman AG, Rodriguez OJ, Verhallen P, and Badimon JJ. High resolution *ex
   vivo* magnetic resonance imaging of *in situ* coronary and aortic atherosclerotic plaque
   in a porcine model. *Atherosclerosis* 2000; 150: 321–329.
10. Toussaint JF, Southern JF, Fuster V, and Kantor HL. T2-weighted contrast for NMR
    characterization of human atherosclerosis. *Arterioscler Thromb Vasc Biol* 1995; 15:
    1533–1542.
11. Toussaint JF, LaMuraglia GM, Southern JF, Fuster V, and Kantor HL. Magnetic
    resonance images lipid, fibrous, calcified, hemorrhagic, and thrombotic components
    of human atherosclerosis *in vivo*. *Circulation* 1996; 94: 932–938.
12. Yuan C, Mitsumori LM, Ferguson MS, Polissar NL, Echelard D, Ortiz G, Small
    R, Davies JW, Kerwin WS, and Hatsukami TS. *In vivo* accuracy of multispectral
    magnetic resonance imaging for identifying lipid-rich necrotic cores and intraplaque
    hemorrhage in advanced human carotid plaques. *Circulation* 2001; 104: 2051–2056.
13. Falk E. Plaque rupture with severe pre-existing stenosis precipitating coronary
    thrombosis: characteristics of coronary atherosclerotic plaques underlying fatal
    occlusive thrombi. *Br Heart J* 1983; 50: 127–134.
14. Richardson PD, Davies MJ, and Born GV. Influence of plaque configuration and
    stress distribution on fissuring of coronary atherosclerotic plaques. *Lance.* 1989; 2:
    941–944.
15. Davies MJ, Richardson PD, Woolf N, Katz DR, and Mann J. Risk of thrombosis
    in human atherosclerotic plaques: role of extracellular lipid, macrophage, and
    smooth muscle cell content. *Br Heart J* 1993; 69: 377–381.
16. Wagner WD, St. Clair RW, Clarkson TB, and Connor JR. A study of atherosclerosis
    regression in *Macaca mulatta*: III. Chemical changes in arteries from animals with
    atherosclerosis induced for 19 months and regressed for 48 months at plasma
    cholesterol concentrations of 300 or 200 mg/dl. *Am J Pathol* 1980; 100: 633–650.
17. Small DM. George Lyman Duff Memorial Lecture: progression and regression of
    atherosclerotic lesions: insights from lipid physical biochemistry. *Arteriosclerosis*
    1988; 8: 103–129.
18. Loree HM, Tobias BJ, Gibson LJ, Kamm RD, Small DM, and Lee RT. Mechanical
    properties of model atherosclerotic lesion lipid pools. *Arterioscler Thromb* 1994;
    14: 230–234.
19. Majno G and Joris I. Apoptosis, oncosis, and necrosis: an overview of cell death.
    Am J Pathol 1995; 146: 3–15.

20. Shah PK, Falk E, Badimon JJ, Fernandez-Ortiz A, Mailhac A, Villareal-Levy G, Fallon JT, Regnstrom J, and Fuster V. Human monocyte-derived macrophages induce collagen breakdown in fibrous caps of atherosclerotic plaques: potential role of matrix-degrading metalloproteinases and implications for plaque rupture. *Circulation* 1995; 92: 1565–1569.
21. Brown DL, Hibbs MS, Kearney M, Loushin C, and Isner JM. Identification of 92-kD gelatinase in human coronary atherosclerotic lesions: association of active enzyme synthesis with unstable angina. *Circulation* 1995; 91: 2125–2131.
22. Malik N, Greenfield BW, Wahl AF, and Kiener PA. Activation of human monocytes through CD40 induces matrix metalloproteinases. *J Immunol* 1996; 156: 3952–3960.
23. Bailes DR, Gilderdale DJ, Bydder GM, Collins AG, and Firmin DN. Respiratory ordered phase encoding (ROPE): a method for reducing respiratory motion artefacts in MR imaging. *J Comput Assist Tomogr* 1985; 9: 835–838.
24. Lanzer P, Botvinick EH, Schiller NB, Crooks LE, Arakawa M, Kaufman L, Davis PL, Herfkens R, Lipton MJ, and Higgins CB. Cardiac imaging using gated magnetic resonance. *Radiology* 1984; 150: 121–127.
25. Simonetti OP, Finn JP, White RD, Laub G, and Henry DA. "Black blood" T2-weighted inversion-recovery MR imaging of the heart. *Radiology* 1996; 199: 49–57.
26. Le Roux P, Gilles RJ, McKinnon GC, and Carlier PG. Optimized outer volume suppression for single-shot fast spin-echo cardiac imaging. *J Magn Reson Imaging* 1998; 8: 1022–1032.
27. Chien D, Atkinson DJ, and Edelman RR. Strategies to improve contrast in turbo FLASH imaging: reordered phase encoding and k-space segmentation. *J Magn Reson Imaging* 1991; 1: 63–70.
28. Foo TK, Bernstein MA, Aisen AM, Hernandez RJ, Collick BD, and Bernstein T. Improved ejection fraction and flow velocity estimates with use of view sharing and uniform repetition time excitation with fast cardiac techniques. *Radiology* 1995; 195: 471–478.
29. Shellock FG and Kanal E. Aneurysm clips: evaluation of MR imaging artifacts at 1.5 T. *Radiology* 1998; 209: 563–566.
30. Nissen SE and Yock P. Intravascular ultrasound: novel pathophysiological insights and current clinical applications. *Circulation* 2001; 103: 604–616.
31. Thieme T, Wernecke KD, Meyer R, Brandenstein E, Habedank D, Hinz A, Felix SB, Baumann G, and Kleber FX. Angioscopic evaluation of atherosclerotic plaques: validation by histomorphologic analysis and association with stable and unstable coronary syndromes. *J Am Coll Cardiol* 1996; 28: 1–6.
32. Patwari P, Weissman NJ, Boppart SA, Jesser C, Stamper D, Fujimoto JG, and Brezinski ME. Assessment of coronary plaque with optical coherence tomography and high-frequency ultrasound. *Am J Cardiol* 2000; 85: 641–644.
33. Weinberger J, Azhar S, Danisi F, Hayes R, and Goldman M. A new noninvasive technique for imaging atherosclerotic plaque in the aortic arch of stroke patients by transcutaneous real-time B-mode ultrasonography: an initial report. *Stroke* 1998; 29: 673–676.
34. Becker CR, Knez A, Ohnesorge B, Schoepf UJ, and Reiser MF. Imaging of noncalcified coronary plaques using helical CT with retrospective ECG gating. *Am J Roentgenol* 2000; 175: 423–424.
35. Fayad ZA, Fuster V, Fallon JT, Jayasundera T, Worthley SG, Helft G, Aguinaldo JG, Badimon JJ, and Sharma SK. Noninvasive *in vivo* human coronary artery lumen and wall imaging using black-blood magnetic resonance imaging. *Circulation* 2000; 102: 506–510.

36. Vallabhajosula S and Goldsmith SJ. 99 mTc-low density lipoprotein: intracellularly trapped radiotracer for noninvasive imaging of low density lipoprotein metabolism *in vivo. Semin Nucl Med* 1990; 20: 68–79.

37. Rudd JH, Warburton EA, Fryer TD, Jones HA, Clark JC, Antoun N, Johnstrom P, Davenport AP, Kirkpatrick PJ, Arch BN, Pickard JD, and Weissberg PL. Imaging atherosclerotic plaque inflammation with [18F]-fluorodeoxyglucose positron emission tomography. *Circulation* 2002; 105: 2708–2711.

38. Pasterkamp G, Falk E, Woutman H, and Borst C. Techniques characterizing the coronary atherosclerotic plaque: influence on clinical decision making? *J Am Coll Cardiol* 2000; 36: 13–21.

39. Corti R, Fuster V, Fayad ZA, Worthley SG, Helft G, Smith D, Weinberger J, Wentzel J, Mizsei G, Mercuri M, and Badimon JJ. Lipid lowering by simvastatin induces regression of human atherosclerotic lesions: two years' follow-up by high-resolution noninvasive magnetic resonance imaging. *Circulation* 2002; 106: 2884–2887.

40. Libby P and Aikawa M. New insights into plaque stabilisation by lipid lowering. *Drugs* 1998; 56: 9–13.

41. Jousilahti P, Vartiainen E, Pekkanen J, Tuomilehto J, Sundvall J, and Puska P. Serum cholesterol distribution and coronary heart disease risk: observations and predictions among middle-aged population in eastern Finland. *Circulation* 1998; 97: 1087–1094.

42. Long-term effectiveness and safety of pravastatin in 9014 patients with coronary heart disease and average cholesterol concentrations: the LIPID trial follow-up. *Lancet* 2002; 359: 1379–1387.

43. West of Scotland Coronary Prevention Study: identification of high-risk groups and comparison with other cardiovascular intervention trials. *Lancet* 1996; 348: 1339–1342.

44. Randomised trial of cholesterol lowering in 4444 patients with coronary heart disease: the Scandinavian Simvastatin Survival Study (4S). *Lancet* 1994; 344: 1383–1389.

45. Blankenhorn DH, Azen SP, Kramsch DM, Mack WJ, Cashin-Hemphill L, Hodis HN, DeBoer LW, Mahrer PR, Masteller MJ, Vailas LI, et al. Coronary angiographic changes with lovastatin therapy: Monitored Atherosclerosis Regression Study (MARS), MARS Research Group. *Ann Intern Med* 1993; 119: 969–976.

46. Ambrose JA and Martinez EE. A new paradigm for plaque stabilization. *Circulation* 2002; 105: 2000–2004.

47. Libby P. Current concepts of the pathogenesis of the acute coronary syndromes. *Circulation* 2001; 104: 365–372.

48. Toussaint JF, Southern JF, Fuster V, and Kantor HL. ^{13}C-NMR spectroscopy of human atherosclerotic lesions: relation between fatty acid saturation, cholesteryl ester content, and luminal obstruction. *Arterioscler Thromb* 1994; 14: 1951–1957.

49. Mohiaddin RH, Firmin DN, Underwood SR, Abdulla AK, Klipstein RH, Rees RS, and Longmore DB. Chemical shift magnetic resonance imaging of human atheroma. *Br Heart J* 1989; 62: 81–89.

50. Pearlman JD, Zajicek J, Merickel MB, Carman CS, Ayers CR, Brookeman JR, and Brown MF. High-resolution ^{1}H NMR spectral signature from human atheroma. *Magn Reson Med* 1988; 7: 262–279.

51. Shinnar M, Fallon JT, Wehrli S, Levin M, Dalmacy D, Fayad ZA, Badimon JJ, Harrington M, Harrington E, and Fuster V. The diagnostic accuracy of *ex vivo* MRI for human atherosclerotic plaque characterization. *Arterioscler Thromb Vasc Biol* 1999; 19: 2756–2761.

52. Kaufman L, Crooks LE, Sheldon PE, Rowan W, and Miller T. Evaluation of NMR imaging for detection and quantification of obstructions in vessels. *Invest Radiol* 1982; 17: 554–560.
53. Herfkens RJ, Higgins CB, Hricak H, Lipton MJ, Crooks LE, Sheldon PE, and Kaufman L. Nuclear magnetic resonance imaging of atherosclerotic disease. *Radiology* 1983; 148: 161–166.
54. Edzes HT and Samulski ET. Cross relaxation and spin diffusion in the proton NMR or hydrated collagen. *Nature* 1977; 265: 521–523.
55. Rapp JH, Connor WE, Lin DS, Inahara T, and Porter JM. Lipids of human atherosclerotic plaques and xanthomas: clues to the mechanism of plaque progression. *J Lipid Res* 1983; 24: 1329–1335.
56. Kucharczyk W and Henkelman RM. Visibility of calcium on MR and CT: can MR show calcium that CT cannot? *Am J Neuroradiol* 1994; 15: 1145–1148.
57. Bradley WG, Jr. MR appearance of hemorrhage in the brain. *Radiology* 1993; 189: 15–26.
58. Yamashita Y, Hatanaka Y, Torashima M, and Takahashi M. Magnetic resonance characteristics of intrapelvic haematomas. *Br J Radiol* 1995; 68: 979–985.
59. Murray JG, Manisali M, Flamm SD, VanDyke CW, Lieber ML, Lytle BW, and White RD. Intramural hematoma of the thoracic aorta: MR image findings and their prognostic implications. *Radiology* 1997; 204: 349–355.
60. Toussaint JF, Southern JF, Fuster V, and Kantor HL. Water diffusion properties of human atherosclerosis and thrombosis measured by pulse field gradient nuclear magnetic resonance. *Arterioscler Thromb Vasc Biol* 1997; 17: 542–546.
61. Skinner MP, Yuan C, Mitsumori L, Hayes CE, Raines EW, Nelson JA, and Ross R. Serial magnetic resonance imaging of experimental atherosclerosis detects lesion fine structure, progression and complications *in vivo*. *Nat Med* 1995; 1: 69–73.
62. Helft G, Worthley SG, Fuster V, Fayad ZA, Zaman AG, Corti R, Fallon JT, and Badimon JJ. Progression and regression of atherosclerotic lesions: monitoring with serial noninvasive magnetic resonance imaging. *Circulation* 2002; 105: 993–998.
63. Helft G, Worthley SG, Fuster V, Zaman AG, Schechter C, Osende JI, Rodriguez OJ, Fayad ZA, Fallon JT, and Badimon JJ. Atherosclerotic aortic component quantification by noninvasive magnetic resonance imaging: an *in vivo* study in rabbits. *J Am Coll Cardiol* 2001; 37: 1149–1154.
64. Worthley SG, Helft G, Fuster V, Zaman AG, Fayad ZA, Fallon JT, and Badimon JJ. Serial *in vivo* MRI documents arterial remodeling in experimental atherosclerosis. *Circulation* 2000; 101: 586–589.
65. Fayad ZA, Fallon JT, Shinnar M, Wehrli S, Dansky HM, Poon M, Badimon JJ, Charlton SA, Fisher EA, Breslow JL, and Fuster V. Noninvasive *in vivo* high-resolution magnetic resonance imaging of atherosclerotic lesions in genetically engineered mice. *Circulation* 1998; 98: 1541–1547.
66. Matschl V, Heverhagen JT, Kalinowski M, Alfke H, Jaensch HJ, Wagner HJ, and Klose KJ. *In vivo* evaluation of an intravascular receiver coil for MRI at 1.0 Tesla. *Vasa* 2001; 30: 9–13.
67. Zimmermann-Paul GG, Quick HH, Vogt P, von Schulthess GK, Kling D, and Debatin JF. High-resolution intravascular magnetic resonance imaging: monitoring of plaque formation in heritable hyperlipidemic rabbits. *Circulation* 1999; 99: 1054–1061.

68. Rogers WJ, Prichard JW, Hu YL, Olson PR, Benckart DH, Kramer CM, Vido DA, and Reichek N. Characterization of signal properties in atherosclerotic plaque components by intravascular MRI. *Arterioscler Thromb Vasc Biol* 2000; 20: 1824–1830.

69. Worthley SG, Helft G, Fuster V, Fayad ZA, Shinnar M, Minkoff LA, Schechter C, Fallon JT, and Badimon JJ. A novel nonobstructive intravascular MRI coil: *in vivo* imaging of experimental atherosclerosis. *Arterioscler Thromb Vasc Biol* 2003; 23: 346–350.

70. Fayad ZA, Nahar T, Fallon JT, Goldman M, Aguinaldo JG, Badimon JJ, Shinnar M, Chesebro JH, and Fuster V. *In vivo* magnetic resonance evaluation of athero- sclerotic plaques in the human thoracic aorta: a comparison with transesophageal echocardiography. *Circulation* 2000; 101: 2503–2509.

71. Coulden RA, Moss H, Graves MJ, Lomas DJ, Appleton DS, and Weissberg PL. High resolution magnetic resonance imaging of atherosclerosis and the response to balloon angioplasty. *Heart* 2000; 83: 188–191.

72. Yuan C, Beach KW, Smith LH, Jr., and Hatsukami TS. Measurement of athero- sclerotic carotid plaque size *in vivo* using high resolution magnetic resonance imaging. *Circulation* 1998; 98: 2666–2671.

73. Hatsukami TS, Ross R, Polissar NL, and Yuan C. Visualization of fibrous cap thickness and rupture in human atherosclerotic carotid plaque *in vivo* with high- resolution magnetic resonance imaging. *Circulation* 2000; 102: 959–964.

74. Yucel EK, Anderson CM, Edelman RR, Grist TM, Baum RA, Manning WJ, Culebras A, and Pearce W. AHA scientific statement: magnetic resonance angio- graphy: update on applications for extracranial arteries. *Circulation* 1999; 100: 2284–2301.

75. Hayes CE, Mathis CM, and Yuan C. Surface coil phased arrays for high-resolution imaging of the carotid arteries. *J Magn Reson Imaging* 1996; 6: 109–112.

76. Summers RM, Andrasko-Bourgeois J, Feuerstein IM, Hill SC, Jones EC, Busse MK, Wise B, Bove KE, Rishforth BA, Tucker E, Spray TL, and Hoeg JM. Evaluation of the aortic root by MRI: insights from patients with homozygous familial hypercholesterolemia. *Circulation* 1998; 98: 509–518.

77. Jaffer FA, O'Donnell CJ, Larson MG, Chan SK, Kissinger KV, Kupka MJ, Salton C, Botnar RM, Levy D, and Manning WJ. Age and sex distribution of subclinical aortic atherosclerosis: a magnetic resonance imaging examination of the Framing- ham Heart Study. *Arterioscler Thromb Vasc Biol* 2002; 22: 849–854.

78. Worthley SG, Helft G, Fayad ZA, Fuster V, Rodriguez OJ, Zaman AG, and Badimon JJ. Cardiac gated breath-hold black blood MRI of the coronary artery wall: an *in vivo* and *ex vivo* comparison. *Int J Cardiovasc Imaging* 2001; 17: 195–201.

79. Botnar RM, Stuber M, Kissinger KV, Kim WY, Spuentrup E, and Manning WJ. Noninvasive coronary vessel wall and plaque imaging with magnetic resonance imaging. *Circulation* 2000; 102: 2582–2587.

80. Yu X, Song SK, Chen J, Scott MJ, Fuhrhop RJ, Hall CS, Gaffney PJ, Wickline SA, and Lanza GM. High-resolution MRI characterization of human thrombus using a novel fibrin-targeted paramagnetic nanoparticle contrast agent. *Magn Reson Med* 2000; 44: 867–872.

81. Flacke S, Fischer S, Scott MJ, Fuhrhop RJ, Allen JS, McLean M, Winter P, Sicard GA, Gaffney PJ, Wickline SA, and Lanza GM. Novel MRI contrast agent for molecular imaging of fibrin: implications for detecting vulnerable plaques. *Circu- lation* 2001; 104: 1280–1285.

82. Johansson LO, Bjornerud A, Ahlstrom HK, Ladd DL, and Fujii DK. A targeted contrast agent for magnetic resonance imaging of thrombus: implications of spatial resolution. *J Magn Reson Imaging* 2001;13: 615–618.

83. Schmitz SA, Winterhalter S, Schiffler S, Gust R, Wagner S, Kresse M, Coupland SE, Semmler W, and Wolf KJ. USPIO-enhanced direct MR imaging of thrombus: preclinical evaluation in rabbits. *Radiology* 2001; 221: 237–243.

84. Zhao M, Beauregard DA, Loizou L, Davletov B, and Brindle KM. Noninvasive detection of apoptosis using magnetic resonance imaging and a targeted contrast agent. *Nat Med* 2001; 7: 1241–1244.

85. Schmitz SA, Taupitz M, Wagner S, Coupland SE, Gust R, Nikolova A, and Wolf KJ. Iron-oxide-enhanced magnetic resonance imaging of atherosclerotic plaques: postmortem analysis of accuracy, inter-observer agreement, and pitfalls. *Invest Radiol* 2002; 37: 405–411.

86. Schmitz SA, Coupland SE, Gust R, Winterhalter S, Wagner S, Kresse M, Semmler W, and Wolf KJ. Superparamagnetic iron oxide-enhanced MRI of atherosclerotic plaques in Watanabe hereditable hyperlipidemic rabbits. *Invest Radiol* 2000; 35: 460–471.

87. Ruehm SG, Corot C, Vogt P, Kolb S, Debatin JF. Magnetic resonance imaging of atherosclerotic plaque with ultrasmall superparamagnetic particles of iron oxide in hyperlipidemic rabbits. *Circulation* 2001; 103: 415–422.

88. Schmitz SA, Taupitz M, Wagner S, Wolf KJ, Beyersdorff D, and Hamm B. Magnetic resonance imaging of atherosclerotic plaques using superparamagnetic iron oxide particles. *J Magn Reson Imaging* 2001; 14: 355–361.

89. Worthley SG, Osende JI, Helft G, Badimon JJ, and Fuster V. Coronary artery disease: pathogenesis and acute coronary syndromes. *Mt Sinai J Med* 2001; 68: 167–181.

90. Corti R, Fayad ZA, Fuster V, Worthley SG, Helft G, Chesebro J, Mercuri M, and Badimon JJ. Effects of lipid-lowering by simvastatin on human atherosclerotic lesions: a longitudinal study by high-resolution, noninvasive magnetic resonance imaging. *Circulation* 2001; 104: 249–252.

8 Nuclear Imaging of the Vulnerable Plaque: Single Photon Emission Computed Tomography (SPECT) and Positron Emission Tomography (PET)

*John Davies, James Rudd, Tim Fryer,
Jonathan Gillard, and Peter Weissberg*

CONTENTS

8.1 INTRODUCTION

Atherosclerosis is a ubiquitous disease in the Western World. After a long asymptomatic phase, it presents either by causing a chronic obstruction to blood flow leading to reversible tissue ischemia as in chronic stable angina or as an acute, often fatal, thrombotic event leading to tissue infarction as in myocardial infarction and stroke. Progression of the disease occurs partly as a result of gradual accumulation of lipid and partly through repeated subclinical episodes of plaque rupture and repair.[1] Thus, plaque rupture is responsible for the most severe manifestations of the disease and for its silent progression.

Research over the past two decades has identified many of the crucial cellular and molecular mechanisms responsible for plaque erosion, rupture, and subsequent thrombosis. It has become clear that plaque composition is a much more important determinant of plaque rupture than plaque size.[2] However, identifying patients at risk of rapid disease progression or plaque rupture events is currently problematic. Algorithms based on Framingham risk factors have considerable predictive value at a population level, but offer little predictive value for individuals, whereas currently used imaging techniques, in particular contrast angiography, provide little information on plaque composition. Furthermore, it is also now clear that atherosclerotic burden is not well reflected by images of vessel lumens.

This has stimulated interest in developing techniques that can identify vulnerable plaques, both to target interventional treatments such as angioplasty and to monitor the effects of systemic treatments aimed at plaque stabilization. Nuclear imaging provides one of the more accurate methods of identifying and quantifying cellular, molecular, and metabolic processes. Over the past two decades, a great deal of interest has focused on the ability of nuclear imaging, using various radiolabelled compounds to identify different characteristics of vulnerable atherosclerotic plaques.

This chapter will briefly outline the important aspects of plaque biology that directly relate to plaque instability and its subsequent detection by nuclear imaging. The basic principles of nuclear imaging will be reviewed followed by a more detailed look at the research and results achieved. A summary covering nuclear imaging and its current and future roles concludes the chapter.

8.2 CELLULAR AND MOLECULAR BIOLOGY OF THE VULNERABLE PLAQUE: IMPORTANT ASPECTS RELATED TO IMAGING

The morphological features of a vulnerable atherosclerotic plaque include a thin fibrous cap, high lipid content, and low fibrous cap thickness-to-lipid core thickness ratio.[2] The most important cellular features are high macrophage contents and low vascular smooth muscle cell (VSMC) numbers.

VSMCs, macrophages, and T lymphocytes comprise the majority of cells within a mature atherosclerotic plaque. VSMCs have important synthetic and healing roles through production of extracellular matrix components that provide the fibrous cap with tensile strength, thereby promoting plaque stability. Inflammatory cells, on the other hand, particularly macrophages, produce matrix degrading enzymes. They are both directly and indirectly cytotoxic to VSMCs and thereby promote plaque instability.[3]

Atherosclerosis is, therefore, a fine balance of inflammation leading to breakdown of plaque ultrastructure and synthesis of extracellular matrix promoting healing. If the balance tips in the direction of inflammation, a plaque is likely to become vulnerable and rupture. If it moves in the direction of synthesis of extracellular matrix, it stabilizes and thrombus formation and subsequent clinical events become much less likely.

8.3 BASIC PRINCIPLES OF NUCLEAR IMAGING

The four sequential components of nuclear imaging are synthesis of a compound labelled with a radioactive isotope (the tracer), injection and cellular uptake of the tracer, detection of the distribution of the tracer over time, and finally the conversion of the data into an image. Ideally, the tracer molecule should be taken up only by the tissue of interest and should be cleared rapidly from the blood pool in order to ensure a maximal target-to-background ratio to allow straightforward identification of the tissue of interest on the resulting image.

With regard to the vulnerable atherosclerotic plaque, it is also important that the chosen tracer is capable of measuring cellular and/or molecular pathways that are likely to yield information regarding the probability of plaque rupture and subsequent clinical events. The two main types of radioactive isotopes used in nuclear imaging are those that emit gamma rays and those that emit positrons.

8.3.1 GAMMA EMISSION NUCLEAR IMAGING

When gamma emitting tracers are injected, the gamma rays produced penetrate the tissues of the body with little if any attenuation. Once they leave the body, they are detected by scintillation crystals housed within a gamma camera which convert the energy into single photons that are subsequently multiplied up to magnify the signal. Computer technology then converts this data into an image that displays the distribution of the tracer compound at a given time postinjection. In order to localize individual decay events, the gamma camera is fitted with a collimator, a series of parallel septa used to selectively interfere with or block those gamma rays not travelling within the desired plane.

All gamma rays detected by the camera can be assumed to have originated along a single plane. The distance between the septa, the length of the septa, and the distance between the subject and camera determine the resolution and sensitivity of the system.

Depending on the detector hardware and computer interface, the resultant image can be either a planar image or a series of cross-sectional images; the latter is better known as single photon emission computerized tomography (SPECT). In order to produce tomographical images, the gamma rays emitted from the subject must be collected in multiple planes. This can be achieved either with a camera that can move through a 180-degree arc around the subject or by placing the subject within a 360-degree ring of detectors.

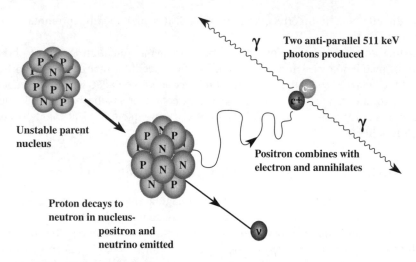

FIGURE 8.1 Positron emission resulting in an annihilation reaction with an electron and subsequent emission of coincidence photons 180 degrees to one another.

8.3.2 POSITRON EMISSION NUCLEAR IMAGING

Radionuclides such as fluorine 18 (^{18}F), decay by releasing positively charged electrons known as positrons. Emitted positrons only travel a very short distance within tissues before colliding with negatively charged electrons. A collision known as annihilation results in the release of energy in the form of a pair of photons emitted at almost 180 degrees to one another (Figure 8.1). Paired photons are subsequently detected almost simultaneously (or "in coincidence") by discrete bismuth germinate scintillation crystals housed within a 360-degree scanner that surrounds the patient.

The information gathered by the detectors can then be reconstructed by computer hardware and software to produce multiple cross-sectional images of the original radionuclide distribution. This technique is known as positron emission tomography (PET). Despite the short distance that the positron travels in tissue before annihilating with an electron, this distance is one of the factors that determine the maximum resolution of PET scanning. In addition, because the two photons are not emitted at exactly 180 degrees to each other, there is a theoretical limit on the spatial resolution of PET.

In practice, however, the finite detector size, scanner sensitivity, and the need to smooth the dataset to limit noise constrain resolution in most clinical settings. PET scans may be performed in two-dimensional (2-D) and three-dimensional (3-D) modes. In 2-D mode, annular rings made of lead or tungsten and known as septa separate the detector rings from each other. This means that photons originating outside the field of view and those that do not travel perpendicular to the axis of the scanner and are rejected, thus maintaining a favorable signal-to-noise ratio.

The sensitivity of the PET scanner can be increased by a factor of up to five times by operating in 3-D mode. In this mode, the septa are withdrawn, allowing the acquisition of decay events between detectors in different planes of the scanner. However, this is done at the expense of a large increase in the amount of scatter and

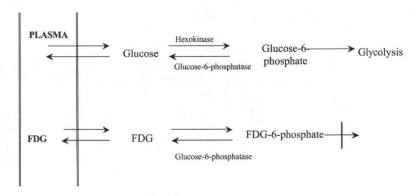

FIGURE 8.2 Metabolic pathway of glucose and ^{18}FDG. ^{18}FDG is taken up from plasma and metabolized via the same pathways as glucose. Once converted to [^{18}F]FDG-6-phosphate, it becomes trapped in the tissue compartment allowing for identification of tissue [^{18}F]FDG uptake by PET.

the detection of other background events, especially from activity outside the field of view. In addition, the computing power required to process data acquired in 3-D mode is much greater than that required for 2-D mode.

Because positron emitters do not exist in nature, they must be manufactured in a dedicated particle accelerator known as a cyclotron. Because of the short half lives of most positron emitters, a cyclotron facility must be near the PET scanner. The exception is ^{18}F which has a relatively long half life (109.8 min). The majority of radiotracers used in PET are based upon carbon, nitrogen, and oxygen atoms because they are biologically important elements and their radioactive versions can be used to study important biological processes *in vivo*. The fourth key positron emitting atom is fluorine-18. ^{18}F can be introduced into the glucose structure in the place of a hydroxyl moiety at the C-2 position in the carbon ring to produce fluorodeoxyglucose ([^{18}F]FDG), a glucose analogue used to image atherosclerosis. This will be discussed in more detail later in the chapter.

Figure 8.2 shows the fate of [^{18}F]FDG after injection into the body. Once inside the cell, both glucose and [^{18}F]FDG undergo the first step in the glycolytic pathway, phosphorylation by the hexokinase enzyme to glucose-6-phosphate and [^{18}F]FDG-6-phosphate, respectively. After this reaction, however, the two molecules have different fates. Glucose is further metabolized down the glycolytic pathway. However, for stoichiometric reasons, [^{18}F]FDG-6-phosphate is not metabolized further. It is a polar molecule and therefore cannot cross the cell membrane. [^{18}F]FDG-6-phosphate can be dephosphorylated by glucose-6-phosphatase, but this enzyme is found at low concentrations in most cells. [^{18}F]FDG thus becomes trapped in cells in quantities that reflect the glucose usage of the cells.[4]

One of the strengths of PET is its ability to perform quantitative studies. In its most basic form, relative quantification means that average values of tracer uptake can be compared in different areas of interest in the region under study. At the other end of the spectrum, absolute quantification allows the determination of physiological parameters (e.g., blood flow, oxygen extraction, glucose uptake, etc.) in absolute units for the tissue of interest

However, qualitative analysis remains the most common form of analysis in clinical PET studies. It involves simple visual inspection and interpretation of PET images without attempts to formulate numerical quantifications. It is widely used in oncological PET to diagnose metastatic disease.

Although PET can provide information regarding important physiological processes, the images often contain very little anatomical detail. Therefore, it can be difficult to relate areas of high tracer uptake to specific anatomical structures. This problem can be overcome by careful co-registration with another imaging modality such as CT or MR, a technique known as image fusion. Recently, dedicated machines with the capability to produce both CT and PET images have been designed to facilitate accurate image fusion.

For vascular imaging, the ideal technique would produce an image with high spatial and contrast resolution to enable tracer uptake by the atherosclerotic plaque to be distinguished from uptake of the blood pool and perivascular structures. However, with current technology, this can only be achieved by reducing detection sensitivity, which invariably leads to an underestimation of tracer uptake into the atherosclerotic plaque and failure to image clinically important lesions. SPECT and PET are widely accepted as the most appropriate nuclear imaging techniques for *in vivo* visualization and quantification of physiological, biochemical, and pharmacological pathways. Such functional imaging has the potential to provide much needed information about cellular and subcellular activities within atherosclerotic plaques.

8.4   IMAGING OF ATHEROTHROMBOSIS WITH GAMMA EMITTING ISOTOPES

Gamma and positron emitting tracers have both been used in attempts to image and quantify important metabolic processes within atherosclerotic plaques. To date, most research has concentrated on SPECT and gamma emitters largely because of the high cost and limited availability of PET.

8.4.1   IMAGING OF ATHEROSCLEROTIC PLAQUE WITH GAMMA EMITTING ISOTOPES

Several components of plaques provide potential targets for radiolabelled tracers. These include cellular components such as macrophages, VSMCs, and endothelial cells, as well as biochemical components such as lipids and molecules responsible for inflammatory cell recruitment. Figure 8.3 provides a summary of potential targets within the atherosclerotic plaque and corresponding radiolabelled ligands that have been developed for imaging, some of which are described in more detail below.

Low density lipoprotein (LDL) accumulates within atherosclerotic plaques where it plays a role in the formation, progression, and destabilization of lesions.[5] LDL has been labelled with various radioisotopes including iodine-123 (^{123}I), technetium-99m (^{99m}Tc), and Indium-111 (^{111}In).[6–11] In a heterogeneous group of asymptomatic and symptomatic patients with combinations of coronary, carotid, iliac, and

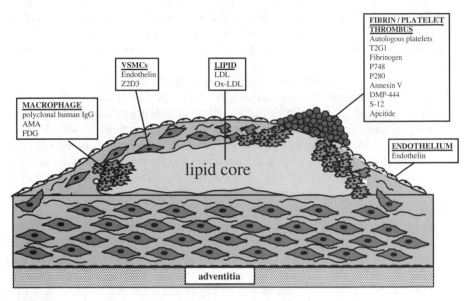

FIGURE 8.3 *(A color version of this figure follows page 112.)* Ruptured atherosclerotic plaque with surface thrombus formation. The text boxes represent substrates labelled with radiotracer molecules related to their targets within the plaque. Further explanation is provided in text. AMA = aminomalonic acid. FDG = fluorodeoxyglucose. LDL = low-density lipoprotein. Ox-LDL = oxidized low-density lipoprotein.

femoral atheroma, uptake of [99mTc] LDL was imaged in 7 of the 17 patients. In the subgroup of patients with carotid atheromas, analysis of endarterectomy specimens 1 day after imaging revealed two to four times greater uptake into lesions rich in macrophages when compared with those containing few macrophages. Histologically, imaged plaques contained abundant macrophages and foam cells whereas plaques providing no images were found to be predominantly fibrocalcific.[9,10] Thus [99mTc] LDL appears to be able selectively to image those plaques with high macrophage and foam cell numbers and therefore may be able to yield vital information regarding plaque vulnerability. Unfortunately, however, this approach is hampered by slow clearance of labelled LDL from the blood, significantly reducing its usefulness to image vulnerable lesions.

Because macrophages take up oxidized LDL much more readily than native LDL,[12–14] attempts have been made to image atherosclerosis using radiolabelled oxidized LDL. A small pilot study of seven patients with symptomatic carotid artery disease revealed uptake of [99mTc] oxidized LDL in 10 of 11 atheromatous lesions, with [99mTc] oxidized LDL target-to-background ratios approximately 1.5 times higher in diseased than in normal carotid arteries.[15] Unfortunately, no comparison was made of symptomatic and asymptomatic lesions and no carotid endarterectomy specimens were collected.

The above studies confirm the potential to image atherosclerotic plaques using radiolabelled lipoproteins. However, the sensitivity of [99mTc] LDL for the detection of atheromatous lesions appears to be low, whereas radiolabelled oxidized LDL has a more favorable pharmacokinetic profile and a higher sensitivity for the detection of plaque. However, no information indicates the ability of the technique to distinguish unstable from stable plaques and therefore its use as a diagnostic tool remains uncertain.

Macrophages within atherosclerotic plaques express cell surface Fc receptors. ^{111}In-labelled polyclonal human immunoglobulin G (IgG) contains an Fc subunit that binds to these macrophage receptors. [111]In polyclonal human IgG has been evaluated in patients with carotid atheromas and it was found to identify 86% of lesions detected by ultrasound.[16] Uptake of ^{111}In-IgG did not correlate with morphology suggestive of a large lipid core on ultrasound. However, ultrasound is not a well validated method of delineating plaque composition and the lack of correlation is as likely to represent the shortcomings of ultrasound as it is the failings of ^{111}In-IgG.

Imaging studies using ^{111}In-IgG on Watanabe heritable hyperlipidemic (WHHL) rabbits with aortic atherosclerosis were unsuccessful due to poor target-to-background ratios.[17] In addition, autoradiographical analysis revealed that uptake was not reduced in rabbits treated with lipid lowering therapy. Taken together, the results suggest that ^{111}In polyclonal IgG is not an appropriate tracer to identify unstable atherosclerotic lesions.

Radiolabels have been produced with the potential to provide indirect measures of macrophage content. One example is the radioiodinated monoclonal antibody against aminomalonic acid (AMA), a molecule vital to monocyte recruitment and foam cell production within atherosclerotic lesions.[18] ^{131}I-AMA was assessed in an experimental rabbit model of atherosclerosis. As with ^{111}In polyclonal human IgG, biodistribution studies revealed significantly increased uptake in diseased aortic tissue when compared with normal tissue, but the slow radiotracer clearance from the circulation meant that *in vivo* imaging of aortic plaque was unsuccessful. Consequently, human studies have not been attempted.

Antibodies directed against other cells and antigens present in atheromatous lesions have been studied. In preliminary experiments, Z2D3 F(ab´)₂ IgM, an antibody fragment that binds to antigen on the surfaces of proliferating VSMCs,[19] has been shown to localize in experimental lesions in rabbits. This paved the way for a small study of 11 patients due to undergo carotid endarterectomies.[20] Planar and SPECT images revealed focal uptake of the antibody in all patients within 4 hr of injection. The location of uptake corresponded with the anatomical location of the plaque as delineated by angiography. Uptake of the tracer was also seen in the contralateral carotid artery of approximately 50% of the patients. Subsequent immunohistochemical analysis of carotid endarterectomy specimens confirmed the uptake of Z2D3 into areas of the plaque rich in smooth muscle cells. The results of this study must be interpreted carefully and in conjunction with current theories regarding plaque instability and rupture. As stated previously, plaque rupture appears to correlate with lesions with thin fibrous caps containing many macrophages and relatively few VSMCs. Therefore, identification of proliferating VSMCs within an atheromatous plaque could indicate recent rupture followed by an adequate healing response. Thus, on the one hand, uptake of Z2D3 could suggest a lesion at high risk of future events given the recent instability of the plaque or it could indicate a lesion with low risk because of an aggressive healing response. Further studies are clearly needed to delineate the utility of this approach which may be better suited to studying vascular response to balloon injury, which is a primarily a smooth muscle proliferative response, than to studying primary atherosclerosis.

In an attempt to image and quantify endothelial dysfunction, a prerequisite for atheroma formation, radiolabelled endothelin peptides have been derived and investigated. Endothelin is produced by smooth muscle and endothelial cells and is upregulated in the presence of endothelial dysfunction. Both iodinated and ^{99m}Tc-labelled endothelin and its derivatives have been shown to accumulate in experimental rabbit atherosclerotic lesions.[21,22] As with Z2D3, uptake of radiolabelled endothelin correlated with the number of VSMCs in the intimal layers of the experimentally induced plaques. No correlation was found between macrophage number and endothelin uptake. To date, no human studies have been published. Since the above experiments involved experimental rabbit lesions produced by intimal balloon injury, human studies could produce different results. It is, therefore, too early to assess the clinical and research utility of this technique.

8.4.2 IMAGING OF THROMBI WITH GAMMA EMITTING ISOTOPES

A different approach to identifying vulnerable plaques is to image superimposed thrombi by targeting their subcomponents with radiolabelled compounds. Figure 8.3 summarizes the radioligands developed to image plaque-associated thrombi.

Imaging approaches have targeted three components of the hemostatic process: platelets, fibrinogen, and fibrinolytic molecules. Studies using radiolabelled autologous platelets in patients with carotid, femoral and aortic atherosclerosis have produced conflicting results.[23–25] However, the studies had important design differences that could explain the discrepancies in outcomes.

In a study of 60 patients, 38 of whom had cerebrovascular events referable to the carotid system, Moriwaki et al. found that ^{111}In-labelled platelet accumulation correlated with overall plaque burden and plaque ulceration as detected by careful B-mode ultrasound examination.[23] In contrast, Minar et al. in a similar study, found no correlation between radiotracer uptake and ultrasound parameters.[24] Perhaps importantly, in the first study, antiplatelet medications were stopped 3 wk prior to imaging which was carried out 48 hr after injection of the radiotracer. In the second study, antiplatelet medications were continued and images were taken 24 to 26 hr postinjection. Both studies used surface ultrasound to identify atherosclerotic lesions, but ultrasound is not a sensitive method of detecting plaque with associated thrombi. We know of no studies that have correlated radiolabelled platelet uptake with plaque histology.

Small pilot studies have been carried out to assess the utility of radiolabelled fibrinogen and fibrin degradation products. However, slow fibrinogen accumulation and low fibrin content in arterial thrombi compared with venous thrombi makes fibrinogen an unpromising candidate for useful clinical imaging of atheroma.[26]

Annexin V is a small protein that binds avidly to a phosphatidylserine moiety on the surfaces of activated platelets and apoptotic VSMCs in the fibrous cap. It has a rapid plasma clearance and, in a porcine model, ^{99m}Tc annexin V has been found to localize to thrombi generated in the left atrium, yielding high thrombus:blood ratios and therefore clear resolution.[27] It potentially could provide a useful noninvasive method of detecting atherosclerosis-associated thrombi, as well as apoptotic VSMCs in the fibrous caps of vulnerable plaques.

Research has identified several radiolabelled antibodies against platelets and fibrin that may have potential to image thrombi on atherosclerotic plaques. For example, monoclonal antibodies against the glycoprotein IIb/IIIa receptor and the membrane glycoprotein GMP-140 on activated platelets have been developed with the intention of imaging thrombi. S-12, an antibody against the GMP-140 glycoprotein, has been radiolabelled with technetium 99m and shown to localize to acute intra-arterial thrombi in animal models.[28] Again human studies are awaited.

Several synthetic peptides that bind to thrombi have been radiolabelled. Most of these target the GPIIb/IIIa receptor on activated platelets. Because of their small size they have the advantage of rapid clearance from the circulation. They are also less likely than immunoglobulin labels to stimulate immune responses.

Rapid uptake of ^{99m}Tc-P748, a synthetic peptide ligand to the GPIIb/IIIa receptor, by thrombi in the carotid arteries of dogs (induced by crush injury) has been demonstrated with very favorable thrombus:blood ratios.[29] ^{99m}Tc-P280 was the first GPIIb/IIIa-binding peptide to be studied in humans.[30] A pilot study of nine patients with carotid atherosclerosis showed uptake of ^{99m}Tc-P280 in 11 of 18 carotid arteries as detected by SPECT imaging. When compared with duplex ultrasound findings, the correlation between the two was modest but, as stated earlier, ultrasound has significant limitations in detecting plaque-associated thrombi.

More recently, Mitchel et al. tested the ability of DMP-444, a new glycoprotein IIb/IIIa platelet inhibitor labelled with ^{99m}Tc, to identify platelet-rich thrombi by nuclear imaging in the coronary arteries of a canine model.[31] They found that markedly positive nuclear images could be obtained and that postmortem studies confirmed the presence of radioactive platelet-rich thrombi. Dogs with very little DMP-444 uptake showed lower postmortem nuclear counts and thrombus weights, a result that reached statistical significance. No DMP-444 human studies have thus far been published.

Similar peptides have been developed and radiolabelled but few studies have been carried out to make them relevant to this review. However, a study investigating ^{99m}Tc-apcitide deserves a mention as it addresses the question of differentiating acute and chronic thrombi, albeit in venous thrombosis.[32] This issue is clearly important in terms of identifying arterial lesions responsible for recent symptoms. 99mTc-apcitide, like the other synthetic peptides mentioned above, binds to the glycoprotein IIb/IIIa receptors expressed on activated platelets. Bates et al. enrolled patients with newly diagnosed first deep vein thrombosis (DVT) and patients with previous DVT. With images interpreted in a blinded fashion, they found that the sensitivity and specificity of ^{99m}Tc-apcitide for differentiating acute and chronic thrombi were 92 and 86%, respectively. These results will hopefully lead to further studies on arterial thrombosis.

Thus, a number of approaches show potential for imaging plaque-associated thrombi. The potential advantage of identifying the presence of surface thrombi is that it might identify plaques that have recently undergone fibrous cap erosion or rupture. Recently ruptured or eroded plaques are at a very high risk of causing future vascular events and, therefore, a technique to identify them would be extremely useful. However, thrombus imaging is unlikely to identify inflamed plaques that have the potential to rupture. Therefore, thrombus imaging is likely to be most useful in identifying lesions responsible for recent vascular events and less likely to be of use in predicting adverse vascular events in patients with asymptomatic atheroma. Thrombus imaging is also unlikely to be able to distinguish thrombi on the surfaces of plaques and those due to hemorrhages from fragile vessels within the bodies of plaques. The distinction is important because the two different plaque events represent different pathological processes and do not necessarily lead to the same clinical outcome.

8.5 IMAGING OF ATHEROSCLEROTIC PLAQUES WITH POSITRON EMITTING ISOTOPES

Positron emission tomography (PET) has certain advantages over conventional gamma camera technology. PET can provide 4- to 5-mm resolution compared with 1- to 1.5-cm resolution for planar and SPECT imaging. This is extremely important for imaging small structures such as atherosclerotic plaques. However, the scanning technology and production of radiolabels is relatively expensive and, because of their short half lives, the isotopes must be synthesized near a scanner. Consequently, PET is not widely available.

8.5.1 Experimental Atherosclerosis

Following the discovery by Kubota et al.[32] that tumor macrophages take up significant amounts of [18F]FDG, interest in using [18F]FDG to image macrophages in atherosclerotic plaques has expanded. Preliminary studies using a rabbit model of atherosclerosis confirmed uptake of [18F]FDG in the regions of the aortic arches in atherosclerotic rabbits fed high cholesterol diets.[33] Normal rabbits did not show uptake above background levels.

Ex vivo analysis of the aortic arch confirmed [18F]FDG uptake in areas of atherosclerosis rich in macrophages. A further study by Lederman et al.[34] using a balloon injury model of atherosclerosis in New Zealand white rabbits confirmed a four-fold increase in [18F]FDG uptake by diseased segments of iliac artery when compared with normal segments. A positron-sensitive fiber optic probe placed in contact with the arterial intima was used to detect [18F]FDG uptake in *ex vivo* iliac artery specimens following injection of [18F]FDG 2 to 4 hr earlier. Subsequent histology confirmed that injured arteries had significantly higher macrophage and smooth muscle cell densities than uninjured arteries.

In recent studies in our laboratory, we found focal areas of [18F]FDG uptake into atherosclerotic lesions in rabbits maintained on high cholesterol diets, with markedly reduced [18F]FDG uptake in the same lesions following cholesterol withdrawal (Rudd et al., unpublished data). These studies taken together provide strong evidence that [18F]FDG-PET has the potential to monitor plaque inflammation *in vivo* and have paved the way for human studies.

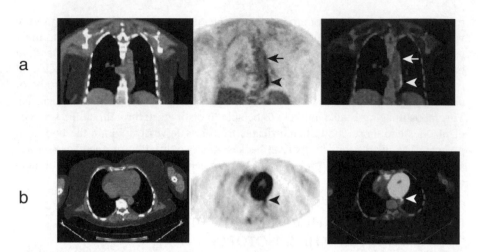

FIGURE 8.4 *(A color version of this figure follows page 112.)* (a) Coronal CT (left), PET (middle), and fused PET/CT (right) images. FDG uptake is seen in the middle and lower descending aorta (arrow and arrowhead). (b) Transaxial CT (left), PET (middle), and fused PET/CT (right) images. [^{18}F]FDG uptake is clearly demonstrated in the aortic wall (arrowhead). (Modified from Tatsumi M. et al., *Radiology*, 229, 831, 2003. With permission.)

8.5.2 HUMAN ATHEROSCLEROSIS

Few studies of [^{18}F]FDG uptake in humans have been reported. Yun et al.[35] reported the incidental observation of vascular [^{18}F]FDG uptake in patients undergoing PET investigation for cancer. Of 137 consecutive patients undergoing PET scanning, approximately 50% had vascular wall uptake of [^{18}F]FDG. Yun et al. made the presumption that the [^{18}F]FDG uptake seen on the scans was representative of atheroma.

Post hoc analysis reported a statistically significant difference in vascular wall [^{18}F]FDG uptake in patients with at least one of the traditional atherogenic risk factors when compared uptakes of patients with no risk factors.[36] Among all risk factors, age was found to be the most significant and consistent factor correlating with vascular [^{18}F]FDG uptake, but hypercholesterolemia also correlated consistently with vascular [^{18}F]FDG levels. More recently, Tatsumi et al. retrospectively evaluated aortic wall [^{18}F]FDG uptake in 85 consecutive oncology patients undergoing whole body scans using a combined PET/CT imaging device.[37] They found that 50 patients had at least one area of [^{18}F]FDG uptake in the thoracic aorta, 14 of whom showed focal [^{18}F]FDG uptake (Figure 8.4).

Patients with [^{18}F]FDG uptake were older, and there were positive correlations with female sex, hyperlipidemia, and documented cardiovascular disease. Interestingly no correlation was noted between aortic wall [^{18}F]FDG uptake and calcification — the latter is a common finding of aging and stable atherosclerosis.

Our group performed the only published human study to date in which the primary aim was to image atherosclerosis with PET. In preliminary studies on excised carotid plaques, we showed that deoxyglucose accumulates in macrophage-rich areas of plaques, suggesting that ^{4}[^{18}F]FDG accumulation rate could be used as a surrogate

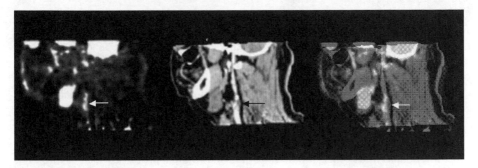

FIGURE 8.5 *(A color version of this figure follows page 112.)* Sagittal images of carotid artery in patient with transient ischemic attack showing FDG accumulation (white arrow) on the [18F]FDG-PET image (left panel), carotid artery stenosis (black arrow) on the CT angiogram (middle panel), and co-localization of [18F]FDG uptake and carotid artery stenosis (white arrow) on the fused image (right panel)

marker of macrophage number and activity. We then tested the ability of [18F]FDG-PET to image inflammation within carotid artery atherosclerotic plaques *in vivo.* Eight patients with symptomatic carotid atherosclerosis underwent [18F]FDG-PET scanning an average of 4 mo after experiencing transient ischemic attacks. Uptake of [18F]FDG was seen in all patients within 3 hr of injection.

Co-registration using CT angiography confirmed that the uptake was located in the regions of atherosclerotic plaques (Figure 8.5).[38] In addition, by drawing a region of interest around the area of stenosis on the CT angiogram and calculating the plaque-to-plasma [18F]FDG concentration on the co-registered PET image, we were able to quantify plaque inflammation. The [18F]FDG accumulation rate was significantly higher in symptomatic than in asymptomatic lesions. We noted no measurable [18F]FDG uptake into normal carotid arteries.

Because it is now widely accepted that plaque macrophage activity is a major determinant of plaque rupture, [18F]FDG-PET could provide a powerful tool for identifying and locating vulnerable plaques. It could also be used to measure the effects of lifestyle and pharmacological intervention on inflammation and macrophage activity within atherosclerotic lesions. [18F]FDG-PET has some limitations. The radiation dose used in the above study was relatively high. However, preliminary data using dynamic imaging with half the dose of the original study indicate that plaques can be imaged 2 hr postinjection (unpublished data).

The use of CT angiography to localize lesions and measure plaque volume is not ideal because it only allows visualization of the vessel lumen and plaque calcification with little detail concerning plaque constituents. It may not allow for the detection of lesions that do not encroach on vessel lumens. This problem is being overcome by co-registering PET with high resolution MRI of the neck.

Finally, because [18F]FDG is taken up by all metabolically active tissues including myocardium, it cannot be used to image coronary atheroma. This will require a more macrophage-specific ligand than [18F]FDG. Currently, the most promising macrophage ligand in clinical use is PK11195 which binds to peripheral benzodiazepine receptors in mitochondrial membranes, particularly in macrophages.[39]

Studies are currently under way to evaluate the potential of this ligand to image atherosclerosis using PET.

PET imaging of atherosclerosis is still very much in its infancy and further studies are needed to confirm the reproducibility of [^{18}F]FDG-PET. If the technique is highly reproducible, then longitudinal studies looking at changes in inflammation over time and after pharmacological interventions could be carried out both in humans and experimental models. Long-term outcome studies will be needed before [^{18}F]FDG-PET can be considered a clinical tool for predicting future risk. Further research should also concentrate on the development of other tracer compounds with the potential to label other important pathophysiological processes such as thrombus formation, intraplaque hemorrhage, lipid deposition, and matrix breakdown.

8.6 CONCLUDING REMARKS

Until recently, imaging technology for atherosclerosis has focused almost entirely on defining anatomical obstructions to flow. However, recent advances in understanding of the cell biology leading to atherosclerosis-related clinical events have highlighted a clear need for imaging techniques that can provide information on plaque composition. X-ray angiography, the current "gold standard" imaging tool in clinical practice, is unable to provide such information. This need is driving research into the development of more informative imaging techniques. Newer imaging modalities such as intravascular ultrasound and magnetic resonance imaging can provide information on plaque composition in some vascular beds, but are unlikely to be able to provide metabolic data on plaque inflammatory cell activity, the major determinant of plaque stability.

Nuclear imaging, in particular PET, has the potential to provide invaluable information on the cellular, metabolic, and molecular compositions of plaques. However, both scanning technology and radiolabelled tracer molecules must be improved in order to produce images of sufficient resolution and quality to allow detection and functional assessment of atherosclerotic lesions in medium to small sized arteries such as those found in the coronary circulation. Recent PET studies in animals and humans suggest that this should be achievable.

REFERENCES

1. Davies M.J., A macro and micro view of coronary vascular insult in ischemic heart disease, *Circulation*, 82, II38, 1990.
2. Davies M.J., Stability and instability: two faces of coronary atherosclerosis: the Paul Dudley White Lecture, 1995, *Circulation*, 94, 2013, 1996.
3. Weissberg P.L., Atherogenesis: current understanding of the causes of atheroma, *Heart*, 83, 247, 2000.
4. Gallagher B.M., Fowler J.S., Gutterson N.I. et al. Metabolic trapping as a principle of radiopharmaceutical design: some factors responsible for the biodistribution of [18F] 2-deoxy-2-fluoro-D-glucose, *J Nucl Med*, 19, 1154, 1978.
5. Ross R., Atherosclerosis — an inflammatory disease, *New Engl J Med*, 340, 115, 1999.

6. Rosen J.M., Butler S.P., Meinken G.E. et al. Indium-111-labeled LDL: a potential agent for imaging atherosclerotic disease and lipoprotein biodistribution, *J Nucl Med*, 31, 343, 1990.

7. Vallabhajosula S., Paidi M., Badimon J.J. et al. Radiotracers for low density lipoprotein biodistribution studies *in vivo*: technetium-99m low density lipoprotein versus radioiodinated low density lipoprotein preparations, *J Nucl Med*, 29, 1237, 1988.

8. Pirich C. and Sinzinger H., Evidence for lipid regression in humans *in vivo* performed by [123]iodine–low density lipoprotein scintiscanning, *Ann NY Acad Sci*, 748, 613, 1995.

9. Lees A.M., Lees R.S., Schoen F.J. et al. Imaging human atherosclerosis with ^{99m}Tc-labeled low density lipoproteins, *Arteriosclerosis*, 8, 461, 1988.

10. Virgolini I., Rauscha F., Lupattelli G. et al. Autologous low-density lipoprotein labelling allows characterization of human atherosclerotic lesions *in vivo* as to presence of foam cells and endothelial coverage, *Eur J Nucl Med*, 18, 948, 1991.

11. Chang M.Y., Lees A.M., and Lees R.S., Time course of ^{125}I-labeled LDL accumulation in the healing, balloon-deendothelialized rabbit aorta, *Arterioscler Thromb*, 12, 1088, 1992.

12. Steinberg D., Parthasarathy S., Carew T.E. et al. Beyond cholesterol: modifications of low density lipoprotein that increase its atherogenicity, *New Engl J Med*, 320, 915, 1989.

13. Steinbrecher U.P., Lougheed M., Kwan W.C. et al. Recognition of oxidized low density lipoprotein by the scavenger receptor of macrophages results from derivatization of apolipoprotein B by products of fatty acid peroxidation, *J Biol Chem*, 264, 15216, 1989.

14. Goldstein J.L., Ho Y.K., Basu S.K. et al. Binding site on macrophages that mediates uptake and degradation of acetylated low density lipoprotein, producing massive cholesterol deposition, *Proc Natl Acad Sci USA*, 76, 333, 1979.

15. Iuliano L., Signore A., Vallabajosula S. et al. Preparation and biodistribution of [99m]technetium labelled oxidized LDL in man, *Atherosclerosis*, 126, 131, 1996.

16. Sinzinger H., Rodriguez M., and Kritz H., Radioisotopic imaging of atheroma, in *Syndromes of Atherosclerosis: Correlations of Clinical Imaging and Pathology*, Fuster V., Ed., Futura Publishing, Armonk, NY, 1996, p. 369.

17. Demacker P.N., Dormans T.P., Koenders E.B. et al. Evaluation of indium-111–polyclonal immunoglobulin G to quantitate atherosclerosis in Watanabe heritable hyperlipidemic rabbits with scintigraphy: effect of age and treatment with antioxidants or ethinylestradiol, *J Nucl Med*, 34, 1316, 1993.

18. Chakrabarti M., Cheng K.T., Spicer K.M. et al. Biodistribution and radioimmunopharmacokinetics of ^{131}I-AMA monoclonal antibody in atherosclerotic rabbits, *Nucl Med Biol*, 22, 693, 1995.

19. Narula J., Petrov A., Bianchi C. et al. Noninvasive localization of experimental atherosclerotic lesions with mouse/human chimeric Z2D3 F(ab´)2 specific for the proliferating smooth muscle cells of human atheroma: imaging with conventional and negative charge-modified antibody fragments, *Circulation*, 92, 474, 1995.

20. Carrio I., Pieri P.L., Narula J. et al. Noninvasive localization of human atherosclerotic lesions with indium 111-labeled monoclonal Z2D3 antibody specific for proliferating smooth muscle cells, *J Nucl Cardiol*, 5, 551, 1998.

21. Dinkelborg L., Hingler C., and Semmier W., Endothelin derivatives for imaging atherosclerosis, *J Nucl Med*, 36, 102P, 1995.

22. Prat L., Torres G., Carrio I. et al. Polyclonal ^{111}In-IgG, ^{125}I-LDL and ^{125}I-endothelin-1 accumulation in experimental arterial wall injury, *Eur J Nucl Med*, 20, 1141, 1993.
23. Moriwaki H., Matsumoto M., Handa N. et al. Functional and anatomic evaluation of carotid atherothrombosis: a combined study of indium-111 platelet scintigraphy and B-mode ultrasonography, *Arterioscler Thromb Vasc Biol*, 15, 2234, 1995.
24. Minar E., Ehringer H., Dudczak R. et al. Indium-111-labeled platelet scintigraphy in carotid atherosclerosis, *Stroke*, 20, 27, 1989.
25. Smyth J.V., Dodd P.D., Walker M.G., Indium-111 platelet scintigraphy in vascular disease, *Br J Surg*, 82, 588, 1995.
26. Mettinger K.L., Larsson S., Ericson K. et al. Detection of atherosclerotic plaques in carotid arteries by the use of ^{123}I-fibrinogen, *Lancet*, 1, 242, 1978.
27. Stratton J.R., Dewhurst T.A., Kasina S. et al. Selective uptake of radiolabeled annexin V on acute porcine left atrial thrombi, *Circulation*, 92, 3113, 1995.
28. Miller D., Radionuclide labeled monoclonal antibody imaging of atherosclerosis and vascular injury, in *Syndromes of Atherosclerosis: Correlations of Clinical Imaging and Pathology*, Fuster V., Ed., Futura Publishing, Armonk, NY, 1996, p. 403.
29. Vallabhajosula S., Technetium-99m-P748 platelet-specific techtide for imaging arterial thrombus: preclinical studies in a canine model of intra-arterial thrombus, *J Nucl Med*, 152P, 1996.
30. Lister-James J., Knight L.C., Maurer A.H. et al. Thrombus imaging with a technetium-99m-labeled activated platelet receptor-binding peptide, *J Nucl Med*, 37, 775, 1996.
31. Mitchel J., Waters D., Lai T. et al. Identification of coronary thrombus with a IIb/IIIa platelet inhibitor radiopharmaceutical, technetium-99m DMP-444: a canine model, *Circulation*, 101, 1643, 2000.
32. Bates S.M., Lister-James J., Julian J.A. et al. Imaging characteristics of a novel technetium Tc 99m-labeled platelet glycoprotein IIb/IIIa receptor antagonist in patients with acute deep vein thrombosis or a history of deep vein thrombosis, *Arch Intern Med*, 163, 452, 2003.
33. Vallabhajosula S., Machac K., Knesaurek J., Imaging atherosclerotic macrophage density by positron emission tomography using F-18-fluorodeoxyglucose (FDG), *J Nucl Med*, 37, 38, 1996.
34. Lederman R.J., Raylman R.R., Fisher S.J. et al. Detection of atherosclerosis using a novel positron-sensitive probe and 18-fluorodeoxyglucose (FDG), *Nucl Med Commun*, 22, 747, 2001.
35. Yun M., Yeh D., Araujo L.I. et al. F-18 FDG uptake in the large arteries: a new observation, *Clin Nucl Med*, 26, 314, 2001.
36. Yun M., Jang S., Cucchiara A. et al. [18]F FDG uptake in the large arteries: a correlation study with the atherogenic risk factors, *Semin Nucl Med*, 32, 70, 2002.
37. Tatsumi M., Cohade C., Nakamoto Y. et al. Fluorodeoxyglucose uptake in the aortic wall at PET/CT: possible finding for active atherosclerosis, *Radiology*, 229, 831, 2003.
38. Rudd J.H., Warburton E.A., Fryer T.D. et al. Imaging atherosclerotic plaque inflammation with [18F]-fluorodeoxyglucose positron emission tomography, *Circulation*, 105, 2708, 2002.
39. Anholt R.R., Pedersen P.L., De Souza E.B. et al. The peripheral-type benzodiazepine receptor: localization to the mitochondrial outer membrane, *J Biol Chem*, 261, 576, 1986.

9 Identification of Vulnerable Plaques: The Role of Thermography

Konstantinos Toutouzas, Sophia Vaina, and Christodoulos Stefanadis

CONTENTS

9.1 INTRODUCTION

The pathophysiological pathways that lead to formation and progression of atherosclerosis are characterized by diversity and complexity. An increasing body of evidence indicates that inflammation plays a pivotal role in this multifactorial process, initiating from the earliest identifiable lesion (fatty streak)[1] to the advanced vulnerable plaque.[2]

Heat is one of the elements characterizing inflammation. Thus, it has been postulated that extensive inflammatory involvement within atherosclerotic plaques results in increased heat production. In the first *ex vivo* study, Casscells et al. demonstrated that heat is released from inflamed plaques by activated macrophages.[3] Samples of carotid artery were taken at endarterectomy from 48 patients and were probed with a thermistor. It was observed that 37% of plaques had substantially warmer regions. Temperature correlated positively with cell density and inversely with the distances of cell clusters from the luminal surfaces. Most cells were macrophages. Infrared thermographic images also revealed heterogeneity in temperature among the plaques.[3]

9.2 CATHETER-BASED DEVICES FOR CORONARY TEMPERATURE MEASUREMENTS

In vivo temperature measurement of the coronary atherosclerotic plaque has become feasible with the use of specially designed thermography catheters.[4–7] The first *in vivo* measurement of human atherosclerotic plaques was performed with a thermography catheter designed and developed in our institution and now manufactured (Medispes SW AG, Zug, Switzerland).[4,5] See Figure 9.1.

A thermistor probe (Microchip NTC, model 100K6MCD368, BetaTHERM), 0.457 mm in diameter, is attached to the distal end of a 138-cm long nonthrombogenic polyurethane shaft. The gold-plated lead wires of the thermistor pass through the main lumen of a catheter and end to a connector at the proximal part. At the distal 20 cm, the catheter has a second lumen for insertion of a guide wire (0.014 in.). The catheter is advanced to the target lesion by a monorail system (Rapid Exchange). Opposite the thermistor is a hydrofoil, specially designed to ensure contact of the thermistor with the vessel wall.

The technical characteristics of the polyamide thermistor include (1) temperature accuracy, 0.05°C; (2) time constant, 300 msec; and (3) spatial resolution, 0.5 mm. The signal from the thermistor catheter is processed to a computer. During temperature measurements, the values are displayed in real time on the screen of the computer (Figure 9.2). All data are stored in the computer for further analysis.

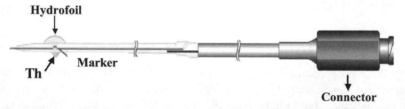

FIGURE 9.1 Coronary thermography catheter. A thermistor (Th) is positioned at the distal part. Opposite the thermistor is a hydrofoil that facilitates the contact of the thermistor with the vessel wall. At the proximal part, the connector for the thermistor lead wires is demonstrated.

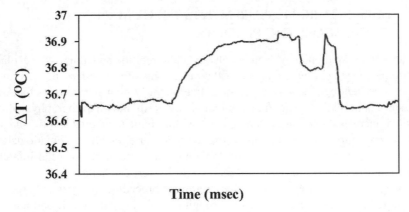

Time (msec)

FIGURE 9.2 Coronary temperature recording with the Epiphany thermography catheter. Temperature measurements at the proximal segment and at the lesion. The recording demonstrates a significant temperature difference between the proximal vessel wall and the lesion (Δ): 0.27°C.

Recently, two more thermography catheters have been introduced into clinical practice.[6] The thermography basket catheter consists of an expandable catheter made of a nitinol system loaded with small and flexible thermocouples (Volcano Therapeutics).[7-9] Another thermography catheter is an over-the-wire system consisting of a functional end that can be engaged by retracting a covering sheath. The distal part has four dedicated thermistors at the distal end and four flexible nitinol strips (each at 90 degrees) that, after engagement, with an expansion width of 9 mm, ensure endoluminal surface contact with the vessel wall. The thermistors are made of 5 k7 bare chips (5 kOhm resistance; curve 7 material), with gold metallization and 40-American wire gauge wires soldered onto the metal; they can perform up to 25 measurements per second and are delivered with a certified accuracy of 0.05°C (Thermocore Medical Systems NV).[6,10]

In addition, a guide wire-based system provides an alternative method with greater spatial resolution and ease of use. A thermocouple sensor (Imetrx Inc.) in the tip of a guide wire couples to a rotary pullback device that enables sampling of temperatures along arterial walls.[11] A pressure–temperature guide wire has been also used *in vivo* (Radi Medical Systems Inc., Sweden) for intracoronary temperature measurements in human atherosclerotic coronary plaques.[12]

An infrared thermography catheter has also been used. The prototype consists of a 4-Fr side viewing catheter capable of imaging temperature of the vessel wall with a 180-degree scope. It has 19 chalcogenide fibers and a wedge-shaped mirror assembly at its tip, which is transparent to infrared radiation and capable of receiving the heat reflected from the arterial wall. The fiber optic catheter is connected to a focal plane array-cooled infrared camera. This catheter is being tested in *ex vivo* settings. [13]

9.3 TEMPERATURE MEASUREMENTS OF HUMAN ATHEROSCLEROTIC PLAQUES

Vascular inflammation may lead to plaque vulnerability and thus induce plaque rupture. Because heat release is one of the main signs of inflammation, detection of temperature heterogeneity within plaques may identify high-risk plaques that demonstrate inflammation. The first clinical study with the thermography catheter revealed increased thermal heterogeneity within human atherosclerotic plaques, while temperature was constant in normal coronary arteries.[5] Symptomatic patients with suffering from stable angina, unstable angina, or acute myocardial infarction were included and sex- and age-matched controls were studied.

Briefly, steps of the coronary thermography procedure were as follows. The thermography catheter was advanced through the guiding catheter. Blood temperature was measured when the thermistor had just emerged from the tip of the guiding catheter so that it would not be in contact with the vessel wall. Temperature measurements were performed in the proximal segment in which intravascular ultrasound (IVUS) indicated no evidence of atherosclerosis. The most frequent temperature of these measurements was assigned as the background value and thereafter temperatures were recorded at the sites of the lesions.

In all patients, measurements were obtained approximately 5 min after contrast infusion. Most atherosclerotic plaques had higher temperatures compared with the proximal vessel wall. The difference between maximum plaque and background temperatures did not correlate with coronary artery stenoses. Greater values in the differences between maximum plaque and background temperatures were observed in patients with unstable angina and acute myocardium infarctions.

Differences between maximum culprit plaque temperature and background temperatures increased progressively from patients with stable angina to those with acute myocardial infarctions. Mean temperature differences between the target lesions and proximal vessel walls in each group were $0.010 \pm 0.020°C$ in normal subjects, $0.153 \pm 0.134°C$ in patients with stable angina, $0.787 \pm 0.360°C$ in patients with unstable angina, and $1.593 \pm 0.704°C$ in patients with acute myocardial infarctions.

Heterogeneity within the region of interest was shown in 20% of patients with stable angina, 40% in patients with unstable angina, and 67% of the patients with acute myocardial infarctions, respectively, whereas no heterogeneity was shown in the control subjects. Heterogeneity within plaques between patients with stable angina, unstable angina, and acute myocardial infarction was different ($p < 0.05$). Multiple regression analysis revealed that C-reactive protein was the only factor significantly associated with the differences between maximum temperature in the region of interest and background temperature ($r^2 = 0.55$; $p < 0.001$).[5]

In this first series of patients in the acute phase of unstable angina or myocardial infarction, increased thermal heterogeneity was noted within the culprit lesions. However, whether this increased temperature at the site of the lesion was prolonged after the acute phase is unknown. Therefore, we studied patients with previous myocardial infarctions and compared the temperature measurements at the culprit lesions with measurements obtained from patients with stable clinical syndromes.

We enrolled patients with previous myocardial infarctions (2 to 4 months) before the measurements and patients with chronic stable angina.

In both groups, the percentage of patients receiving statins was similar. The mean value of temperature difference between the culprit lesion and the proximal vessel wall was higher in patients with previous myocardial infarctions than in those with chronic stable angina (0.22 ± 0.24°C versus 0.12 ± 0.10°C; p <0.05). Thus, thermal heterogeneity is prolonged at least 4 mo after the acute phase and remains increased compared to patients with chronic stable angina.[14] The impact of a prolonged period of vulnerability assessed by coronary thermography, on clinical outcomes in this study group needs to be determined by a prospective study of a large number of patients.

9.3.1 THERMOGRAPHY AND INFLAMMATION

In order to investigate the role of inflammation in heat production, we measured culprit plaque temperature and acute phase reactants such as serum amyloid A and C-reactive protein in patients with coronary heart disease suffering from stable angina, unstable angina, or acute myocardial infarction and matched controls without coronary artery disease.[15]

A positive correlation was found between temperature differences and C-reactive protein (r = 0.796; p = 0.01) as well as temperature differences and serum amyloid A levels (r = 0.848; p = 0.01) in the whole study population. Furthermore, multiple regression analysis revealed that C-reactive protein (B = 12.794; p <0.01) and serum amyloid A were the only factors significantly associated with plaque temperature.[15]

Other markers of inflammation were also correlated with coronary plaque temperature. We studied 25 patients (12 had recent myocardial infarctions and 13 had unstable angina) and 10 sex- and age-matched controls without coronary artery disease. A good correlation was found between temperature difference of the culprit plaque and the proximal vessel wall and the concentration of vascular cell adhesion molecules (r = 0.53; p = 0.01). A correlation with soluble intercellular adhesion molecule-1 did not reach statistical significance.[16]

We also explored the role of inflammation in a study population that included 29 patients who had recent myocardial infarctions (2 to 4 mo before the measurements) and 26 patients with chronic stable angina. In the total study, the temperature difference between the culprit atherosclerotic plaque and the proximal vessel wall was positively correlated with C-reactive protein (R = 0.50; p <0.01), interleukin-6 (R = 0.58; p <0.01), and soluble intercellular adhesion molecule-1 (R = 0.40; p = 0.03) levels.[14]

Akasaka et al. investigated the relation of thermal heterogeneity recorded with the Radi wire and histological findings.[12] Intracoronary temperature and histology of specimens obtained by directional atherectomy were compared in 34 stenotic lesions of 32 patients with stable and unstable angina. Coronary plaque temperature was significantly higher in plaques with macrophage infiltration (0.37 ± 0.15 versus 0.11 ± 0.10°C; p <0.01). A cutoff value of 0.19°C was demonstrated to predict macrophage infiltration histologically with a sensitivity of 80% and a specificity of

96%.[12] Similar results were reported in a prospective study that correlated inflammatory markers measured from atherectomy specimens with coronary plaque temperature in patients undergoing directional coronary atherectomies.[17]

9.3.2 THERMOGRAPHY AND MORPHOLOGICAL CHARACTERISTICS

Preliminary studies have shown a correlation between morphological and functional characteristics of culprit atherosclerotic lesions, assessed by intravascular ultrasound and coronary thermography, respectively.[9,18] We studied 55 patients with coronary artery disease. All patients underwent intravascular ultrasound examination and coronary thermography. Twenty-nine patients had class IB and IIB unstable angina and 26 had chronic stable angina. Patients of both groups were similar in age, reference vessel size, and percent diameter stenosis. Positive remodeling was more common in the group with unstable syndrome compared to the stable angina group (58.6% versus 34.6%). Conversely, negative remodeling was more common in the stable angina group (65.4% versus 41.4%). Patients with unstable angina showed increased culprit plaque temperatures compared to patients with chronic stable angina ($0.30 \pm 0.25°C$ versus $0.12 \pm 0.09°C$; $p = 0.001$). Patients with positive remodeling showed increased plaque temperatures compared to those with negative remodeling ($0.33 \pm 0.26°C$ versus $0.11 \pm 0.07°C$; $p < 0.0001$). Additionally, we found a good correlation between temperature difference and remodeling index ($p = 0.001$; $R = 0.43$).

9.3.3 TEMPERATURE MEASUREMENTS AND BLOOD FLOW

In vivo coronary temperature measurements are influenced by several factors. A mismatch in results has been observed between *ex vivo* and *in vivo* studies. *Ex vivo* studies demonstrated higher temperature measurements compared to *in vivo* studies[3] and this discrepancy may be due to the effect of blood flow.

We recently showed that *in vivo* temperature measurements are influenced by coronary flow.[19,20] Eighteen patients with effort angina were studied. Temperature measurements were performed at the proximal vessel walls and at the lesions before, during, and after complete interruption of blood flow by inflation of a balloon. The temperature difference between the proximal vessel wall temperature and the maximal temperature during and after complete interruption of flow was $0.012 \pm 0.01°C$ and $-0.006 \pm -0.01°C$ ($p < 0.001$), respectively. Temperature difference between the atherosclerotic plaque and the proximal vessel wall increased by $60.5 \pm 14.1\%$ during blood flow interruption. Most importantly, the increase was more substantial in patients who demonstrated no thermal heterogeneity at baseline under flow. This subgroup shows a $76.0 \pm 8.4\%$ increase. These results indicated that coronary flow exerts a cooling effect on thermal heterogeneity that may lead to underestimation of heat production locally.[19]

This observation may explain the discrepancy between the *in vivo* and *ex vivo* temperature measurements. The impact of blood flow on temperature measurements should be considered, especially in lesions producing moderate stenoses because blood flow is reduced or even completely interrupted in significant occlusive lesions

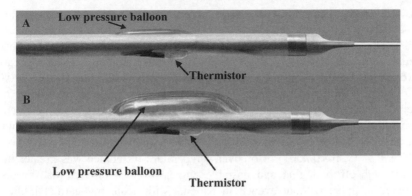

FIGURE 9.3 A: Balloon thermography catheter. The thermistor is opposite the deflated balloon. B: The balloon is inflated for the interruption of the flow while the thermistor is opposed to the vessel wall. (From Stefanadis, C. et al., *Catheter Cardiovasc. Interv.*, 58, 344, 2003. With permission.)

and, therefore, the recorded temperature is more accurate. The cooling effect must be eliminated from current technology unless only severe lesions are studied. The catheter-based thermistor delivery system is, therefore, valuable in examining significant lesions, but it seems to underestimate the temperature differences of small to moderate lesions. New catheters by which temperature is recorded without the need of contact of the sensor with the arterial wall may resolve this limitation of current technology.

In an effort to eliminate the effect of blood flow on *in vivo* plaque temperature measurements, we designed a new balloon thermography catheter (Figure 9.3).[20] The technical characteristics of the thermistor are identical to those of the coronary thermography catheter. Opposite the thermistor is a noncompliant semiballoon. Progressive inflation of the balloon in low atmospheres interrupts blood flow without dilatation of arterial walls. In a preliminary study in 10 patients with effort angina, temperature was recorded at the proximal vessel walls and at the lesions before, during, and after complete interruption of blood flow. It was observed, that plaque temperature was increased by almost 60% during balloon inflation.[20]

9.3.4 TEMPERATURE OF CULPRIT ATHEROMATOUS PLAQUE AS A PROGNOSTIC MARKER

Several experimental and clinical studies revealed that percutaneous coronary intervention in inflamed plaques is associated with unfavorable clinical and angiographic outcomes.[21–26] In clinical settings, inflammatory involvement has been assessed by indexes measured in the peripheral blood and also by atherectomy specimens.

We recorded temperatures of culprit atheromatous plaques in humans before scheduled percutaneous coronary interventions and evaluated the impact of local temperatures on clinical mid-term outcome.[27] The study population included patients with effort angina and with unstable or acute myocardial infarction undergoing successful percutaneous coronary intervention. All patients were prospectively followed for the occurrence of death, myocardial infarction, and target lesion revascularization

The temperature difference between the atherosclerotic plaques and the nondiseased vessel walls increased progressively from effort angina to acute myocardial infarction (0.13 ± 0.18°C, 0.63 ± 0.26°C, and 0.94 ± 0.58°C, respectively; p <0.01). After a median follow-up period of 17.88 ± 7.16 months, 21 patients suffered major adverse cardiac events including three deaths. Temperature difference between the culprit atheromatous plaque and the proximal vessel wall was greater in patients with adverse cardiac events than in patients without events (0.939 ± 0.49 versus 0.428 ± 0.42°C; p <0.0001). Moreover, temperature difference was greater in the patients with effort angina and unstable angina with adverse cardiac events as compared to those without events. In patients with acute myocardial infarction, temperature difference was greater, although it did not reach significant statistical difference.

Cox regression analysis after adjustment for several clinical and angiographic factors revealed that temperature difference was a strong predictor of adverse cardiac events during the follow-up period (OR [odds ratio] 2.14; 95% confidence interval, 1.31 to 6.85; p = 0.043). Sensitivity and specificity analyses showed that the threshold of the temperature difference value (cutoff point) above which the risk for an adverse outcome after the intervention significantly increased was 0.5°C. The sensitivity for this cutoff point was 86% and the specificity was 60% for predicting future adverse cardiac events.

When the study population was categorized according to the cutoff value of temperature difference, the incidence of adverse cardiac events in patients with temperature differences 0.5C was greater (41%) compared to patients without increased thermal heterogeneity (7%). A Cox survival plot adjusted for temperature difference and stratified for the cutoff point showed a clear relationship between temperature difference and event-free survival.[27] However, these results do not prove a causal relationship between increased temperature of atherosclerotic plaques and adverse cardiac events. Nevertheless, they are indicative for considering strategies to stabilize atherosclerotic plaques after percutaneous coronary interventions.

9.4   FROM VULNERABLE PLAQUE TO VULNERABLE PATIENT

9.4.1   CORONARY THERMOGRAPHY FOR WIDESPREAD INFLAMMATION

The early identification of global high-risk patients for adverse cardiovascular events is more important than ever, as such patients can now be effectively treated. It has been shown that in a number of patients with coronary artery disease, active inflammatory processes are present in atherosclerotic plaques.[2,28,29] It was recently observed that inflammation is not only a local phenomenon restricted to culprit atherosclerotic plaques; particularly in patients with acute coronary events, inflammation is widespread in the coronary arteries.[30–32]

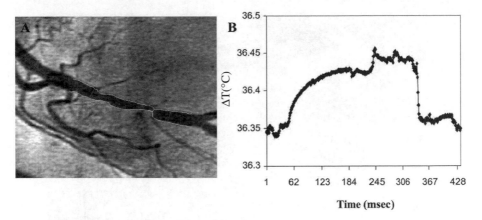

FIGURE 9.4 A: Coronary angiogram of nonculprit lesion at right coronary artery (70% stenosis at the distal segment. B: Temperature difference (Δ) at nonculprit lesion = 0.11°C.

In a preliminary study evaluating the basket thermography catheter, Webster et al. found "hot spots" proximal or distal to culprit lesions. This was the first study showing that thermal heterogeneity was not restricted to angiographically significant lesions and may be widespread in the coronary arterial tree.[7] In order to investigate the presence of increased thermal heterogeneity in multiple lesions in the same patient, we studied 21 patients with two or more lesions. In all these patients, the culprit lesions were identified by noninvasive techniques. Temperature measurements were performed at the culprit lesions and at nonculprit lesions that presented stenoses above 60%. In culprit lesions, the mean temperature difference between the lesion and the healthy vessel wall was 0.12 ± 0.15°C and in nonculprit lesions was 0.12 ± 0.13°C (p = 0.91); see Figure 9.4. In 32 of 42 lesions, the temperature difference between the lesion and the healthy vessel wall was greater than 0.05°C. Of the ten lesions in which thermal heterogeneity was not detected (<0.05°C), six were culprit lesions and four were nonculprit. Interestingly, 50% of the study group showed higher temperature differences in nonculprit lesions compared to culprit lesions, indicating that heat production is not limited to culprit lesions.

9.4.2 BEYOND THE VULNERABLE PLAQUE: CORONARY SINUS THERMOGRAPHY

These findings challenge the concept of a single vulnerable plaque in acute coronary syndromes. Therefore, techniques are required not only to detect vulnerable plaques, but also to detect vulnerable patients. In a recent study, we hypothesized that widespread inflammation may result in increased temperature in the coronary sinus, as blood is drained from the left coronary artery.[33,34] We sought to use a new coronary sinus thermography catheter to investigate whether patients with significant stenoses in left coronary arteries showed increased blood temperature differences between the coronary sinus and right atrium compared to patients with significant stenoses in right coronary artery and subjects without angiographically visible lesions.[33,34]

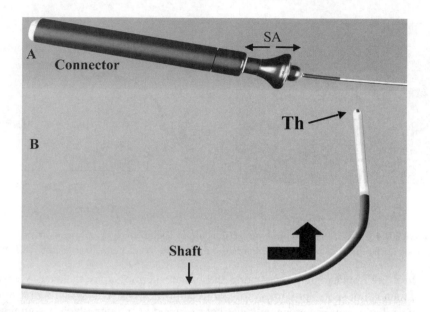

FIGURE 9.5 A: Coronary sinus thermography catheter. The steering arm (SA) with a connector for the thermistor (Th) lead wires is attached to the proximal part of the catheter. B: Distal 7 cm of the shaft of the catheter consists of a soft nonthrombogenic material. Manipulation of the steering arm proximally allows the distal end of the catheter to be curved (black arrow). (From Stefanadis, C. et al., *Am. J. Cardiol.*, 93, 207, 2004. With permission.)

The thermography catheter (7F, Medispes SW AG, Zug, Switzerland) is shown in Figure 9.5. A steering arm with a connector for the thermistor lead wires is attached to the proximal part of the catheter. The steering arm passes through a lumen of the catheter and is attached to its tip. The distal 7 cm of the shaft of the catheter consist of a soft nonthrombogenic material. The thermistor lead wires end at the connector and pass through another lumen of the catheter. A thermistor probe[5,27] is positioned at the center of the tip of the catheter. Manipulation of the steering arm proximally enables the distal end of the catheter to be curved (0 to 180 degrees).

The study population consisted of patients with significant lesions only in left coronary arteries with stenoses (27 patients) or only in right coronary arteries (20 patients) and 23 healthy subjects without coronary artery disease. All patients with coronary artery disease had unstable angina. Significant lesions were defined as stenoses ≥70%. Subjects without coronary artery disease were selected based on the absence of any luminal narrowing. To ensure accurate positioning of the coronary sinus thermography catheter, during the diagnostic catheterization a prolonged recording of the venous phase was obtained. By manipulation of the steering arm at the proximal end, the distal end of the catheter was curved and the tip was positioned approximately 3 cm from the coronary sinus orifice. Thereafter, the catheter was withdrawn into the mid-right atrium.

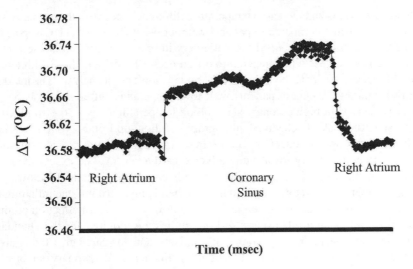

FIGURE 9.6 Temperature measurements with a coronary sinus thermography catheter. Temperature difference (Δ) between coronary sinus and right atrium = 0.16°C.

The mean blood temperature obtained in the coronary sinus and right atrium was designated as the temperature of coronary sinus and right atrium, respectively (Figure 9.6). The temperature difference was designated as the mean blood temperature of the coronary sinus minus mean blood temperature of right atrium. The mean blood temperature was lower in the right atrium compared to the coronary sinus in patients with coronary artery disease. The temperature difference was greater in patients with coronary artery disease compared to the control group (left coronary artery: 0.27 ± 0.10 versus right coronary artery: 0.18 ± 0.08 versus control: 0.09 ± 0.07°C; p <0.001).[34]

The widespread inflammatory activation in patients with unstable angina was shown by demonstrating that in both groups of patients, either with lesions only in the left coronary artery or in the right coronary artery, the temperature difference between the coronary sinus and the right atrium was greater compared to the control subjects. Thus, the increase of coronary sinus blood temperature was independent of the location of the lesion.

This study group was also clinically followed up to track any adverse cardiac events to investigate the impact of coronary sinus thermography on clinical outcome. The majority of these patients were treated by percutaneous intervention and the remainder were treated either by coronary artery bypass grafting or by medical therapy. Clinical follow-up was obtained after a median follow-up of 8.7 ± 3 months. The occurrences of death, Q wave and nonQ myocardial infarction, and any lesion revascularization during the follow-up period were also analyzed. The control group experienced no adverse events.

In patients with coronary artery disease, nine adverse cardiac events were recorded. One patient died after coronary artery bypass surgery. Two patients suffered from acute myocardial infarction due to angiographically proven closure of the target vessel; six patients underwent repeat revascularization procedures. Patients with adverse events had increased temperature differences between the coronary sinus and the right atrium compared to patients without events ($0.35 \pm 0.11°C$ versus $0.20 \pm 0.08°C$; p<0.01). We grouped the patients with coronary artery disease into the same category as those with temperature differences <0.25°C and those with temperature differences ≥0.25°C according to the applied cutoff point analysis. The incidence of adverse cardiac events in patients with low temperature differences was 34.78% and in patients with high coronary sinus blood temperature was 4.16% (p <0.01).[35]

Despite the lack of scheduled angiographic follow-up in this group of patients, the impact of coronary sinus temperature measurement seems to provide significant evidence of vulnerability for a future adverse cardiac event. The exact mechanism involved in the rise of coronary sinus blood temperature is still unknown. The changes in metabolic factors observed in an ischemic myocardium, the inflammatory activation, or the alterations in coronary blood flow may have an effect on coronary sinus blood temperature. However, several studies are required for the elucidation of the responsible pathophysiologic mechanisms and the strategies that may be considered for the stabilization of patients with increased coronary sinus blood temperature. All these issues need to be further investigated in large prospective studies.

In an effort to explore the pathophysiologic substrate leading to increased coronary sinus blood temperature, we demonstrated that temperature difference between coronary sinus and right atrium blood was well correlated with markers of inflammation. The study included 47 patients with coronary artery disease and 23 healthy subjects. In all patients, C-reactive protein and fibrinogen were measured and temperature measurements were performed. Plasma levels of C-reactive protein and fibrinogen were well correlated with temperature differences between coronary sinus and right atrium blood (R = 0.29, p = 0.02; R = 0.26, p = 0.04, respectively).

These studies showed that coronary sinus thermography may provide information regarding patient vulnerability. New studies, however, with greater numbers of patients are required to investigate the role of coronary sinus thermography in identifying vulnerable patients.

9.5   THERMOGRAPHY-GUIDED SELECTION OF TREATMENT

It is becoming increasingly apparent that prevention is as important or even more important than healing plaque rupture. Current therapeutic strategies could be directed primarily to high-risk atheromatous plaques, as available technology allows us to study in detail and promptly identify the anatomical and functional abnormalities of atherosclerotic plaques.

9.5.1   EXPERIMENTAL STUDIES

Animal studies revealed that atherosclerotic plaques can be modified.[10,36] Mounting evidence indicates that the administration of statins results in plaque stabilization.[37] Statins appear to exert pleiotropic effects beyond their efficiency in cholesterol lowering. They seem to produce direct antiatherogenic effects on the arterial vessel walls through mechanisms unrelated to or only indirectly dependent on lowering of plasma lipid levels via anti-inflammatory effects or lowering of plaque oxidized low density lipoproteins.[38]

The effects of diet and statins on atherosclerotic plaque thermal heterogeneity were recently studied.[10] Twenty New Zealand rabbits were randomized to either normal or cholesterol-rich diets for 6 mo. In all animals, intravascular ultrasound and temperature measurements of the surface of aortic arches and descending aortae were performed. Thereafter, the rabbits were either euthanized, and their aortas analyzed histologically or they received normal diets for additional 3 mo and underwent repeat intravascular ultrasound and thermography before euthanasia followed by histological evaluation. In those animals euthanized after receiving high lipid diets, histology revealed that plaques were composed of fibromuscular tissue and contained foam cells of macrophage origin. Temperature heterogeneity was markedly elevated and correlated with plaque thickness. After 3 mo of cholesterol lowering, plaque thickness remained unchanged, but temperature heterogeneity was significantly decreased. This paralleled plaque histology, which showed marked losses of macrophages. The findings of this study demonstrated the relation between local temperature and total macrophage concentration and, furthermore, that *in vivo* temperature heterogeneity of rabbit atherosclerotic plaques is determined by plaque composition.[10]

In a human study in which we evaluated the effects of statins on atherosclerotic plaque temperature, thermal heterogeneity was lower in patients treated with statins.[39] The study population included 72 patients with effort angina, unstable angina, or acute myocardial infarction. Approximately half of the study population received statins for more than 4 wk; the remainder did not receive statins. Statistical analysis showed that the mean value of temperature difference between the culprit atherosclerotic plaque and the proximal vessel wall was higher in the untreated group compared to the statin-treated group. Moreover, the favorable effect of decreased heat production from the culprit atherosclerotic plaque was present in all clinical syndromes including stabilized patients and also patients with acute coronary syndromes. Multivariate analysis showed that treatment with statins was an independent factor for temperature variation.[39]

It has been also observed that treatment with statins has a favorable effect on culprit plaque temperatures in patients with previous myocardial infarctions.[14] In a recent study including patients with previous myocardial infarctions (2 to 4 months earlier) and chronic stable angina, patients with recent myocardial infarctions treated with statins showed only a trend toward higher plaque temperature compared to treated patients with chronic stable angina ($0.41 \pm 0.35°C$ versus $0.19 \pm 0.20°C$; p = 0.11). On the contrary, patients with previous myocardial infarctions who were not treated with statins had significantly higher temperatures compared to untreated patients with chronic stable angina ($0.76 \pm 0.70°C$ versus $0.27 \pm 0.01°C$, p <0.01).[14]

9.6 FUTURE PERSPECTIVES

Coronary thermography has revealed that inflammation can be locally identified. However, clinical evidence has been obtained from already symptomatic patients with significant lesions, but small and intermediate lesions have not been evaluated. The limitations of the current technology include the need for contact of the sensors with the atheromatous lesion and the impacts of several factors such as blood flow on temperature measurements. In order to extend the application of coronary thermography and make it a valuable tool for the assessment of nonsignificant lesions, the development of sensors without the requirement for contact with the plaque is essential.

Coronary sinus thermography is a new diagnostic tool that may help identify vulnerable patients. However, further studies are needed to clarify the significance of elevated coronary sinus blood temperature in different subgroups of patients with coronary artery disease. The technique may also prove useful in evaluating existing or future treatment modalities. Measurement of coronary sinus blood temperature could be expanded beyond coronary artery disease in order to investigate other pathophysiological conditions such as hypertrophic or dilated cardiomyopathy.

9.7 CONCLUDING REMARKS

Plaque rupture is probably the most important mechanism underlying the sudden onset of an acute coronary event. Plaques rich in soft extracellular lipids and macrophages are possibly more prone to rupture. One of the most significant targets of current research is early identification of vulnerable sites that are potentially at risk of rupture in order to prevent the sequel of events that may lead to this devastating outcome.

Inflammation within the atherosclerotic plaques may be detected by identifying temperature heterogeneity within the culprit lesions. Thermography may be used in the future for the detection of local or systemic inflammatory involvement, and thus allow early identification of patients at increased risk and selection of therapies that will reduce risks for future adverse cardiac events.

REFERENCES

1. Stary, H.C. et al. A definition of initial, fatty streak, and intermediate lesions of atherosclerosis. *Circulation* 1994; 89: 2462–2478.
2. van der Wal, A.C. et al. Site of intimal rupture or erosion of thrombosed coronary atherosclerotic plaques is characterized by an inflammatory process irrespective of the dominant plaque morphology. *Circulation* 1994; 89: 36–44.
3. Casscells, W. et al. Thermal detection of cellular infiltrates in living atherosclerotic plaques: possible implications for plaque rupture and thrombosis. *Lancet* 1996; 347: 1447–1451.
4. Stefanadis, C. and Toutouzas, P. *In vivo* local thermography of coronary artery atherosclerotic plaques in humans. *Ann Intern Med* 1998; 129: 1079–1080.
5. Stefanadis, C. et al. Thermal heterogeneity within human atherosclerotic coronary arteries detected *in vivo*: a new method of detection by application of a special thermography catheter. *Circulation* 1999; 99: 1965–1971.
6. Van Langenhove, G. et al. First controlled human intracoronary thermography trial to detect vulnerable plaque. *Circulation* 2002; 106: II 657.

7. Webster, M. et al. Intracoronary thermography in stable and unstable coronary disease. *Circulation* 2002; 106: II 657.

8. Naghavi, M. et al. New developments in the detection of vulnerable plaque. *Curr Atheroscler Rep* 2001; 3:125–135.

9. Wijns, W. et al. Worldwide experience on safety and feasibility of a novel intra-coronary thermography system in patients with stable and unstable angina. *Circulation* 2003; 108: 1920.

10. Verheye, S. et al. *In vivo* temperature heterogeneity of atherosclerotic plaques is determined by plaque composition. *Circulation* 2002; 105: 1596–1601.

11. Courtney, B. et al. *In vitro* surface temperature images from a guidewire-based thermography system. *Circulation* 2002; 106: 2921.

12. Akasaka, T. et al. Increase in plaque temperature reflects macrophage infiltration in coronary stenotic lesions: intracoronary temperature measurement and histological assessment. *Circulation* 2003; 108: IV 373.

13. Madjid, M. et al. Thermal detection of vulnerable plaque. *Am J Cardiol* 2002; 90: 36L–39L.

14. Toutouzas, K. et al. Patients after acute myocardial infarction have for a prolonged period increased thermal heterogeneity in culprit atherosclerotic lesions: additional effect of statins on plaque stabilization. *J Am Coll Cardiol* 2003; 41: 1010–1048.

15. Stefanadis, C. et al. Heat production of atherosclerotic plaques and inflammation assessed by the acute phase proteins in acute coronary syndromes. *J Mol Cell Cardiol* 2000; 32: 43–52.

16. Vaina, S. et al. Correlation of soluble cell adhesion molecule expression and heat production of atherosclerotic plaques. *Eur Heart J* 2002; 4 (Suppl.): 291.

17. Toutouzas, K. et al. Correlation of coronary plaque temperature with inflammatory markers obtained from atherectomy specimens in humans. *Am J Cardiol* 2003; 92: 476.

18. Toutouzas, K. et al. Correlation of IVUS characteristics with temperature of the culprit lesion: new insights in arterial remodeling. *Eur Heart J* 2001; 22: 591.

19. Stefanadis, C. et al. Thermal heterogeneity in stable human coronary atherosclerotic plaques is underestimated *in vivo*: the "cooling effect" of blood flow. *J Am Coll Cardiol* 2003; 41: 403–408.

20. Stefanadis, C. et al. New balloon-thermography catheter for *in vivo* temperature measurements in human coronary atherosclerotic plaques: novel approach for thermography? *Catheter Cardiovasc Interv* 2003; 58:344–350.

21. Chan, A.W. et al. Relation of inflammation and benefit of statins after percutaneous coronary interventions. *Circulation* 2003; 107: 1750–1756.

22. Danenberg, H.D., et al. Systemic inflammation induced by lipopolysaccharide increases neointimal formation after balloon and stent injury in rabbits. *Circulation* 2002; 105:2917–2922.

23. Gaspardone, A. et al. Predictive value of C-reactive protein after successful coronary-artery stenting in patients with stable angina. *Am J Cardiol* 1998; 82: 515–518.

24. Patti, G. et al. Prognostic value of interleukin-1 receptor antagonist in patients undergoing percutaneous coronary intervention. *Am J Cardiol* 2002; 89: 372–376.

25. Pietersma, A. et al. Late lumen loss after coronary angioplasty is associated with the activation status of circulating phagocytes before treatment. *Circulation* 1995; 91:1320–1325.

26. Walter, D.H. et al. Preprocedural C-reactive protein levels and cardiovascular events after coronary stent implantation. *J Am Coll Cardiol* 2001; 37: 839–846.

27. Stefanadis, C. et al. Increased local temperature in human coronary atherosclerotic plaques: an independent predictor of clinical outcome in patients undergoing a percutaneous coronary intervention. *J Am Coll Cardiol* 2001; 37:1277–1283.

28. Moreno, P.R. et al. Macrophage infiltration in acute coronary syndromes: implications for plaque rupture. *Circulation* 1994; 90: 775–778.

29. Naruko, T. et al. Neutrophil infiltration of culprit lesions in acute coronary syndromes. *Circulation* 2002; 106: 2894–2900.

30. Cusack, M.R. et al. Systemic inflammation in unstable angina is the result of myocardial necrosis. *J Am Coll Cardiol* 2002; 39: 1917–1923.

31. Buffon, A. et al. Widespread coronary inflammation in unstable angina. *New Engl J Med* 2002; 347: 5–12.

32. Spagnoli, L.G. et al. Multicentric inflammation in epicardial coronary arteries of patients dying of acute myocardial infarction. *J Am Coll Cardiol* 2002; 40: 1579–1588.

33. Toutouzas, K. et al. Significant atherosclerotic lesions in left coronary artery are associated with increased temperature in coronary sinus compared to only right coronary artery disease. *Circulation* 2002; 106:II 533.

34. Stefanadis, C. et al. Temperature of the blood in the coronary sinus and right atrium in patients with and without coronary artery disease. *Am J Cardiol* 2004; 93: 207–210.

35. Toutouzas, K. et al. Increased coronary sinus blood temperature is a predictor for adverse cardiac events: mid-term follow-up. *Eur Heart J* 2003; 23: 624.

36. Helft, G. et al. Progression and regression of atherosclerotic lesions: monitoring with serial noninvasive magnetic resonance imaging. *Circulation* 2002; 105: 993–998.

37. Krone, W. and Muller-Wieland, D. Lipid lowering therapy and stabilization of atherosclerotic plaques. *Thromb Haemost* 1999; 82 (Suppl. 1): 60–61.

38. Koh, K.K. Effects of statins on vascular wall: vasomotor function, inflammation, and plaque stability. *Cardiovasc Res* 2000; 47: 648–657.

39. Stefanadis, C. et al. Statin treatment is associated with reduced thermal heterogeneity in human atherosclerotic plaques. *Eur Heart J* 2002; 23: 1664–1669.

10 Treatment of Vulnerable Plaques: Current and Future Strategies

Leonard Kritharides, David Brieger,
S. Benedict Freedman, and Harry C. Lowe

CONTENTS

10.1 DETECTION OF PATIENTS WITH VULNERABLE PLAQUES (VPs)

10.1.1 INTRODUCTION

Unstable angina pectoris and myocardial infarction (MI) are mediated by a variable combination of endothelial surface defects of atherosclerotic lesions, mural hematomas, and luminal thromboses included in the category of type VI lesions.[1] Most, but not all such plaques, are lipid-rich and have thin caps (so-called vulnerable plaque or VPs). However, 20 to 30% of plaques associated with clinical coronary instability are not ruptured, rather are fibrotic or calcified, with subendothelial inflammation or erosion underlying thrombosis.[2–4] In addition, intraplaque hemorrhage related to neo-vascularization, and macrophage infiltration secondary to red cell deposition may also contribute to plaque vulnerability[5,6] and may require different preventative approaches from those with primarily erosive–thrombotic etiologies. The characteristics of different kinds of VPs may become relevant for designing patient-specific treatment strategies. A recent review categorized criteria for vulnerability as major and minor; the most important criteria are summarized in Table 10.1.[3,4]

We face major questions in developing treatments of VPs according to pathological etiologies. For example, should we delineate between inflammatory states with predominant lymphocyte activation and those with predominant monocyte

TABLE 10.1
Suggested Major Criteria for Defining Vulnerable Plaque

Active inflammation with monocytes/macrophages and/or T-lymphocytes
Thin cap with large lipid core
Endothelial denudation with superficial platelet aggregation
Fissured plaque
Stenosis >90%

Data from Naghavi, M. et al. Circulation 108, 1664–1472, 2003; Naghavi, M. et al. Circulation 108, 1772–1778, 2003.

infiltration or neutrophil infiltration? How will systemic features, such as thrombo-genicity of blood, systemic inflammation, and regional plaque characteristics, such as lipid content, be integrated and prioritized when they exist in various combinations? Will clinical or imaging classification algorithms analogous to those required for the diagnosis of rheumatic fever[7] need to be established to identify major and minor criteria of risk of rupture or thrombosis? Most importantly, how will quite distinct causes of VP (e.g., intraplaque hemorrhage versus endothelial erosion-causing platelet aggregation) be identified so as to target specific therapy?

Worsening of clinical symptoms is currently our main method of identification of patients at high risk of MI. This allows, at best, insensitive detection of at-risk patients. Invasive techniques may permit evaluation of individual lesions within the coronary tree, but the application of these techniques will be restricted to subjects who have otherwise been recognized as having increased risks because of both cost and risk to the patient required for coronary artery imaging. Moreover, if systemic rather than local factors predominate, treatments of patients and their systemic risk factors or inflammatory responses may be more important than local treatment of individual plaques.

In this chapter, we review current treatment of vulnerable patients, recognizing that current treatment algorithms can only identify patients with acute coronary syndromes (ACSs), and recognizing that such patients are likely to have combinations of ruptured and vulnerable plaques (VPs). Within each treatment domain, we comment, where possible, on implications for future therapeutic strategies for VP. In addition, we separately introduce novel and potentially important strategies such as treatment with high density lipoproteins (HDLs) and local gene therapy. Given that clinical management is intrinsically linked to diagnosis, we begin by briefly summarizing current and potential diagnostic stratification of vulnerable patients.

10.1.2 AT-RISK PATIENTS AND MYOCARDIAL ISCHEMIA

Although it has long been recognized that patients with increasing or unstable angina pectoris are at increased risk of MI, it is also known that the first presentation of coronary disease in over 40% of adults will be an unheralded MI.[8] In this situation, MI represents progression from VP to ruptured plaque and to complete occlusion without warning. Postmortem and angiographic studies indicate that plaque ruptures are often clinically silent, and that much progression of coronary disease represents repeated rupture and healing of plaques. Thus, reliance on the development or deterioration of clinical symptoms must grossly underestimate the incidence of plaque rupture. The correlate of this is that VPs, of which only a proportion will rupture, can never be reliably detected by clinical presentation alone.

Functional studies that detect myocardial ischemia require hemodynamically significant, flow limiting, stenosis of the coronary artery. Most VPs are not hemodynamically significant, and most MIs derive from stenoses of less than 50% (see earlier chapters). Strategies to detect asymptomatic disease by routine stress testing at fixed intervals (e.g., every year), are by definition restricted to the detection of hemodynamically severe lesions and to arbitrary random sampling required of fixed interval screening.

10.1.3 BIOCHEMICAL MARKERS

Biochemical markers of plaque instability may permit noninvasive detection of patients at greatest risk of coronary events. It is, however, important to distinguish between their use as markers of increased risk in large population studies and their ability to predict or preclude cardiac events in individual patients. The ability to exclude a significant risk of short-term cardiac event is at least as important as the ability to detect those at highest risk, and it is important to be able to express such results in terms of absolute risk, i.e., number of events per hundred patients per annum, in order to justify specific treatment.

The usefulness of biochemical detection and risk stratification will be heavily dependent on the safety and efficacy of treatments, developing or yet to be developed (see below), that ideally will target specific pathologies identified using such markers. This is even more critical in the setting for treatment of nonruptured individual VPs since only a small proportion of these ever cause clinical complications.

Inflammation is clearly of relevance to the initiation and complications of atherosclerosis (see Reference 9 and and earlier chapters). A number of plasma inflammatory markers have been proven to predict subsequent major cardiac events in patients presenting with acute coronary syndromes (i.e., with already ruptured or eroded plaques). These include white cell count, fibrinogen, lipoprotein-associated phospholipase A2, C-reactive protein (CRP), CD40 ligand, troponin T, nitrotyrosine, and myeloperoxidase (MPO).[10–15] Of these, troponin T is understood to be a measure of myocardial injury. CRP, CD40 ligand, and MPO may be involved in generating the inflammatory response. Nitrotyrosine serves as measure of protein damage secondary to inflammatory and oxidative processes.

CRP, CD40 ligand, and MPO have been most intensively studied, have independent prognostic values, and have the ability to predict risk of later plaque rupture distant from the time of sampling. This suggests they may detect inflammation occurring within as-yet-unruptured vulnerable plaques (i.e., true VPs). The strongest direct evidence of this comes from a study in unstable patients demonstrating depletion of neutrophil MPO (neutrophil activation) in coronary arteries without ruptured plaques, implying detection of inflammation in unruptured VPs.[16]

None of the biomarkers to date can be considered specific for atherosclerosis as all are elevated in a number of inflammatory or oxidant states. Future biomarkers of vulnerable plaque may combine tissue specificity with pathological process. For example, oxidant stress is widely recognized as active in atherosclerotic lesions, from the earliest stages of development of fatty streaks to the exacerbation of inflammation and to plaque rupture and damage by MPO. Biomolecules from within atherosclerotic lesions such as haptoglobin,[17] products of oxidation such as nitrotyrosine, oxysterols, cholesteryl ester hydroxides, phospholipid hydroxyalkenals, and lipid moieties that bind to circulating antibodies against oxidized low density lipoproteins (oxLDLs) may all have potential as useful markers.[18–20]

Autoantibodies to modified lipids and proteins may be promising sources of novel diagnostic markers based on studies of autoantibodies to oxLDLs. Circulating autoantibodies to oxLDLs have been shown to localize to atherosclerotic lesions in animal models.[21] The levels of these antibodies increase during acute coronary syndromes, indicating their potential role as markers of plaque vulnerability.[22] Moreover, they may reveal key aspects of the atherosclerotic pathology since lipid moieties in oxLDLs bind beta 2-glycoprotein 1 and are thus recognized by anti--2-glycoprotein antibodies.[23] In addition, mimicry between epitopes of oxLDLs and pneumococcal antigens has revealed a potential to prevent atherosclerosis using pneumococcal vaccination.[24]

10.1.4 IDENTIFICATION OF INDIVIDUAL VULNERABLE PLAQUES

Circulating biomarkers can at best only identify patients who have VPs somewhere in their coronary trees. Thus, local treatment of individual VPs by percutaneous coronary intervention (PCI) or other strategy (see below) would require identification of the VP and this would most likely require invasive investigation. These issues have been addressed elsewhere in this book, but key points are worth reiterating in the context of patient management.

Coronary angiography can detect plaques that have ruptured and are nonocclusive. but VPs cannot be reliably detected by angiography before signs of rupture. Intravascular ultrasound (IVUS), optical coherence tomography, near infrared spectroscopy,[25] and thermography have been discussed in more detail in earlier chapters and reviewed elsewhere.[26] Each technique offers decided and specific advantages over angiography. All share with angiography the risks of invasive coronary cannulation and are therefore unlikely to be used for routine screening of populations. However, each method could be used as an adjunct to angiography in the highest risk groups of patients already warranting such investigation. Key to the application of these technologies will be the development of practical algorithms applying these methods to appropriate patient groups. As a minimum, for patients to warrant IVUS, OCT, or thermography, some validated systemic marker of high risk, acute clinical presentation, or otherwise suspicious angiogram would be required.

Magnetic resonance imaging (MRI) and computerized tomography (CT) scans are of great interest because they are noninvasive but they cannot at this time identify VPs in a coronary tree. MRI is particularly attractive technique because of its soft tissue resolution, but it remains problematic from the view of detection of coronary plaque composition. Recent developments using iron oxide are promising because they appear to detect iron-loaded macrophages in atherosclerotic cores[27] and may permit targeting of these cells.

10.2 CURRENT THERAPEUTICS: LOCAL AND SYSTEMIC APPROACHES

10.2.1 INTRODUCTION

Current treatment of VPs and ruptured plaques without MI attempts to reduce thrombotic and inflammatory activity in the plaque and reduce the risk of extending to MI. This process is sometimes referred to as *passivation*.[28] A number of established treatments target specific aspects of the thrombotic or inflammatory response, and some of these along with their theoretical targets are summarized in Table 10.2. Although numerous potential therapeutic targets exist, we will draw attention to the most important or emergent targets in the remainder of this chapter.

10.2.2 PERCUTANEOUS CORONARY INTERVENTION (PCI OR PTCA) AND SURGERY

PCI is the current principal nonpharmacological treatment for VP for patients presenting with acute coronary syndromes (ACSs).[29] The ACS of nonST elevation myocardial infarction (NSTEMI) and acute ST elevation myocardial infarction (AMI) results from thrombosis at a preexisting VP lesion, often secondary to acute plaque rupture.[30,31] Three principal mechanisms are thought to contribute to the ability of PCI to stabilize plaque in this context: (1) mechanical disruption of thrombus; (2) increasing lumen diameter and coronary flow; and (3) direct plaque compression and sealing of plaque dissection.[33]

10.2.2.1 PCI for NonST Elevation Myocardial Infarction (NSTEMI)

Early trials of PCI for NSTEMI ACS failed to show a greater benefit than medical therapy.[34,35] However, following the introduction of IIb/IIIa receptor antagonists and the widespread use of coronary stents, PCI has been increasingly adopted.[36] The FRISC II trial randomized 2457 ACS patients (57% NSTEMI) to early invasive versus conservative treatment strategies.[37] This resulted in 71% of the invasive group and 9% of the conservative treatment group undergoing revascularization within 10 days of presentation, with 61 to 70% of PCI patients receiving stents.

The primary endpoint of death or nonfatal MI at 6 mo was reached by 9.4% of the invasive group compared to 12.1% of the conservative group (p = 0.031).[37] Angina (22 versus 39%; p <0.001) and readmissions (14 versus 24%; p <0.001) were also significantly reduced.[37] In the TACTICS TIMI (thrombolysis in myocardial infarction) 18 trial, 2220 ACS patients (37% NSTEMI) treated medically, including treatment with the IIb/IIIa receptor antagonist tirofiban for 48 hr, were randomized to an invasive versus conservative strategy, with 83 to 86% of PCIs involving

TABLE 10.2
Established and Potential Treatment Targets

Targets for Plaque Passivation	Treatment
Established Targets	
Lipid-rich core, hyperlipidemia	Lipid lowering agents (statins, fibrates, nicotinic acid)**
Platelet activation	Aspirin, glycoproteinIIb/IIIa inhibitors
Thrombosis	Heparins
Plaque sealing, restoration of flow	PCI and stenting
Potential Targets	
Angiotensin II (AII) receptor*	ACE inhibitors/AII antagonists
Proteases	Protease inhibitors
Inflammatory mediators, cytokines	Antibodies, competitive ligands
Tissue factor	Viper venom, inactive VIIa peptide
Complement	Decay accelerator protein
Oxidant stress or oxidation products (oxLDL, HOCl, ONOO⁻, OH⁻, MPO)	Prevent or inhibit oxidation, immunize against oxLDL
Endothelial dysfunction and activation	Restore eNOS activity
PPAR-α, -γ, -δ, and cofactors	PPAR ligands and agonists
Macrophage infiltration and proliferation	Decrease monocyte homing; promote macrophage apoptosis
SMC survival; collagen deposition	Promote collagen deposition; inhibit SMC apoptosis

* AII receptors have roles in endothelial dysfunction, VCAM-1 expression, and generation of reactive oxygen species (ROS) that may contribute to plaque destabilization. ACE-inhibitors and A-II antagonists are currently prescribed, but on the basis of clinical data showing improved outcomes primarily in the treatment of hypertension and favorable effects on ventricular remodelling. Thus the use of these agents specifically for plaque stabilization is speculative.

** Lipid-lowering agents have extensive *in vitro* and *in vivo* evidence supporting their ability to restore endothelial function and reduce inflammation in tissues and in the circulation; they are primarily indicated currently for their use in reducing LDLc or triglycerides.

stents.[38] The 6-mo primary endpoint of combined death, nonfatal MI, and ACS requiring hospital readmission was reduced for the invasive strategy group (15.9 versus 19.4%; p = 0.025). RITA 3 randomized a slightly lower risk group of 1810 patients with unstable angina to a similar invasive versus conservative strategy in addition to standard medical therapy including enoxaparin (18% NSTEMI).[39]

Revascularization rates were lower (44 versus 10% at 10 days), but the overall outcome was similar to the TACTICS trial, with a composite endpoint of death, MI, readmission or revascularization for angina reduced in the invasive group (9.6 versus 14.5%; p = 0.001). These and other data showing particular benefit for higher risk subgroups with elevated troponins and ST depression on ECG[40,41] have contributed to the widespread approach of early PCI for NSTEMI for facilities in a position to provide this service.

10.2.2.2   PCI for Acute Myocardial Infarction (AMI)

AMI is usually the result of thrombotic vessel occlusion, often secondary to ruptured vulnerable atherosclerotic plaque, and has been long viewed as an ideal target for a therapy inducing mechanical disruption of thrombus, plaque compression, and sealing of dissection.[42,43] Treatment of AMI can therefore be considered in a discussion of treatment of VP, but is done so here only briefly, due to the amount of literature already available on this topic.[44]

The evolution of therapy toward an invasive strategy of PCI for AMI has in many ways mirrored the changes for NSTEMI. PCI is now increasingly recognized as a superior alternative to thrombolysis for the acute treatment of AMI and is the subject of much recent discussion.[42] Initial trials of immediate angioplasty used following thrombolysis for AMI were disappointing, with high rates of recurrent ischemia and hemorrhagic complications. However, the subsequent introduction of IIb/IIIa receptor antagonists and coronary stents has been thought to address residual thrombus and plaque dissection respectively, using direct PCI without thrombolysis in a number of trials.[42] While IIb/IIIa receptor antagonist and coronary stent uses are now widespread, it is noteworthy that in a contemporary trial setting, angioplasty alone (without IIb/IIIa receptor antagonist or stent use) performed by experienced operators to treat AMI is still associated with excellent outcomes, with 30-day mortality reported as low as 1.1 to 2.7%.[45]

10.2.2.3   PCI for VP

PCI for the preemptive stabilization of nonobstructive but vulnerable plaque is currently an area of much debate and ongoing research.[28] This approach has been advocated if such lesions produce symptoms or signs of ischemia,[46] although no clinical trial data yet supports it. More recently, such preemptive treatment has also been proposed for nonobstructive asymptomatic but vulnerable lesions.[47]

This would represent a paradigm shift within clinical cardiovascular practice although at least three significant problems are inherent with this strategy. First, are the present difficulties in the identification of VPs. Although systemic serologic markers of VP are being investigated, much recent interest has focused on imaging individual lesions of VP.[48] Imaging modalities can be broadly described as invasive and noninvasive, and are discussed in detail in earlier chapters and briefly above in this chapter. The currently available invasive and noninvasive modalities have limited utility in VP identification, but a number of research tools show particular promise, including the optically based method known as optical coherence tomography (OCT).[49] This technique has the facility to identify lipid pool and fibrous cap thickness. and its ability to elucidate the degree of macrophage infiltration has also been proposed.[50] The area of VP identification is likely to see significant research efforts in the coming years.[48]

The second significant issue is distant disease. While by definition the nonobstructive but asymptomatic VP lesion is at future risk of becoming a culprit lesion, the pan-coronary state of heightened activation in patients with acute coronary syndromes is attracting increasing recognition.[51] Angiographic evidence of multiple complex coronary lesions is present in up to 39.5% of patients with ACS,[52] and as many as 79% of patients presenting with ACS have yielded IVUS evidence of multiple ruptured plaques at sites distal to the presumed culprit lesion.[53] In this light, the VP lesion that causes clinical sequelae can be viewed as a focal manifestation of an underlying systemic process.[54] Efforts to prevent progression of a single VP lesion are likely to have only limited clinical efficacy in this context. The term *vulnerable patient* has been proposed to describe this systemic process.[3,4]

A third issue is the long-standing problem of in-stent restenosis (ISR). The stenting of nonobstructive VP would turn many lesions into obstructive and symptomatic lesions of ISR.[28] Paradoxically, and as an aside, these ISR lesions would have many features more consistent with stable plaque including thick neointimal areas,[32] although whether this might translate to less morbidity is unclear. It has been suggested that sirolimus and other drug-eluting stents will overcome this issue, given their low rates of ISR demonstrated to date.[55,56] Of interest, however, is the observation that sirolimus is associated with increased vascular wall apoptosis following angioplasty of the pig coronary artery,[57] a potential disadvantage if such a preemptive strategy is used.

10.2.2.4 Surgery

Coronary artery bypass surgery (CABG) is a well established treatment for stable symptomatic coronary atherosclerosis, with particular benefits observed in patients with multivessel disease, left ventricular impairment, and with the use of internal mammary artery conduits. Given the stable clinical status of the majority of patients in these trials, the atherosclerotic coronary lesions bypassed are likely to have been stable, fibrous lesions. Although it is likely that many of these patients would have developed VPs and that CABG, therefore, conferred some survival benefit in subjects with VPs, this can only be inferred.

Data indicating that CABG diminishes risks that VP will subsequently cause clinical sequelae, particularly in the era of PCI and potent antiplatelet combinations, are limited. Indeed, some evidence indicates that CABG in the setting of acute coronary syndromes with ECG changes confers a higher morbidity and mortality risk[58] though CABG has been proposed as treatment for AMI.[59] In general, emergent CABG is reserved for unstable patients who are critical ill, such as those with significant left main stem stenosis, cardiogenic shock,[60] and other associated mechanical complications.

10.2.3 Antiplatelet Agents

As platelets initiate intravascular thrombosis, therapies directed against platelet activation and aggregation may prevent thrombus propagation following rupture of a VP and following the development of erosion on the surface of a plaque in a vulnerable patient. Therapies directed against platelets may also reduce inflammation. Although this hypothesis has not been directly tested, evidence suggests that anti-inflammatory actions contribute to the effectiveness of these treatments in the months following an acute coronary presentation. In this case, these drugs may stabilize nonruptured vulnerable plaques rather than simply prevent thrombosis on the culprit site that precipitated the acute event. Data supporting the use of these agents largely relates to their use in patients with acute coronary syndromes, i.e., ruptured plaques, rather than uncomplicated VPs.

10.2.3.1 Aspirin

Cyclooxygenases 1 and 2 (Cox-1 and Cox-2) have been identified in arterial walls. Cox-1 is present in both normal and diseased arteries; Cox-2 is localized to macrophage cells in atherosclerotic lesions.[61] Cox-1 inhibition, but less consistently Cox-2 inhibition retards development of atherosclerosis in animal models.[62] Aspirin is an irreversible inhibitor of cyclooxygenase at low doses relatively specific for Cox-1[63] and is the most widely used antiplatelet agent. Low doses of aspirin therapy are effective in preventing long-term vascular events and death in patients with ACS.[64]

The Antithrombotic Trialists' Collaboration reported that high doses of 500 to 1500 mg aspirin daily (that are more gastrotoxic) are no more effective than low doses of 75 to 150 mg in preventing vascular events in patients with known atherosclerosis.[65] Although it is generally believed that at these lower doses, aspirin does not produce any significant anti-inflammatory effect, there is some evidence to the contrary. In LDL receptor-deficient mice, low-dose aspirin administration is associated with reduced macrophage content of atherosclerotic plaque and suppression of inflammatory cytokine (intercellular adhesion molecule 1, membrane cofactor protein 1, and tumor necrosis factor-) production.[66] In the Physicians' Health Study, aspirin reduced the relative risk of MI by 60% for subjects in the highest quartile of plasma CRP and by only 14% for subjects in the lowest quartile,[67] indicating at least an interaction between baseline inflammation and aspirin efficacy.

Aspirin may exert anti-inflammatory effects via a number of additional potential routes. Most obviously, the formation of monocyte–platelet aggregates promotes monocyte activation, and inhibition of aggregate formation by aspirin inhibits monocyte activation.[68] Further, aspirin has been shown to reduce neutrophil activation in subjects with coronary disease,[69] inhibit IL-7 release from platelets,[70] and inhibit inflammation-induced endothelial dysfunction.[71] Importantly, statins and aspirin appear to have distinct and complementary anti-inflammatory effects, as statins, but not aspirin, inhibit CRP-induced monocyte MCP-1 secretion.[72] Aspirin does not reduce the expression of CD40 ligand on platelets,[73,74] indicating that additional routes of platelet and leukocyte inactivation are required in VP. Nevertheless, these observations suggest that aspirin may both inhibit platelet activation and suppress inflammation in patients with VPs.

10.2.3.2 Thienopyridines

Ticlopidine and clopidogrel are thienopyridines that inhibit adenosine diphosphate (ADP)-induced platelet aggregation. Ticlopidine has the uncommon but potentially lethal side effects of neutropenia, thrombotic thrombocytopenic purpura, and aplastic anemia that have limited its routine use. Clopidogrel, a newer thienopyridine, has effectively replaced ticlopidine for all indications. It acts by irreversibly binding and inactivating the P2Y ADP receptors, antagonizing ADP-induced inhibition of adenylyl cyclase, affecting intracellular signalling and protein phosphorylation.

Although the impacts of the thienopyridines on processes that are likely to contribute to plaque vulnerability have not been widely studied, clopidogrel has been shown to reduce platelet expression of CD40 ligand,[75] thereby potentially influencing inflammation as well as inhibiting platelet activation and aggregation. The CURE (clopidogrel in unstable angina to prevent recurrent events) trial was a randomized, double blind, placebo-controlled trial enrolling 12,562 patients and comparing clopidogrel with placebo in patients who presented with acute coronary syndromes without ST elevations.[76] Patients were followed for a median of 9 mo. The primary endpoint, a composite of cardiovascular death, nonfatal MI, or stroke, was reduced in the patients in the clopidogrel group relative to those on placebo (9.3 versus 11.4%; relative risk (RR) = 0.8; p <0.001).

The rates of this outcome were lower both within the first 30 days after randomization (relative risk = 0.79; 95% confidence interval = 0.67 to 0.92) and between 30 days and the end of the study (relative risk = 0.82; 95% confidence interval = 0.70 to 0.95). While it is anticipated that the difference in events within the first month was most likely to have been due to the potent effect of platelet suppression on thrombus accumulation at the site of the recently ruptured plaque, these plaques are usually healed within 6 wk of the event.[77] Later clinical episodes are, therefore, commonly assumed to reflect ruptures of additional VPs. Continued later benefit of clopidogrel may be therefore be due to its impact on VPs on other sites in the coronary tree

The PCI–CURE prespecified subgroup analysis of the CURE trial comprised 2658 patients with nonST elevation MIs who underwent PCIs.[76] This study compared pretreatment (median 10 days prior to PCI) and long-term (mean 8 mo) therapy with clopidogrel with placebo with open label administration of clopidogrel for 4 wk following PCI. The result was a 30% reduction in the primary composite endpoint of cardiovascular death, MI, or urgent target vessel revascularization (TVR) within 30 days of PCI, attributable to pretreatment with clopidogrel. This was likely directly related to the suppression of platelet activation at the time of the coronary intervention. Between 30 days and the end of follow-up, the trend was toward lower death rate of MI in the clopidogrel group than in the placebo group, possibly indicating stabilization of vulnerable plaques rather than the original (now largely stented) culprit lesions.

The CREDO (clopidogrel for the reduction of events during observation) study compared 4 wk of clopidogrel to clopidogrel pretreatment plus long-term (1 year) treatment after PTCA.[78] The primary composite endpoint of death, MI, or stroke at 1 yr was reduced in the pretreatment/long-term clopidogrel arm (8.5 versus 11.5%; p = 0.02). Treatment with clopidogrel from day 29 following PCI to 1 yr was associated with a further 37% relative risk reduction of this composite endpoint (p = 0.04). These cumulative data suggest that the thienopyridines may modify VPs remote from stented lesions, and clearly yield benefits above those achieved by aspirin alone.

10.2.3.3   Platelet GP IIb/IIIa Inhibitor Therapy

Activated glycoprotein (GP) IIb/IIIa receptors on the surfaces of platelets mediate the final common pathway of platelet aggregation, binding fibrinogen and von Willebrand factor and cross-linking adjacent platelets. The three parenteral forms of this therapy approved by the United States Food & Drug Administration to date are abciximab (Reopro, Centocor, Malvern, PA USA), eptifibatide (Integrilin, Millennium-COR Therapeutics, San Francisco, CA, USA), and tirofiban (Aggrastat, Merck, White House Station, NJ, USA).

A meta-analysis of 31,402 patients enrolled in six placebo-controlled, randomized trials of this therapy in patients with nonST elevation ACS demonstrated an 8.5% relative reduction (11.5 versus 10.7%; $p = 0.005$) in death or nonfatal MI to 30 days.[79] None of the individual trials showed a dramatic benefit and the majority of the benefit occurred in those who opted for early PCIs. Administration of platelet GP IIb/IIIa inhibitor therapy at the time of PCI is associated with substantial clinical benefit in patients with ACS and those with stable angina. A recent systematic overview of GP IIb/IIIa inhibitor therapy administered at the time of PCI demonstrated mortality benefits at 30 days, 6 months, and longer.[80] However the only single agent with adequate data to demonstrate long term (1 to 3 years) survival benefit is abciximab.[79]

A 22% relative reduction in mortality (6.4% placebo versus 5.0% abcixcmab) was observed in a pooled analysis of approximately 6000 patients enrolled in placebo-controlled randomized trials of abciximab administration during PCI. Clinical benefit in late follow-up was most marked in patients who presented with ACSs. Interestingly, the magnitude of benefit of abciximab therapy has also been found to be greatest in those with the highest levels of soluble CD40 ligand (sCD40L).[81] This, combined with an effect for a significant period of time subsequent to the ACS presentation with plaque rupture, suggests that part of the clinical benefit of abciximab may be ascribed to anti-inflammatory activity.

In a retrospective analysis of the EPIC (evaluation of c7E3 for the prevention of ischemic complications) trial angioplasty cohort, patients assigned to abciximab showed significant suppression of both interleukin (IL)-6 and CRP levels 48 hr after PCI when compared to those who received placebo treatments.[82] No evidence of rebound or reelevation of inflammatory cytokines was found in the 4 wk following PCI. The durability of the inflammatory effects of abciximab may be ascribed to its long effective half life. This may be related to its ability to redistribute to other platelets following dissociation from the GPIIb/IIIa receptors or to actions on nonplatelet GPIIb/IIIa receptors. Eptifibatide has also been demonstrated to suppress IL-6, CRP, and sCD40L during drug infusion, although recurrent elevation of CRP was observed within 24 hr of eptifibatide discontinuation.[83]

Recently, a cytoprotective function has been demonstrated for abciximab. In addition to binding the IIb/IIIa receptor, the antibody can bind other integrins including CD11b/CD18 (MAC-1) receptors on leukocytes. Activated macrophages within atherosclerotic plaques appear to mediate vascular smooth muscle cell death through a mechanism modulated by the CD11b/CD18 (MAC-1) receptor.[84]

In vitro studies show that physiologic concentrations of abciximab suppress vascular smooth muscle cell death in a similar fashion to that afforded by a direct antibody against the MAC-1 receptor. The addition of eptifibatide or tirofiban provides no benefit with respect to smooth muscle cell preservation, suggesting that it is independent of IIb/IIIa antagonism. Thus, part of the long-term mortality benefit observed following abciximab administration after PCI may be due to the stabilization of VP mediated through prevention of macrophage-induced smooth muscle cell apoptosis.

10.2.4 ANTICOAGULANTS AND ANTITHROMBOTICS

Thrombin inhibition is closely linked to suppression of the inflammatory consequences of plaque rupture. Products of thrombosis, including thrombin, cause vascular smooth muscle cells to augment IL-6 production, inducing an acute phase response with hepatic synthesis of fibrinogen, plasminogen activator inhibitor (PAI-1), and CRP.[85] Thus, the products of coronary thrombosis serve to amplify inflammatory responses that may contribute to the destabilization of other vulnerable plaques as discussed elsewhere.

Indirect inhibition of thrombin with unfractionated heparin has a proven role in the prevention of MI in patients with ACS,[86] but has been largely superseded by enoxaparin, a low molecular weight heparin. The superiority of enoxaparin relative to unfractionated heparin in medically treated patients was demonstrated in the ESSENCE (efficacy and safety of subcutaneous enoxaparin in nonQ wave myocardial coronary events) and TIMI (thrombolysis in myocardial infarction) 11B randomized trials.[87,88] Whatever the contributions of different mechanisms to the greater efficacy of low molecular weight heparin, treatment for several days following presentation with ACS seems to be sufficient as in TIMI 11B, and treatment beyond this time was not associated with any additional clinical benefit.

The greater efficacy of enoxaparin over unfractionated heparin may relate to the former agent's more potent action on the proximal component of the coagulation cascade, factor Xa, or, more likely, the more favorable pharmacokinetic profile of the anticoagulant activity of low molecular weight heparin. The anti-inflammatory activities of both drugs may have additional differences. In a randomized comparison with unfractionated heparin, enoxaparin suppressed neutrophil-induced elastase release and complement activation more effectively in a simulated extracorporeal circulation.[89] It is possible that the persistence of low molecular weight products with anticoagulant activities following administration of enoxaparin mediate this prolonged therapeutic effect.[90] The impacts of these small molecules on inflammatory activities have not been addressed.

10.2.5 LIPID LOWERING DRUGS AND THEIR PLEIOTROPIC EFFECTS

10.2.5.1   HMG CoA-Reductase Inhibitors (Statins) Reduce the Incidence of Myocardial Infarction

The best studied class of lipid lowering medications are the HMG CoA-reductase inhibitors, also known as statins. The primary clinical pharmacological function of statins is to inhibit HMG CoA-reductase (in the liver) which results in reduced hepatic cholesterol synthesis and consequent up-regulation of hepatic LDL receptor (LDLr) expression and LDL clearance.[91] By up-regulating LDLr expression, statins increase clearance of LDL cholesterol (LDLc), lower LDLc, and significantly reduce cardiovascular morbidity and mortality in populations at high risk of coronary events.[92]

Statin therapy is established as a fundamental component of the prevention of plaque rupture. Compelling angiographic studies indicate that angiographic regression can be promoted by statins alone or especially by combining statins with nicotinic acid, and can be correlated with reduction in cardiac events.[93] Lowering LDLc by HMG CoA-reductase inhibitors (statins) has consistently reduced the incidence of coronary events. The landmark 4S study was the first major statin study to show reduction in cardiovascular mortality and all-cause mortality.[92] This benefit has been observed in a number of large, well designed, randomized controlled studies, most recently including subjects without hyperlipidemia.[94] The benefit is linearly related to the reduction in LDLc and, to date, appears continuous across all levels of LDLc, without signs of threshold effect.[95,96]

Importantly, benefits are seen in patients with and without prior myocardial infarctions, although the absolute benefit (number of lives saved) is greater for secondary prevention populations. Improvements in endothelial function are rapid after starting statins.[97] but clinical benefit (prevention of MI) usually requires a minimum of 6 to 12 mo of treatment.[96] Accelerated benefit has been seen in patients who have been started on atorvastatin during acute coronary syndromes.[98]

10.2.5.2 Pleiotropic Effects of Statins

HMG CoA-reductase inhibitors block cholesterol synthesis through interference with the mevalonate pathway (reviewed by Waldman and Kritharides[99]). Downstream metabolites of mevalonic acid such as geranylgeranyl pyrophosphate and farnesyl pyrophosphate are important for isoprenylation of cellular proteins involved in regulation of cellular growth, cell-to-cell signalling, and apoptosis (including G proteins ras, rho, rac). The ubiquitous mevalonate pathway and the range of molecules potentially affected by isoprenoid synthesis implies that modulation of this pathway can have far-reaching consequences. A number of studies suggest that diverse pleiotropic properties other than the lowering of LDLc by statins may be of biological importance. Statins also appear to exert effects that are quite independent of the mevalonate pathway.

It is important to note that lowering plasma cholesterol by any means causes a range of plaque stabilizing and anti-inflammatory effects including reduced matrix metalloproteinase activity and increased collagen content of atherosclerotic plaques.[100] Similarly, while statins acutely improve endothelial function, the acute lowering of LDLc by apheresis produces immediate improvement in endothelial function.[101] Nevertheless, statins do have diverse, important biological effects that warrant brief review.

10.2.5.3   Statins and Inflammation

Statins lower CRP,[102] suggesting a direct anti-inflammatory effect. Interestingly, this occurs without alteration of circulating IL-6, suggesting a direct effect rather than an effect secondary to the reduction of IL-6. In some studies, the extent of lowering of CRP correlated with the degree of lowering of LDLc.[103] Effective reduction in CRP has also been seen in the setting of ACS.[104]

In secondary prevention studies, statins have been shown to benefit most those with elevated CRP levels.[105] The adverse prognosis conferred by elevations in inflammatory markers such as CRP and serum amyloid A after MI may be overcome by the use of statins.[10,105] This result is analogous to the effect of aspirin in primary prevention studies.[67] The greater benefit in those with elevated CRP may indicate that statins exert their benefit by lowering CRP or by directly inhibiting inflammatory processes. However, as the improvement in clinical outcome with statins typically follows years of treatment, and the reduction of CRP is very rapid, the stabilization of patients at risk is unlikely to be simply due to immediate anti-inflammatory effects. Perhaps CRP, as a marker of inflammation and a predictor of adverse outcome, may predict those patients at highest risk of plaque rupture, and identify those for whom lowering of LDLc and reducing plaque lipid and macrophage content may exert greatest benefit.

A particularly important recent finding was that statins directly regulate inducible major histocompatibility complex class II (MHC-II) response *in vitro*.[106] MHC-II molecules are involved in the activation of T lymphocytes, and the expression of MHC-II in endothelial cells and monocytes is inducible by interferon (IFN)-. This inducible expression of MHC-II is prevented by statins by virtue of direct inhibition of the promoter of transactivator molecule CIITA. This effect is independent of the lowering of LDLc and of the mevalonate pathway, suggesting an entirely novel immunomodulatory mechanism. Although it is unclear whether this observation is an important contributor to the effects of statins in humans *in vivo*, the mechanism of this effect may reveal novel therapeutic or pharmaceutical targets.

Inflammatory and thrombotic processes are commonly linked and are likely to be causally linked in VPs. For example, CRP increases tissue factor expression in monocytes–macrophages.[107] Statins concurrently lower inflammatory and thrombotic factors in the circulation[108] and inhibit CRP-induced MCP-1 expression by monocytes,[72] and this phenomenon is not simply explained by the extent of LDL lowering.[109]

It may relate to changes in plaque, such as diminished tissue factor expression[110,111] or diminished cytokine-induced endothelial expression of CD40 ligand,[112] an effect that is mevalonate-independent. Modulation of CD40 ligand expression is likely to be of some relevance, as it is elevated in patients with diabetes[113] and is an independent predictor of MI and death in patients with unstable coronary disease.[15]

10.2.5.4 Statins, Endothelial Function, and eNOS

Statins improve endothelial function in normocholesterolemic men.[114] The effects of statins on endothelial function are rapid.[97] Simvastatin enhances the migration and proliferation of endothelial cell progenitors, probably via rapidly activation of Akt protein kinase.[115] This may restore endothelial integrity and improve dysfunction. Statins increase eNOS protein levels and activity in atherosclerosis by post-transcriptional mechanisms, and this may exert favorable effects on endothelial and platelet function.[96,116,117] Importantly, statins inhibit hypoxia-mediated down-regulation of eNOS, and this is reversed by treatment with mevalonate, indicating that this effect is HMG CoA-reductase-dependent.[118]

One novel cytoprotective action of statins on endothelial cells was recently identified, whereby statins reduced complement-mediated endothelial injury by promoting endothelial expression of complement inhibitory protein decay-accelerating factor.[119] This was inhibited by L-mevalonate and geranylgeranyl pyrophosphate. Thus is HMG CoA reductase-dependent and independent of NO activity. This property may represent a bridging of anti-inflammatory and endothelium-preserving properties of statins.

10.2.5.5 Effects in Atherosclerotic Tissue Relevant to VP

The ability to stabilize plaque is often referred to as passivation, and the process appears to be promoted by statins and other antithrombotic agents.[28] The anti-inflammatory effects of statins in atherosclerotic plaque are well described and have recently been extended to primate studies.[120] In a recent study, despite matching for plasma cholesterol, statins reduced tissue macrophage content, IL1β, and VCAM-1, and increased collagen content relative to animals matched for plasma cholesterol by restriction of dietary intake.

Statins reduce early growth response gene product (Egr-1) expression in atherosclerotic plaques in apolipoprotein E knockout (apoE KO) mice.[111] Egr-1 is important for the expression of platelet-derived growth factor (PDGF) which is critical for cellular migration in atherosclerotic lesions, local expression of which is stimulated by stimulation of the angiotensin II receptor[121,122] (see gene therapy section below). Statins also inhibit angiotensin II-mediated signal transduction via modulating transcription factors c-jun and c-fos[123] and inhibit PDGF-BB-mediated smooth muscle cell (SMC) migration and proliferation.[124,125] Given the role of the angiotensin II receptor in atherosclerotic lesion progression and in generation of reactive oxygen species, inhibition of downstream effects of angiotensin-II activation may be important for inhibition of proliferative, oxidative, and inflammatory components of atherosclerotic lesion development.

10.2.5.6 Lessons from Statins in Designing Future Therapies: Angiogenesis

Future treatments may be derived from the effects of statins. It is not clear whether new approaches should target individual processes or effectors, or whether they should continue to target general upstream mediators as do the statins. For example, if statins exert their most important effects by inhibiting protein myristoylation or farnesylation as part of the mevalonate pathway, is it reasonable to target these processes deliberately and selectively, or is it more reasonable to target more specific downstream targets that may reduce the potential for harm? Good examples of these complex treatment targets are neovascularization and angiogenesis.

Statins inhibit angiogenesis[126] by inhibiting the geranylgeranylation of rhodamine A (RhoA). Inhibition of plaque neovascularization may be important for reducing macrophage infiltration in atherosclerotic lesions.[127] Neovascularization may also be involved in plaque hemorrhage.[5] Interestingly, statins have also been suggested to promote angiogenesis in the setting of ischemia, and promote recruitment of endothelial cell precursors.[115,128]

The apparent inconsistency of these results may relate to the precise context of statin therapy and the presence or absence of local myocardial ischemia that may be a key permissive regulator of statin-induced angiogenesis. This may also provide a unique autoregulatory control mechanism for targeted neovascularization by statins which may be difficult to achieve by administration of downstream effectors of angiogenesis such as vascular endothelial growth factor (VEGF), which could be harmful.

Because statins exert so many potentially favorable effects, it is in our view impossible to delineate which of these are suitable for selective targeted therapy. Given the unequivocal clinical benefit derived from the lowering of plasma cholesterol, any derived or novel targeted therapies will certainly need to be additive to the use of statins.

10.2.6 FIBRATES AND PPAR AGONISTS

A range of other lipid lowering agents are either in clinical use or are in advanced stages of clinical development and it is beyond the scope of this chapter to discuss them.[129] They include peroxisome proliferator activator receptor (PPAR) agonists, and combination therapies. Fibrates lower triglycerides by increasing expression of lipoprotein lipase (LPL) and decreasing production of very low density lipoprotein (VLDL) and apoCIII. Fibrates are of greatest current interest as they have been shown to reduce cardiovascular events (and thus plaque rupture) in patients with impaired insulin sensitivity and elevated triglycerides. The extent of benefit approximately correlates with the elevation of HDL (VAHITS).[130] This may relate to the effects of triglyceride lowering, HDL raising, or direct effects of fibrates on inflammatory processes that are inhibited by their activation of PPARs (see below).

Fibrates, like statins, reduce CRP and soluble CD40 ligand levels in plasma and acutely improve endothelial function.[131] PPARs have broader implications for understanding links between inflammation and atherosclerosis, future therapies, and the potential beneficial effects of statins. They are discussed in somewhat more detail below.

10.3 NOVEL TREATMENT STRATEGIES

10.3.1 PPAR Agonists

PPARS are nuclear receptors that function as ligand-activated transcription factors and are expressed by all major cells involved in atherosclerosis.[132] They are responsible for the expression of groups of genes involved in cholesterol metabolism (for example, adenosine triphosphate (ATP)-binding cassette transporter 1 (ABCA1), apolipoprotein A-I (apoA-I), LPL, apoCIII, and apoE), inflammation [especially nuclear factor (NF)-κB-dependent pathways], and glucose/lipid metabolism (lowering plasma triglycerides, increasing HDL cholesterol, and improving insulin sensitivity).[132,133] Of the three major subtypes of PPARs, PPAR-α and PPAR-γ are the most widely studied; PPAR-δ has recently been studied in more detail.

Activated PPARs heterodimerize with activated retinoid-X-receptor (RXR) before binding to peroxisome proliferator response elements (PPREs) in the promoter regions of target genes and thereby induce gene expression. Recently, PPAR-α and PPAR-γ activators have been noted to up-regulate scavenger receptor B (SRB)-1 and ABCA1 expression[134] and to inhibit cholesteryl ester accumulation in macrophages.[135,136] As PPAR agonists induce macrophage apoptosis,[137] they may serve as natural therapeutic targets for plaque stabilization. However, it is possible that effective targets for plaque stabilization may not need to be PPAR ligands, as RXR and LXR agonists are also antiatherogenic.[138]

10.3.1.1 PPAR-α

PPAR-α is highly expressed in tissues that readily catabolize free fatty acids, such as fat, liver, and heart, and contributes to the regulation of genes responsible for fatty acid esterification and oxidation. The fibrate class of lipid lowering drugs such as gemfibrozil and fenofibrate are low-affinity agonists of PPAR-α. While their PPAR agonist activity contributes to their lipid lowering and antiatherogenic properties, newer selective agents with greater PPAR affinities may exert very profound anti-inflammatory lipid lowering effects.[139] Gemfibrozil, one of the major currently available fibrates, has been shown to reduce cardiovascular events in patients with impaired insulin sensitivity and elevated triglycerides, and the extent of benefit correlates with the degree of elevation of HDL.[130] There appear to be differences between fibrates in their regulation of key lipoprotein genes in different tissues[140] and these may be due to differential PPAR cofactor recruitment or differential affinity of binding to PPAR-α.

Literature describing the potential effects of PPAR-α agonists in atherosclerotic plaques has almost uniformly indicated that they should inhibit proinflammatory and proatherosclerotic processes. PPAR-α ligands inhibit human aortic SMC production of IL-6 and Cox-2 via repression of NF-κB.[141] Adhesion molecule expression by endothelial cells and tissue factor expression in human monocytes are inhibited by agonists of PPAR-α,[142–144] and these are both therapeutic targets for stabilization of inflamed and prothrombotic VPs. Whether differences in the extent or location of PPAR activation or effects on HDLs and triglycerides between fibrates and other

PPAR-α agonists will translate into differences in clinical outcomes will be important for the targeting of novel antiatherosclerotic, plaque-stabilizing treatments.

10.3.1.2 PPAR-γ

PPAR-γ is predominantly expressed in adipose tissues, adrenal glands, and spleens. In adipose tissue, PPAR-γ has roles in adipocyte differentiation (promoting lipid storage) and glucose metabolism. Importantly, mutations in PPAR-γ are associated with insulin resistance and hypertension.[145] Thiazolidinediones (glitazones, a generic class of PPAR-γ agonists) have been used to improve glucose and lipid control in patients with diabetes and are generally believed to have great potential to directly modify inflammatory processes within atherosclerotic plaques. Of some importance for the biology of VPs, PPAR-γ is expressed in human atherosclerotic plaques and is markedly up-regulated in activated macrophages.[146,147]

Such up-regulation permits PPAR-γ ligands such as endogenous ligand 15d-PGJ2 and other pharmacological ligands to inhibit the expression of iNOS, gelatinase B, and SRA which have roles in lesional oxidative stress, proteolysis, and lipoprotein uptake, respectively and also inhibit the production of inflammatory cytokines by macrophages.[148] PPAR-γ may also diminish inflammation by acting on circulating leukocytes, as indicated by a recent study showing that glitazones reduce expression of the MCP-1 receptor, C-C chemokine receptor 2 (CCR2), in both lesional and circulating monocytes[149] and reduce plasma levels of soluble CD40 ligands in diabetics.[113]

Anti-inflammatory effects appear to be mediated at least in part by inhibition of the transcription factors AP-1, STAT, and NF-κB. PPAR-α was not, in contrast to PPAR-γ, significantly expressed in activated macrophages,[146,147] perhaps suggesting that the most important macrophage-specific effects in VPs are more likely to be achieved by PPAR-γ ligands rather than PPAR-α ligands.

PPAR-γ agonists have been shown to inhibit SMC proliferation and migration,[150] which may be advantageous with respect to atherosclerosis progression and restenosis after angioplasty. However, PPAR-γ agonists have also been shown to induce caspase-mediated apoptosis.[151] Thus, the consequences of PPAR agonism may depend on the precise clinical context — a property that is favorable against post-angioplasty restenosis may be unfavorable in a patient with evidence of plaque instability. PPAR-γ agonists also inhibit endothelial cell migration,[152] a property that may be favorable or unfavorable, depending on whether such migration contributed to endothelial recovery after local injury and inflammation or contributed to angiogenesis that can promote plaque instability. Recent studies indicate that PPAR-γ agonists inhibit angiogenesis, inhibiting VEGF-induced choroidal neovascularization.[153]

10.3.1.3 PPAR-δ

PPAR-δ (synonymous with PPAR-β), unlike PPAR-α and PPAR-γ, does not have clinical agonists currently available, and its role has remained speculative. Recent studies suggest that PPAR-δ expression in macrophages increases expression of

MCP-1, IL-1, and matrix metalloproteinase (MMP)-9 and can thus be expected to be both proinflammatory and proatherosclerotic. However, ligand activation of PPAR-δ exerts the opposite, anti-inflammatory effects.[154]

The biochemistry of this complex process has only recently been revealed. It appears that upon ligand binding to PPAR-δ, the transcriptional repressor of inflammation known as BCL-6 is released, causing suppression of inflammation. Thus, transfection of PPAR-δ into PPAR-δ-deficient cells can promote inflammation by binding BCL-6, but ligand binding of PPAR-δ can inhibit inflammation because of BCL6 release. Because VLDL appears to be a regulator of PPAR-δ activity and because LPL generates fatty acid ligands of PPAR-α, PPAR-γ, and PPAR-δ as a result of lipolysis,[155] the PPARs may be key mediators of the inflammatory response seen in hypertriglyceridemia and states with elevated free fatty acids such as diabetes.

This is indirectly supported by the observation that LPL activity is inversely related to the extent of coronary disease.[156] However, given that free fatty acid concentrations are elevated in diabetes and are important (adverse) prognostic predictors of cardiovascular death,[157] favorable manipulation of PPAR biology may be much more complex than simply increasing the bioavailability of free fatty acids in plasma or in artery walls.

10.3.1.4 Combinations of Statins and Fibrates and Implications for PPARs

Fibrates are sometimes combined with statins in clinical practice to achieve superior control of hypertriglyceridemia and LDLc. The two classes of agents exert very different effects on lipoprotein kinetics, most notable being that only fibrates increase apoA-I synthesis and secretion.[158] The produce other potential synergies at a more molecular level. While fibrates directly bind and activate PPAR-α, statins activate PPAR and RXR transcription indirectly by inhibiting the formation of cholesterol and other precursor polar sterols via the HMG CoA-reductase pathway.[159] The indirect effects of statins are mediated via inhibition of Rho and permit synergy between the two classes of drugs.[160] These studies suggest that a combination of these drugs may provide synergistic up-regulation of antiatherosclerotic clusters of genes regulated by PPARs and RXRs.

10.3.2 ACCELERATED PLAQUE REGRESSION AND STABILIZATION USING HIGH DENSITY LIPOPROTEIN (HDL) AND HDL-LIKE MOLECULES

10.3.2.1 HDL and Atherosclerosis

Plasma concentrations of HDL cholesterol are inversely related to the risk and extent of coronary heart disease, and HDL has typically been a better discriminator of those with coronary disease than LDL.[161–163] Although certain isolated populations such as those with congenital cholesteryl ester transfer protein (CETP) deficiency who face increased risk of CHD despite increased HDL, the protective association of HDL and low rates of CHD holds in most populations. In part, the inverse relationship of

HDL and atherosclerosis or coronary events is attributable to coexistence of low HDL with the proatherogenic risk factors of the metabolic syndrome — central obesity, elevated triglycerides, impaired insulin sensitivity, and small dense LDLs.[164]

Some have suggested that low HDL in conjunction with other changes in lipoprotein profile may be secondary to systemic inflammation, and that some of the inverse relationship of HDL and coronary artery disease (CAD) may relate to suppression of HDL during systemic inflammation.[165] However, the predictive value of CRP appears at least in part independent of HDL.[166] Most importantly, overwhelming evidence in animal models now indicates that HDL is directly antiatherogenic, that it does not simply act as a stable marker of other pathogenic risk factors, and that it is a suitable target for direct elevation by pharmacological means or infusion.[167,168]

Some of the most convincing early animal data concerning directly antiatherogenic effects of HDL came from studies infusing HDL into rabbits or overexpressing human apoA-I in atherosclerosis-prone apoE-deficient mice.[169,170] Importantly, apoA-I, the main protein component of HDL, has also been shown to cause regression of preformed atherosclerosis[171] and to cause remarkably rapid clearance of macrophages and macrophage lipids from preformed plaques.[172] The mechanisms by which HDL exerts its protective effects have been intensively studied, but remain unclear.

10.3.2.2 HDL: Mechanisms of Action

The most widely studied process by which HDL is felt to inhibit or regress atherosclerosis is reverse cholesterol transport (RCT), whereby cholesterol is removed from peripheral cells by HDL or its component molecules and then delivered to the liver for excretion in the bile. The presence of RCT in humans is supported by studies showing excretion of sterols in the bile following infusion of apoA-I–phospholipid discs.[173,174]

In RCT, lipid-poor apoA-I is understood to be a major initial acceptor of cellular cholesterol, and this initial removal of cellular cholesterol is dependent upon the activity of the ATP-binding cassette transporter ABCA1.[175,176] Genetic anomalies in ABCA1 mediate a rare low HDL state known as Tangier disease, which is characterized by hypoalphalipoproteinemia and premature atherosclerosis. Subjects with lesser degrees of dysfunction of ABCA1 have been identified as having low HDL and increased risk of CAD.[177]

ABCA1 expression is increased by cholesterol loading and involves oxysterol-dependent activation of LXR and RXR transcription factors.[178] The clearance of cholesterol once removed from peripheral cells is dependent on transfer reactions in the plasma mediated by lecithin cholesterol acyl transferase (LCAT) and CETP, and then uptake by the liver.[179] Several target genes involved in the regulation of cholesterol metabolism are regulated by LXR and RXR and include apoE, ABCA1, LPL, and CETP.[178]

Clearance of cholesterol from LDL and HDL by the liver is relevant to this process and involves the selective uptake of cholesteryl ester by SRB-1[180] and the excretion of biliary sterols by the expression of ABCG5 and ABCG8.[181] SRB-1 is also likely to play a role in facilitating cholesterol mobilization from peripheral stores.[182] Although over-expression of SRB-1 lowers plasma HDLc, its role in mediating net clearance of cholesterol from tissues is supported by accelerated atherosclerosis with cardiac ischemia in mice deficient in SRB-1.[183] Because several key components of the reverse cholesterol transport pathway are regulated by ligands for LXR and RXR, these may be suitable targets for future therapies, and there is some indication they can be modulated by PPAR ligands.

RCT-independent processes are also suggested for HDL. These include direct anti-inflammatory properties of HDL at the level of endothelium (suppressing TNF-α-mediated up-regulation of VCAM-1 and ICAM-1),[184] antioxidant capacities of HDL,[185,186] monocyte activation (blocking contact-mediated activation of monocytes by T lymphocytes[187]) and monocyte traffic, and inhibiting the homing of macrophages into atherosclerotic lesions.[185,188] The last process may be particularly important for the acute stabilization of inflamed VPs.

10.3.2.3 Prospects for Therapeutic Administration of Exogenous HDL or HDL-Like Molecules

ApoA-I Milano is a variant of apoA-I which is associated with longevity and reduced rates of coronary disease.[189] ApoA-I Milano has been shown to promote atheroma regression in animal studies.[172,190] More recently, apoA-I Milano–phospholipid complexes (resembling nascent HDL) reduced atheroma volume in humans with acute coronary syndromes after five weekly injections.[191]

The mechanism of benefit was not elucidated as changes in plasma lipoprotein cholesterol concentrations, CRP or other markers of systemic inflammation were not described. Nevertheless, this result is impressive as proof of principle. Although remarkable, the rapid response is compatible with recent studies in mice.[171,172] The absence of comparative data with native apoA-I prevents any conclusions to be drawn regarding the relative potency of particles containing native apoA-I and apoA-I Milano in inducing regression or egress of macrophages and thus plaque stabilization.

ApoA-I has not been tested as an antiatherogenic. As a naturally occurring molecule, its potential as a commercially successful agent may be limited. However, peptides containing α helices that can act as apoA-I mimics and efficiently remove cellular cholesterol have been successfully synthesized, and appear to inhibit atherosclerosis development in animals.[192–194] Small molecule mimetics can apparently exert such therapeutic effects when given orally[194] and this may greatly enhance the application of this technology in humans.

10.3.2.4 Prospects for Targeted Elevation of HDL by Pharmacological Agents

An alternative to direct administration of HDL or its component molecules in humans is elevating HDL by pharmacological means. Potential strategies for this include over-expression of apoA-I, LCAT, or ABCA1 or inhibition of CETP. Increased expression of apoA-I is already possible via PPAR-α agonists such as fenofibrate, which directly increases apoA-I transcription in the liver. Newer PPAR-α agonists with greater specificity and affinity for PPAR-α may be expected to achieve this with even greater efficacy. Alternatively, targeted apoA-I gene over-expression as achieved in animals has potential, but must overcome the potential adverse effects of sustained adenoviral or retroviral infection.

Pharmacological agents that increase ABCA1 activity are currently being sought and are most likely to initially target the LXR pathway that regulates ABCA1 expression. However, this approach has potential theoretical problems. Any benefit of therapeutic ABCA1 over-expression may require very efficient hepatic clearance of cholesterol. Otherwise, enhanced mobilization of cholesterol via ABCA1 (from peripheral tissue stores and even from liver) could theoretically increase the risk of atherosclerosis if plasma cholesterol increases. Most importantly, the association between cellular ABCA1 activity and plasma HDL levels appears strongest at very low levels of HDL, contributing less to HDL concentration at higher, more "normal" levels of HDL.[195] This may mean that simple over-expression of ABCA1 in patients with normal or only mildly depressed HDL may exert more modest effects on plasma HDL than restoring normal expression in states of marked deficiency or dysfunction might suggest.

The most immediately amenable approach to substantially increasing HDL will involve the use of pharmacological CETP inhibitors currently in Stage II trials.[196] CETP promotes the transfer of cholesteryl esters from HDL species to apolipoprotein B-containing lipoproteins including VLDL, remnants, and LDL. A genetic deficiency of CETP is associated with increased HDL levels; thus, inhibition of CETP is considered a reasonable therapeutic strategy for increasing HDL. CETP inhibitors have achieved elevation of HDL in animal studies and results of human intervention trials are awaited with interest. Critical to this evaluation will be the identification of whether all HDL elevation achieved by these agents is beneficial, whether sub-types of HDL must be elevated, or whether hepatic cholesterol clearance mechanisms must also be independently regulated during such treatment.

10.3.3 ANTIAPOPTOTIC THERAPY

Apoptosis, a term introduced in 1972,[197] describes the process of "programmed cell death"[198] and is discussed more fully in previous chapters dealing with pathogenesis. Cell apoptosis is distinguished from cell necrosis by a number of morphological, biochemical, and structural features, including cell shrinkage, nuclear fragmentation, and chromatin condensation.[199] Recent interest focuses on the concept that targeting the apoptotic process in the context of VP will have therapeutic potential based on two main groups of observations.

First, considerable data implicate apoptosis in the pathogenesis of VP and acute plaque rupture. Acute plaque rupture is associated with thinning of the atherosclerotic fibrous cap, particularly to <65 μm.[200] Acute ruptures may occur at the plaque shoulders, zones with comparatively fewer SMCs and increased macrophage content. Increased SMC apoptosis is evident in lesions from patients with unstable, compared to stable, angina and it has been suggested that SMC apoptosis may lead to cap thinning and ultimately plaque rupture.[201]

The second observation is that recent precedents suggest that modification of apoptosis may have therapeutic potential in a cardiovascular context.[198,202] Inhibition of bcl-x gene expression increases apoptosis in vascular lesions and is associated with inhibition of neointimal formation.[203] Over-expression of insulin-like growth factor-1 in mouse cardiomyocytes results in reduced apoptosis and reduced ventricular dilatation and hypertrophy.[204] Apoptosis regulation in the processes of restenosis and myocardial infarction would, therefore, appear to provide possible therapeutic avenues.

Targeting the apoptotic process in the context of VP is, however, not straightforward. The cell type in which apoptosis occurs is of crucial importance. While SMC apoptosis may promote plaque instability, macrophage apoptosis may actually promote the reverse by decreasing macrophage activity and collagen breakdown and enhancing fibrous cap integrity.[205] Adding to the complexity, macrophages adjacent to the lipid cores form the largest proportion of apoptotic cells in advanced atherosclerotic lesions and macrophage apoptosis is also found at the sites of plaque rupture[206] although the role of macrophages in plaque rupture remains unclear. Approaches regulating apoptosis in the context of VP will have to be delivered very precisely to VP lesions in terms of both anatomical site and cell type.

Phototherapy (PT) following the administration of motexafin lutetium (MLu) is proposed as a targeted means of inducing localized macrophage apoptosis as a possible treatment of VP.[207,208] MLu is synthetic porphyrin that selectively localizes in metabolically active inflammatory cells such as macrophages in atherosclerotic plaques and alters redox states.[209] When exposed to far red light, MLu facilitates the generation of oxygen radicals that in turn induce macrophage apoptosis. Far red light can be delivered to coronary or peripheral vessels, and in phase I human trials this approach appears well tolerated in isolation or following coronary stenting.[208,210]

Questions as to mechanisms of action and clinical utility, however, are still unanswered because increases in macrophage apoptosis are accompanied by increased levels of smooth muscle cell apoptosis[207,208] — a process that potentially increases plaque vulnerability. Based on the delicate balance of SMC and macrophage apoptosis in plaque stability and the probable inability of PT to be selectively delivered to certain tissue types, this approach requires further development. In addition, although PT can be applied locally and at multiple sites, the present requirement for preadministration of MLu 18 to 24 hr prior to PT is somewhat cumbersome. Nevertheless, this technique appears likely to undergo further evaluation.

10.3.4 Proteases

The integrity of the fibrous cap is in part dependent on collagen and extracellular matrix (ECM). Vascular SMCs synthesize both collagen and ECM, and turnover rates of both of these may increase in atherosclerotic vessels.[211] ECM is comprised of fibrillar collagen, (principally types I and III, but also types IV, V, and VI), proteoglycans, and elastin. A reduction of synthesis of these structural elements may reduce fibrous cap tensile strength and contribute to plaque instability; likewise, agents promoting synthesis may be expected to stabilize plaque.

Increased matrix degrading activity associated with macrophages, vascular smooth muscle cells, and T lymphocytes has been described in unstable atherosclerotic plaques. Among the principal mediators of extracellular matrix degradation are the MMPs. Fibrillar collagen types I and III, are the major structural components conferring tensile strength to the fibrous caps and the expression and enzymatic activities of a number of MMPs capable of digesting these collagen types are increased in atherosclerotic plaques of patients with unstable angina.[212]

MMPs are secreted as inactive zymogens (pro-MMPs), subsequently activated by proteolysis involving urokinase-generated plasmin, a deficiency of which decreases aneurysm formation and medial degradation in atherosclerosis-prone mice.[213,214] MMPs are inhibited by tissue inhibitors (TIMPs). TIMPs have important roles in inhibiting angiogenesis and in regulating MMP activities.[215]

The inflammatory environment that characterizes VPs promotes expression and/or activity of MMPs. In macrophages and very smooth muscle cells (VSMCs), TNF-α and IL1 up-regulate the expression of MMP-9.[216,217] In neutrophils, transcription of the MMP-9 gene can be up-regulated via stimulation by IL-8 or TNF-α.[218] The interaction of T lymphocytes with VSMCs through CD40 and its ligand up-regulates the expression of several MMPs in VSMCs.[219] Chemotactic factors including IL-8 and the ligation of receptors on the surfaces on neutrophils induce degranulation of MMP-9 from neutrophils.[220] Thus, MMPs are potent enzymes capable of destabilizing VP, with augmented activity in the inflammatory state that accompanies ACS.

Studies in genetically engineered mice have provided unexpected insights into the role of MMPs in plaque development and rupture. In general, MMP deficiency achieved in knockout animals has either not affected or has increased atherosclerosis, but reduced aneurysm formation, which is the hallmark phenotype of medial degeneration. For example, MMP-3 inactivation was found to preserve atherosclerosis but diminished aneurysm formation.[221]

The development of a strain of apoE knockout mice prone to plaque rupture[222] provided a background into which additional genetic modifications of the MMP family could be introduced. Recent presentation of preliminary data (C.L. Jackson, European Society of Cardiology, 2003) indicated that eliminating MMP-1 or MMP-7 had no impact on plaque characteristics in these animals. Eliminating MMP-9 resulted in doubling of plaque size and a doubling in the frequency of plaque rupture, suggesting that this gelatinase might be important in plaque healing and, remarkably, protect against rupture. In contrast, deficiency of MMP-12 apparently resulted in smaller, more stable plaques, suggesting that at least in the mouse model, MMP-12 may contribute to plaque vulnerability and may be a potential therapeutic target for VPs.

In patients with abdominal aortic aneurysms, administration of tetracycline-derived antibiotics (which inhibit both the synthesis and activity of MMPs) for 7 days preoperatively resulted in suppression of macrophage expression of MMP-9 mRNA and activation of pro-MMP-2 in the aortic wall.[223] Ongoing studies are investigating the pathological impact of this therapy over a longer term. Limitations to the application of direct inhibitors of MMPs include their role in the normal remodelling of tissues such as myocardium[224] and their potential role in restricting the extent of atherosclerosis. If part of the effect of MMPs is mediated via their ability to promote angiogenesis,[225] alternative strategies for preventing angiogenesis may reduce the need to apply direct inhibitors of these agents in VPs.

10.3.5 TISSUE FACTOR (TF)

TF is a surface-bound glycoprotein normally not exposed to the circulation. Its exposure to plasma proteins results in the binding of factor VII to TF and activation of TF–factor VIIa complexes catalyzes activation of factor X and eventually results in the formation of thrombin. TF is present in subendothelial smooth cells in artery walls, vascular adventitia, and activated monocytes.[226] CRP, platelet-derived growth factor, and cytokines such as IFN-γ stimulate monocyte TF expression, as does the binding of T lymphocytes to CD40 receptors on monocytes and macrophages.

Platelets and neutrophils have also been reported to express TF. TF antigens and activities have been demonstrated in atherosclerotic lesions,[227] and are particularly enriched in the necrotic cores and in cellular regions. TF typically colocalizes with TFPI (a pathway inhibitor), and exposure of blood to TF expressed in subendothelial or inflammatory tissues is thought to be a major factor in mediating coronary thrombosis. In summary, TF is likely to contribute to thrombotic sequelae in two respects. First, it may contribute to initiation of plaque thrombosis as a result of activation of circulating monocytes. Second, it is likely to be a major factor in determining the extent of luminal thrombosis following plaque rupture and the exposure of subendothelial tissues to circulating coagulant factors.

Conventional treatments reduce TF expression and activity. Heparin increases plasma TFPI activity.[228] Lipid lowering by diet or by statins reduces TF expression and cell apoptosis in plaques.[111,229,230] Although beyond the scope of this review, it is worth noting that specific inhibition of the TF pathway may permit prevention of adverse thrombosis without causing systemic bleeding. Such approaches include factor VIIa antagonism (using active site-inactivated recombinant factor VIIa), monoclonal antibodies to TF, and modified (inactive) recombinant TF used as an antagonist of membrane-bound TF.[226] Others have successfully investigated rTFPI, and a peptide with similar mode of action to TFPI nematode anticoagulant protein c2 (NAPc2) are also in trials.[231]

10.3.6 ANTIBIOTICS

The possibility of an association between infectious agents and cardiovascular disease has been recognized for over a decade, prompting trials of specific antibiotics as potential preventative agents capable of reducing plaque vulnerability.[211,252] Most data are available for the bacterium *Chlamydiae pneumoniae* although cytomegalovirus (CMV) and *Helicobacter pylori* have also been implicated. Proposed mechanisms by which infectious agents may promote plaque vulnerability include general effects of acute or chronic inflammation and more specific direct effects of infectious agents on vessel walls, such as endothelial injuries and SMC dysfunctions.[233]

Serologic evidence of *Chlamydiae pneumoniae* was initially observed in association with human coronary atherosclerosis and AMI.[234] Subsequently, *C. pneumoniae* was identified within human atherosclerotic plaques by a variety of techniques including immunohistochemistry for *C. pneumoniae* protein, polymerase chain reaction for *C. pneumoniae* DNA, and direct culture of *C. pneumoniae* from atheromatous plaque material.[235,236] That *C. pneumoniae* is of biologic importance is suggested by multiple studies demonstrating activation of numerous cytokines, growth factors, and adhesion molecules implicated in the atherosclerotic response.[232,237]

These basic studies prompted initial clinical investigations examining pathogenetic mechanisms of *C. pneumoniae* and possible mechanisms of action of antibiotic therapies. Endothelial dysfunction has been shown to be related to *C. pneumoniae* infection and its effects were reduced with antibiotic treatment.[232] Neointimal proliferation as measured by intimal and medial thickness in the context of carotid artery disease was increased in *C. pneumoniae* seropositive patients; effects were reduced by roxithromycin over a 2-yr follow-up.[238] Neointimal proliferation in the context of in-stent restenosis was also reduced by roxithromycin but only in patients with high-titer anti-*C. pneumoniae* antibodies.[239]

One effect of reducing plaque vulnerability — at least as measured by reductions in clinical events in patients with atherosclerosis treated by *C. pneumoniae* targeting antibiotics — has not yet however, been realized by larger scale clinical trials. Azithromycin (given for 4 days) was compared to a placebo in 1439 patients with ACS or AMI and found to show no effects in reducing clinical events at 6 mo.[240] Zithromax, a similar agent (given weekly for 11 wk) was compared to a placebo in 7747 patients with prior AMIs and elevated *C. pneumoniae* titers and found to have no benefit at 2 yr.[232] Although *C. pneumoniae* has a potential role in atherosclerosis development, particularly via its effects on cell proliferation, no specific evidence points to its involvement in VPs. While ongoing trials continue to examine prolonged antibiotic treatments in higher risk patient subsets, the importance and relevance of this role at a clinical level remain speculative.

10.3.7 GENE THERAPY

The first clinical trials of gene therapy for cardiovascular disease started over a decade ago, and while vulnerable plaque (VP) was an early proposed target,[241] the ultimate utility of gene therapy in a vascular context is much debated.[242,243] Gene therapy may defined as the modulation of gene function, either by direct introduction (transfer) of genes or by gene modification, generally by oligonucleotides and related molecules.

The prototypical use for vascular gene therapy is restenosis.[244] In many ways, restenosis is an ideal target because the precise site and time of onset of the pathogenetic process are known and the vessel is already instrumented, thus facilitating delivery. For the most part, VPs do not share these advantages. The lesion sites may be difficult to identify; the timing of rupture is imprecise, and vessels are generally not instrumented. Nevertheless, gene therapy for VP has benefited from a number of investigations made in the context of restenosis, in two broad areas: gene delivery and gene targets.

For more than a decade, vascular gene therapy delivery methods have centered on the use of balloon catheters[245] that allow local delivery by a variety of means, but have been hampered by low efficiencies, and in many cases, the induction of injury responses. More recently, stent-based gene delivery has been achieved. This was initially shown for green fluorescent protein (GFP) plasmid DNA incorporated into a polylactic–polyglycolic acid (PGLA) polymer emulsion on a stainless steel stent delivered to normal pig coronary arteries.[246] Transfection efficiency was initially low, however, on the order of 1% of neointimal SMCs.[246] Transfection efficiency has improved with the use of antibody-tethered adenoviruses.[247] More recently, plasmid DNA delivered via a novel denatured collagen PGLA stent coating has achieved transfection in up to 10% of neointimal SMCs.[248] These latter results suggest that clinically meaningful gene transfer may be possible using a stent-based approach.

An overwhelming number of gene targets have been proposed for gene therapy approaches for restenosis,[249,250] probably reflecting our incomplete understanding of their relative importance. Broadly, these include growth factors and cytokines, transcription factors, cell cycle regulators, enzymes, and related molecules. Many of these may also be pertinent in the context of VP. In particular, are the efforts intended to reduce oxidant injury or induce atherosclerosis? Paradoxically, however, a number of gene targets proposed for restenosis reduction may even be detrimental in the setting of VP. These include inducing apoptosis by fas ligand delivery[251] and reducing SMC proliferation using a variety of means.

Gene modification approaches used for restenosis may also be applied for VP with similar caveats related to gene transfer methods. Antisense or decoy methods of inhibiting SMC proliferation, useful as anti-restenosis methods,[252,253] may be detrimental for VP. Conversely, catalytic antisense or DNAzyme approaches have been proposed, One example is targeting transcription factor Egr-1 implicated in macrophage apoptosis,[254] present in the fibrous caps of atherosclerotic lesions,[255] and successfully targeted in other contexts.[256,257] Despite these difficulties, the advances in stent-based delivery and increasing knowledge of the molecular mechanisms of VP development mean that gene therapy approaches for VP are likely to see continued investigation.

10.4 CONCLUDING REMARKS

Although our understanding of the pathology of VP is now far advanced compared with what was known even 5 to 10 years ago, our application of this knowledge is lagging. Practical application of novel treatments will inevitably have to compromise between theoretical ideals and the realities of cost and potential complications of treatment. Nevertheless, monitoring of patients by plasma markers and improved VP imaging within coronary arteries should combine with novel drug and molecular targets to reduce the risks of patients presenting with potentially life-threatening myocardial infarctions.

ABBREVIATIONS

FRISC, Fast Revascularization during Instability in Coronary Artery Diseases; ICAM, Intracellular Adhesion Molecule; RITA, Randomized Intervention Treatment of Angina; TACTICS, Treat Angina with Aggrastat and determine Cost of Therapy with an Invasive or Conservative Strategy; VAHITS, Veterans Affairs High-Density Lipoprotein Cholesterol Intervention Trial; VCAM, vascular cell adhesion molecule.

REFERENCES

1. Stary, H.C. Natural history and histological classification of atherosclerotic lesions: an update, *Arterioscler Thromb Vasc Biol* 20, 1177–1178, 2000.
2. Maseri, A. and Fuster, V. Is there a vulnerable plaque? *Circulation* 107, 2068–2071, 2003.
3. Naghavi, M. et al. From vulnerable plaque to vulnerable patient: a call for new definitions and risk assessment strategies, part I, *Circulation* 108, 1664–1472, 2003.
4. Naghavi, M. et al. From vulnerable plaque to vulnerable patient: a call for new definitions and risk assessment strategies, part II, *Circulation* 108, 1772–1778, 2003.
5. Kolodgie, F.D. et al. Intraplaque hemorrhage and progression of coronary atheroma, *New Engl J Med* 349, 2316–2325, 2003.
6. Lutgens E. et al. Atherosclerotic plaque rupture: local or systemic process? *Arterioscler Thromb Vasc Biol* 23, 2123–2130, 2003.
7. Marcus, R.H. et al. The spectrum of severe rheumatic mitral valve disease in a developing country: correlations among clinical presentation, surgical pathologic findings, and hemodynamic sequelae, *Ann Intern Med* 120, 177–183, 1994.
8. Lloyd-Jones, D.M. et al. Lifetime risk of developing coronary heart disease, *Lancet* 353, 89–92, 1999.
9. Libby, P., Ridker, P.M., and Maseri, A. Inflammation and atherosclerosis, *Circulation* 105, 1135–1143, 2002.
10. Ridker, P.M. et al. Inflammation, pravastatin, and the risk of coronary events after myocardial infarction in patients with average cholesterol levels: Cholesterol and Recurrent Events (CARE) Investigators, *Circulation* 98, 839–844, 1998.
11. Sabatine, M.S. et al. Relationship between baseline white blood cell count and degree of coronary artery disease and mortality in patients with acute coronary syndromes: a TACTICS-TIMI 18 substudy, *J Am Coll Cardiol* 40, 1761–1768, 2002.
12. Packard, C.J. et al. Lipoprotein-associated phospholipase A2 as an independent predictor of coronary heart disease: West of Scotland Coronary Prevention Study Group, *New Engl J Med* 343, 1148–1155, 2000.
13. Baldus, S. et al. Myeloperoxidase serum levels predict risk in patients with acute coronary syndromes, *Circulation* 108, 1440–1445, 2003.
14. Shishehbor, M.H. et al. Association of nitrotyrosine levels with cardiovascular disease and modulation by statin therapy, *JAMA* 289, 1675–1680, 2003.
15. Varo, N. et al. Soluble CD40L: risk prediction after acute coronary syndromes, *Circulation* 108, 1049–1052, 2003.
16. Buffon, A. et al. Widespread coronary inflammation in unstable angina, *New Engl J Med* 347, 5–12, 2002.

17. Matuszek, M.A. et al. Haptoglobin elutes from human atherosclerotic coronary arteries: a potential marker of arterial pathology, *Atherosclerosis* 168, 389–396, 2003.

18. Kritharides, L. et al. A method for defining the stages of low-density lipoprotein oxidation by the separation of cholesterol- and cholesteryl ester oxidation products using HPLC, *Anal Biochem* 213, 79–89, 1993.

19. Matsuura, E. et al. Autoantibody-mediated atherosclerosis, *Autoimmun Rev* 1, 348–353, 2002.

20. Hoff, H.F. et al. Phospholipid hydroxyalkenals, *Arterioscler Thromb Vasc Biol* 2003, 275–282, 2003.

21. Tsimikas, S. and Shaw, P.X. Non-invasive imaging of vulnerable plaques by molecular targeting of oxidized LDL with tagged oxidation-specific antibodies, *J Cell Biochem Suppl* 39, 138–146, 2002.

22. Tsimikas, S. et al. Temporal increases in plasma markers of oxidized low-density lipoprotein strongly reflect the presence of acute coronary syndromes, *J Am Coll Cardiol* 41, 360–370, 2003.

23. Matsuura, E. et al. Atherogenic autoantigen: oxidized LDL complexes with beta 2-glycoprotein I, *Immunobiology* 207, 17–22, 2003.

24. Binder, C.J. et al. Pneumococcal vaccination decreases atherosclerotic lesion formation: molecular mimicry between *Streptococcus pneumoniae* and oxidized LDL, *Nat Med* 9, 736–743, 2003.

25. Chen, J. et al. *In vivo* imaging of proteolytic activity in atherosclerosis, *Circulation* 105, 2766–2771, 2002.

26. Naghavi, M. et al. New developments in the detection of vulnerable plaque, *Curr Atheroscler Rep* 3, 125–135, 2001.

27. Litovsky, S. et al. Superparamagnetic iron oxide-based method for quantifying recruitment of monocytes to mouse atherosclerotic lesions *in vivo*: enhancement by tissue necrosis factor-alpha, interleukin-1-beta, and interferon-gamma, *Circulation* 107, 1545–1549, 2003.

28. Monroe, V.S. et al. Pharmacologic plaque passivation for the reduction of recurrent cardiac events in acute coronary syndromes, *J Am Coll Cardiol* 41 (Suppl.), 23S–30S, 2003.

29. Timmis A.D. Plaque stabilisation in acute coronary syndromes: clinical considerations, *Heart* 89, 1268–1272, 2003.

30. Cercek B. et al. Effect of short-term treatment with azithromycin on recurrent ischaemic events in patients with acute coronary syndrome in the Azithromycin in Acute Coronary Syndrome (AZACS) trial: a randomised controlled trial. *Lancet* 361, 809–813, 2003.

31. Shah P.K. Pathophysiology of coronary thrombosis: role of plaque rupture and plaque erosion, *Progr Cardiovasc Dis* 44, 357–368, 2002.

32. Ambrose, J.A. and Martinez, E.E. A new paradigm for plaque stabilization, *Circulation* 105, 2000–2004, 2002.

33. Ahmed, J.M. et al. Mechanism of lumen enlargement during intracoronary stent implantation: an intravascular ultrasound study, *Circulation* 102, 7–10, 2000.

34. TIMI Investigators. Effects of tissue plasminogen activator and a comparison of early invasive and conservative strategies in unstable angina and non-Q-wave myocardial infarction: results of the TIMI IIIB trial thrombolysis in myocardial ischemia, *Circulation* 89, 1545–1556, 1994.

35. Boden, W.E. and Pepine, C.J. Introduction to optimizing management of non-ST-segment elevation acute coronary syndromes: harmonizing advances in mechanical and pharmacologic intervention, *J Am Coll Cardiol* 41 (Suppl.), 1S–6S, 2003.

36. Sheridan, P.J. and Crossman, D.C. Critical review of unstable angina and non-ST elevation myocardial infarction, *Postgrad Med J* 78, 717–726, 2002.
37. FRISC II Investigators. Invasive compared with non-invasive treatment in unstable coronary-artery disease: FRISC II prospective randomised multicentre study, *Lancet* 354, 708–715, 1999.
38. Cannon, C.P. et al. Comparison of early invasive and conservative strategies in patients with unstable coronary syndromes treated with the glycoprotein IIb/IIIa inhibitor tirofiban, *New Engl J Med* 344, 1879–1887, 2001.
39. Fox, K.A. et al. Interventional versus conservative treatment for patients with unstable angina or non-ST-elevation myocardial infarction: the British Heart Foundation Randomized Intervention Trial of Unstable Angina, *Lancet* 360, 743–751, 2002.
40. Degertekin M. et al. Persistent inhibition of neointimal hyperplasia after sirolimus-eluting stent implantation: long-term (up to 2 years) clinical, angiographic, and intravascular ultrasound follow-up, *Circulation* 106, 1610–1613, 2002.
41. Solomon D.H. et al. Use of risk stratification to identify patients with unstable angina likeliest to benefit from an invasive versus conservative management strategy, *J Am Coll Cardiol* 38, 969–976, 2001.
42. Keeley, E.C., Boura, J.A., and Grines, C.L. Primary angioplasty versus intravenous thrombolytic therapy for acute myocardial infarction: a quantitative review of 23 randomised trials, *Lancet* 361, 13–20, 2003.
43. Lowe, H.C. et al. Pharmacologic reperfusion therapy for acute myocardial infarction, *J Thromb Thrombolysis* 14, 179–196, 2002.
44. Topol, E.J. et al. Multi-year follow-up of abciximab therapy in three randomized, placebo-controlled trials of percutaneous coronary revascularization, *Am J Med* 113, 1–6, 2002.
45. Stone, G.W. et al. Comparison of angioplasty with stenting, with or without abciximab, in acute myocardial infarction, *New Engl J Med* 346, 957–966, 2002.
46. Arampatzis, C.A. et al. Images in cardiovascular medicine: detection of a vulnerable coronary plaque: a treatment dilemma, *Circulation* 108, 34–35, 2003.
47. Popma, J.J., Kuntz, R.E., and Baim, D.S. A decade of improvement in the clinical outcomes of percutaneous coronary intervention for multivessel disease, *Circulation* 106, 1592–1594, 2002.
48. MacNeill, B.D. et al. Intravascular modalities for detection of vulnerable plaque: current status, *Arterioscler Thromb Vasc Biol* 23, 1333–13442, 2003.
49. Yabushita, H. et al. Characterization of human atherosclerosis by optical coherence tomography, *Circulation* 106, 1640–1645, 2002.
50. Bouma, B.E. et al. Evaluation of intracoronary stenting by intravascular optical coherence tomography, *Heart* 89, 317–320, 2003.
51. Valgimigli, M. et al. Serum from patients with acute coronary syndromes displays a proapoptotic effect on human endothelial cells: a possible link to pan-coronary syndromes, *Circulation* 107, 264–270, 2003.
52. Goldstein, J.A. et al. Multiple complex coronary plaques in patients with acute myocardial infarction, *New Engl J Med* 343, 915–922, 2000.
53. Rioufol, G. et al. Multiple atherosclerotic plaque rupture in acute coronary syndrome: a three-vessel intravascular ultrasound study, *Circulation* 106, 804–808, 2002.
54. Lutgens, E. et al. Atherosclerotic plaque rupture: local or systemic process? *Arterioscler Thromb Vasc Biol* 23, 2123–2130, 2003.
55. Morice, M.C. et al. A randomized comparison of a sirolimus-eluting stent with a standard stent for coronary revascularization, *New Engl J Med* 346, 1773–1780, 2002.

56. Popma, J.J., Kuntz, R.E., and Baim, D.S. A decade of improvement in the clinical outcomes of percutaneous coronary intervention for multivessel coronary artery disease, *Circulation* 106, 1592–1594, 2002.

57. Roque, M. et al. Modulation of apoptosis, proliferation, and p27 expression in a porcine coronary angioplasty model, *Atherosclerosis* 153, 315–322, 2000.

58. Golding, L.A. et al. Emergency revascularization for unstable angina, *Circulation* 58, 1163–1166, 1978.

59. DeWood, M.A. et al. Medical and surgical management of early Q wave myocardial infarction. I. Effects of surgical reperfusion on survival, recurrent myocardial infarction, sudden death and functional class at 10 or more years of follow-up, *J Am Coll Cardiol* 14, 65–77, 1989.

60. Hochman, J.S. et al. Early revascularization in acute myocardial infarction complicated by cardiogenic shock: should we emergently revascularize occluded coronaries for cardiogenic shock? *New Engl J Med* 341, 625–634, 1999.

61. Stemme, V. et al. Expression of cyclo-oxygenase-2 in human atherosclerotic carotid arteries, *Eur J Vasc Endovasc Surg* 20, 146–152, 2000.

62. Pratico, D. et al. Acceleration of atherogenesis by Cox-1-dependent prostanoid formation in low density lipoprotein receptor knockout mice, *Proc Natl Acad Sci USA* 98, 3358–3363, 2001.

63. de Gaetano, G., Donati, M.B., and Cerletti, C. Prevention of thrombosis and vascular inflammation: benefits and limitations of selective or combined COX-1, COX-2 and 5-LOX inhibitors, *Trends Pharmacol Sci* 24, 245–252, 2003.

64. Theroux, P., Antiplatelet and antithrombotic therapy in unstable angina, *Am J Cardiol* 68, 92B–98B, 1991.

65. Antithrombotic Trialists' Collaboration. Collaborative meta-analysis of randomised trials of antiplatelet therapy for prevention of death, myocardial infarction, and stroke in high risk patients, *Br Med J* 324, 71–86, 2002.

66. Cyrus, T. et al. Effect of low-dose aspirin on vascular inflammation, plaque stability, and atherogenesis in low-density lipoprotein receptor-deficient mice, *Circulation* 106, 1282–1287, 2002.

67. Ridker, P.M. et al. Inflammation, aspirin, and the risk of cardiovascular disease in apparently healthy men, *New Engl J Med* 336, 973–979, 1997.

68. May, A.E. et al. Reduction of monocyte–platelet interaction and monocyte activation in patients receiving antiplatelet therapy after coronary stent implantation, *Eur Heart J* 18, 1913–1920, 1997.

69. Egger, G. et al. Blood polymorphonuclear leukocyte activation in atherosclerosis: effects of aspirin, *Inflammation* 25, 129–135, 2001.

70. Damas, J.K. et al. Interleukin-7-mediated inflammation in unstable angina: possible role of chemokines and platelets, *Circulation* 107, 2670–2676, 2003.

71. Kharbanda, R.K. et al. Prevention of inflammation-induced endothelial dysfunction: a novel vasculo-protective action of aspirin, *Circulation* 105, 2600–2604, 2002.

72. Pasceri, V. et al. Modulation of C-reactive protein-mediated monocyte chemoattractant protein-1 induction in human endothelial cells by anti-atherosclerosis drugs, *Circulation* 103, 2531–2534, 2001.

73. Cipollone, F. et al. Preprocedural level of soluble CD40L is predictive of enhanced inflammatory response and restenosis after coronary angioplasty, *Circulation* 108, 2776–2782, 2003.

74. Stumpf, C. et al. Enhanced levels of CD154 (CD40 ligand) on platelets in patients with chronic heart failure, *Eur J Heart Fail* 5, 629–637, 2003.

75. Hermann, A. et al. Platelet CD40 ligand (CD40L): subcellular localization, regulation of expression, and inhibition by clopidogrel, *Platelets* 12, 74–82, 2001.
76. Mehta, S.R. et al. Effects of pretreatment with clopidogrel and aspirin followed by long-term therapy in patients undergoing percutaneous coronary intervention: the PCI-CURE study, *Lancet* 358, 527–533, 2001.
77. Willerson, J.T. et al. Specific platelet mediators and unstable coronary artery lesions: experimental evidence and potential clinical implications, *Circulation* 80, 198–205, 1989.
78. Steinhubl, S.R. et al. Early and sustained dual oral antiplatelet therapy following percutaneous coronary intervention: a randomized controlled trial, *JAMA* 288, 2411–2420, 2002.
79. Roffi, M. et al. Platelet glycoprotein IIb/IIIa inhibition in acute coronary syndromes: gradient of benefit related to the revascularization strategy, *Eur Heart J* 23, 1441–1448, 2002.
80. Karvouni, E., Katritsis, D.G., and Ioannidis, J.P. Intravenous glycoprotein IIb/IIIa receptor antagonists reduce mortality after percutaneous coronary interventions, *J Am Coll Cardiol* 41, 26–32, 2003.
81. Heeschen, C. et al. Soluble CD40 ligand in acute coronary syndromes, *New Engl J Med* 348, 1104–1111, 2003.
82. Lincoff, A.M. et al. Abciximab suppresses the rise in levels of circulating inflammatory markers after percutaneous coronary revascularization, *Circulation* 104, 163–1637, 2001.
83. Merino-Otermin, A. et al. Eptifibatide blocks the increase in C-reactive protein concentration after coronary angioplasty, *Rev Esp Cardiol* 55, 186–189, 2002.
84. Seshiah, P.N. et al. Activated monocytes induce smooth muscle cell death: role of macrophage colony-stimulating factor and cell contact, *Circulation* 105, 174–180, 2002.
85. Aikawa, M. et al. An HMG-CoA reductase inhibitor, cerivastatin, suppresses growth of macrophages expressing matrix metalloproteinases and tissue factor *in vivo* and *in vitro*, *Circulation* 103, 276–283, 2001.
86. Theroux, P. et al. Aspirin versus heparin to prevent myocardial infarction during the acute phase of unstable angina, *Circulation* 88, 2045–2048, 1993.
87. Cohen, M. et al. A comparison of low-molecular-weight heparin with unfractionated heparin for unstable coronary artery disease: efficacy and safety of subcutaneous enoxaparin: Non-Q-Wave Coronary Events Study Group, *New Engl J Med* 337, 447–452, 1997.
88. Antman, E.M. et al. Enoxaparin prevents death and cardiac ischemic events in unstable angina/non-Q-wave myocardial infarction: results of thrombolysis in myocardial infarction (TIMI) 11B trial, *Circulation* 100, 1593–1601, 1999.
89. Gikakis, N. et al. Effect of factor Xa inhibitors on thrombin formation and complement and neutrophil activation during *in vitro* extracorporeal circulation, *Circulation* 94 (Suppl.), 341–346, 1996.
90. Brieger, D. and Dawes, J. Characterisation of persistent anti-Xa activity following administration of the low molecular weight heparin enoxaparin sodium (Clexane), *Thromb Haemost* 72, 275–280, 1994.
91. Brown, M.S. and Goldstein, J.L., A receptor-mediated pathway for cholesterol homeostasis, *Science* 232, 34–47, 1986.
92. Scandinavian Simvastatin Survival Study (4S). Randomised trial of cholesterol lowering in 4444 patients with coronary heart disease, *Lancet* 344, 1383–1389, 1994.

93. Brown, B.G. et al. Simvastatin and niacin, antioxidant vitamins, or the combination for the prevention of coronary disease, *New Engl J Med* 345, 1583–1592, 2001.

94. MRC/BHF Heart Protection Study. Cholesterol lowering with simvastatin in 20,536 high-risk individuals: a randomised placebo-controlled trial, *Lancet* 360, 7–22, 2002.

95. Kastelein, J.J., The future of best practice, *Atherosclerosis* 143, 17–21, 1999.

96. Law, M.R., Wald, N.J., and Rudnicka, A.R. Quantifying effect of statins on low density lipoprotein cholesterol, ischemic heart disease, and stroke: systemic review and meta-analysis, *Br Med J* 326, 1–7, 2003.

97. Laufs, U. et al. Rapid effects on vascular function after initiation and withdrawal of atorvastatin in healthy, normocholesterolemic men, *Am J Cardiol* 88, 1306–1307, 2001.

98. Waters, D.D. Early pharmacologic intervention and plaque stability in acute coronary syndromes, *Am J Cardiol* 88, 30K–36K, 2001.

99. Waldman, A. and Kritharides, L. The pleiotropic effects of HMG-CoA reductase inhibitors: their role in osteoporosis and dementia, *Drugs* 63, 139–152, 2003.

100. Aikawa, M. et al. Lipid lowering promotes accumulation of mature smooth muscle cells expressing smooth muscle myosin heavy chain isoforms in rabbit atheroma, *Circ Res* 83, 1015–1026, 1998.

101. Tamai, O. et al. Single LDL apheresis improves endothelium-dependent vasodilatation in hypercholesterolemic humans, *Circulation* 95, 76–82, 1997.

102. Jialal, I. et al. Effect of hydroxymethyl glutaryl coenzyme a reductase inhibitor therapy on high sensitive C-reactive protein levels, *Circulation* 103 (15), 1933–1935, 2001.

103. Ansell, B.J. et al. hsCRP and HDL effects of statins trial (CHEST): rapid effect of statin therapy on C-reactive protein and high-density lipoprotein levels: clinical investigation, *Heart Dis* 5, 2–7, 2003.

104. Kinlay, S. et al. High-dose atorvastatin enhances the decline in inflammatory markers in patients with acute coronary syndromes in the MIRACL study, *Circulation* 108, 1560–1566, 2003.

105. Sacks, F.M. and Ridker, P.M. Lipid lowering and beyond: results from the CARE study on lipoproteins and inflammation. Cholesterol and recurrent events, *Herz* 24, 51–56, 1999.

106. Kwak, B. et al. Statins as a newly recognized type of immunomodulator, *Nat Med* 6, 1399–1402, 2000.

107. Cermak, J. et al. C-reactive protein induces human peripheral blood monocytes to synthesize tissue factor, *Blood* 82, 513–520, 1993.

108. Di Garbo, V. et al. Nonlipid, dose-dependent effects of pravastatin treatment on hemostatic system and inflammatory response, *Eur J Clin Pharmacol* 56, 277–284, 2000.

109. Gaddam, V., Li, D.Y., and Mehta, J.L. Anti-thrombotic effects of atorvastatin: an effect unrelated to lipid lowering, *J Cardiovasc Pharmacol Ther* 7, 247–253, 2002.

110. Baetta, R. et al. Fluvastatin reduces tissue factor expression and macrophage accumulation in carotid lesions of cholesterol-fed rabbits in the absence of lipid lowering, *Arterioscler Thromb Vasc Biol* 22, 692–698, 2002.

111. Bea, F. et al. Simvastatin inhibits expression of tissue factor in advanced atherosclerotic lesions of apolipoprotein E deficient mice independently of lipid lowering: potential role of simvastatin-mediated inhibition of Egr-1 expression and activation, *Atherosclerosis* 167, 187–194, 2003.

112. Wagner, A.H. et al. 3-hydroxy-3-methylglutaryl coenzyme A reductase-independent inhibition of CD40 expression by atorvastatin in human endothelial cells, *Arterioscler Thromb Vasc Biol* 22, 1784–1789, 2002.

113. Varo, N. et al. Elevated plasma levels of the atherogenic mediator soluble CD40 ligand in diabetic patients: a novel target of thiazolidinediones, *Circulation* 107, 2664–2269, 2003.

114. Wassmann, S. et al. HMG-CoA reductase inhibitors improve endothelial dysfunction in normocholesterolemic hypertension via reduced production of reactive oxygen species, *Hypertension* 37, 1450–1457, 2001.

115. Llevadot, J. et al. HMG-CoA reductase inhibitor mobilizes bone marrow-derived endothelial progenitor cells, *J Clin Invest* 108, 399–405, 2001.

116. Laufs, U. et al. Upregulation of endothelial nitric oxide synthase by HMG CoA reductase inhibitors, *Circulation* 97, 1129–1135, 1998.

117. Laufs, U. et al. Atorvastatin upregulates type III nitric oxide synthase in thrombocytes, decreases platelet activation, and protects from cerebral ischemia in normocholesterolemic mice, *Stroke* 31, 2442–2449, 2000.

118. Laufs, U., Fata, V.L., and Liao, J.K. Inhibition of 3-hydroxy-3-methylglutaryl (HMG)-CoA reductase blocks hypoxia-mediated down-regulation of endothelial nitric oxide synthase, *J Biol Chem* 272, 31725–31729, 1997.

119. Mason, J.C. et al. Statin-induced expression of decay-accelerating factor protects vascular endothelium against complement-mediated injury, *Circ Res* 91, 696–703, 2002.

120. Sukhova, G.K., Williams, J.K., and Libby, P., Statins reduce inflammation in atheroma of nonhuman primates independent of effects on serum cholesterol, *Arterioscler Thromb Vasc Biol* 22, 1452–1458, 2002.

121. Khachigian, L.M. and Collins, T. Early growth response factor 1: a pleiotropic mediator of inducible gene expression, *J Mol Med* 76, 613–616, 1998.

122. Day, F.L. et al. Angiotensin II (ATII)-inducible platelet-derived growth factor A-chain gene expression is p42/44 extracellular signal-regulated kinase-1/2 and Egr-1-dependent and mediated via the ATII type 1 but not type 2 receptor: induction by ATII antagonized by nitric oxide, *J Biol Chem* 274, 23726–23733, 1999.

123. Kreuzer, J. et al. Effects of HMG-CoA reductase inhibition on PDGF- and angiotensin II-mediated signal transduction: suppression of c-Jun and c-Fos in human smooth muscle cells *in vitro*, *Eur J Med Res* 4, 135–143, 1999.

124. Weiss, R.H., Ramirez, A., and Joo, A. Short-term pravastatin mediates growth inhibition and apoptosis, independently of Ras, via the signaling proteins p27Kip1 and P13 kinase, *J Am Soc Nephrol* 10, 1880–1890, 1999.

125. Kohno, M. et al. Inhibition of migration and proliferation of rat vascular smooth muscle cells by a new HMG-CoA reductase inhibitor, pitavastatin, *Hypertens Res* 25, 279–285, 2002.

126. Park, H.J. et al. 3-hydroxy-3-methylglutaryl coenzyme A reductase inhibitors interfere with angiogenesis by inhibiting the geranylgeranylation of RhoA, *Circ Res* 91, 143–150, 2002.

127. Moulton, K.S. et al. Inhibition of plaque neovascularization reduces macrophage accumulation and progression of advanced atherosclerosis, *Proc Natl Acad Sci USA* 100, 4736–4741, 2003.

128. Vasa, M. et al. Increase in circulating endothelial progenitor cells by statin therapy in patients with stable coronary artery disease, *Circulation* 103, 2885–2890, 2001.

129. Bays, H. and Stein, E.A. Pharmacotherapy for dyslipidaemia: current therapies and future agents, *Expert Opin Pharmacother* 4, 1901–1938, 2003.

130. Rubins, H. et al. Gemfibrozil for the secondary prevention of coronary heart disease in men with low levels of high-density lipoprotein cholesterol, *New Engl J Med* 341, 410–418, 1999.

131. Wang, T.D. et al. Efficacy of fenofibrate and simvastatin on endothelial function and inflammatory markers in patients with combined hyperlipidemia: relations with baseline lipid profiles, *Atherosclerosis* 170, 315–323, 2003.

132. Plutzky, J. PPARs as therapeutic targets: reverse cardiology? *Science* 302, 406–407, 2003.

133. Fruchart, J.C., Duriez, P., and Staels, B. Peroxisome proliferator-activated receptor-alpha activators regulate genes governing lipoprotein metabolism, vascular inflammation and atherosclerosis, *Curr Opin Lipidol* 10, 245–257, 1999.

134. Chinetti, G. et al. CLA-1/SR-BI is expressed in atherosclerotic lesion macrophages and regulated by activators of peroxisome proliferator-activated receptors, *Circulation* 101, 2411–2417, 2000.

135. Chinetti, G. et al. Peroxisome proliferator-activated receptor alpha reduces cholesterol esterification in macrophages, *Circ Res* 92, 212–217, 2003.

136. Chinetti, G. et al. PPAR-alpha and PPAR-gamma activators induce cholesterol removal from human macrophage foam cells through stimulation of the ABCA1 pathway, *Nat Med* 7, 53–58, 2001.

137. Chinetti, G. et al. Activation of proliferator-activated receptors alpha and gamma induces apoptosis of human monocyte-derived macrophages, *J Biol Chem* 273, 25573–25580, 1998.

138. Claudel, T. et al. Reduction of atherosclerosis in apolipoprotein E knockout mice by activation of the retinoid X receptor, *Proc Natl Acad Sci USA* 98, 2610–2615, 2001.

139. Fruchart, J.C., Staels, B., and Duriez, P. PPARs, metabolic disease and atherosclerosis, *Pharmacol Res* 44, 345–352, 2001.

140. Staels, B. et al. Fibrates influence the expression of genes involved in lipoprotein metabolism in a tissue-selective manner in the rat, *Arterioscler Thromb* 12, 286–294, 1992.

141. Staels, B. et al. Activation of human aortic smooth-muscle cells is inhibited by PPAR-alpha but not by PPAR-gamma activators, *Nature* 393, 790–793, 1998.

142. Marx, N. et al. PPAR-alpha activators inhibit cytokine-induced vascular cell adhesion molecule-1 expression in human endothelial cells, *Circulation* 99, 3125–3131, 1999.

143. Marx, N. et al. PPAR-alpha activators inhibit tissue factor expression and activity in human monocytes, *Circulation* 103, 213–219, 2001.

144. Plutzky, J. The potential role of peroxisome proliferator-activated receptors on inflammation in type 2 diabetes mellitus and atherosclerosis, *Am J Cardiol* 92, 34J–41J, 2003.

145. Barroso, I. et al. Dominant negative mutations in human PPAR-gamma associated with severe insulin resistance, diabetes mellitus and hypertension, *Nature* 402, 880–883, 1999.

146. Ricote, M. et al. Expression of the peroxisome proliferator-activated receptor gamma (PPAR-gamma) in human atherosclerosis and regulation in macrophages by colony stimulating factors and oxidized low density lipoprotein, *Proc Natl Acad Sci USA* 95, 7614–7619, 1998.

147. Ricote, M. et al. The peroxisome proliferator-activated receptor-gamma is a negative regulator of macrophage activation, *Nature* 391, 79–82, 1998.

148. Jiang, C., Ting, A.T., and Seed, B. PPAR-gamma agonists inhibit production of monocyte inflammatory cytokines, *Nature* 391, 82–86, 1998.

149. Ishibashi, M. et al. Antiinflammatory and antiarteriosclerotic effects of pioglitazone, *Hypertension* 40, 687–693, 2002.
150. Kintscher, U. et al. PPAR-alpha inhibits TGF-beta-induced beta-5 integrin transcription in vascular smooth muscle cells by interacting with Smad4, *Circ Res* 91, 35–44, 2002.
151. Bruemmer, D. et al. Regulation of the growth arrest and DNA damage-inducible gene 45 (GADD45) by peroxisome proliferator-activated receptor gamma in vascular smooth muscle cells, *Circ Res* 93, 38–47, 2003.
152. Goetze, S. et al. Leptin induces endothelial cell migration through Akt, which is inhibited by PPAR-gamma ligands, *Hypertension* 40, 748–754, 2002.
153. Murata, T. et al. Peroxisome proliferator-activated receptor-gamma ligands inhibit choroidal neovascularization, *Invest Ophthalmol Vis Sci* 41, 2309–2317, 2000.
154. Lee, C.H. et al. Transcriptional repression of atherogenic inflammation: modulation by PPAR-delta, *Science* 302, 453–457, 2003.
155. Ziouzenkova, O. et al. Lipolysis of triglyceride-rich lipoproteins generates PPAR ligands: evidence for an antiinflammatory role for lipoprotein lipase, *Proc Natl Acad Sci USA* 100, 2730–2735, 2003.
156. Kastelein, J.J. et al. Lipoprotein lipase activity is associated with severity of angina pectoris: REGRESS Study Group, *Circulation* 102, 1629–1633, 2000.
157. Jouven, X. et al. Circulating nonesterified fatty acid level as a predictive risk factor for sudden death in the population, *Circulation* 104, 756–761, 2001.
158. Watts, G.F. et al. Differential regulation of lipoprotein kinetics by atorvastatin and fenofibrate in subjects with the metabolic syndrome, *Diabetes* 52, 803–811, 2003.
159. Inoue, I. et al. Fibrate and statin synergistically increase the transcriptional activities of PPAR-alpha/RXR-alpha and decrease the transactivation of NF-kappa-B, *Biochem Biophys Res Commun* 290, 131–139, 2002.
160. Martin, G. et al. Statin-induced inhibition of the Rho-signaling pathway activates PPAR-alpha and induces HDL apoA-I, *J Clin Invest* 107, 1423–1432, 2001.
161. Jenkins, P.J., Harper, R.W., and Nestel, P.J., Severity of coronary atherosclerosis related to lipoprotein concentration, *Br Med J* 2, 388–391, 1978.
162. Genest, J.J. et al. Prevalence of risk factors in men with premature coronary artery disease, *Am J Cardiol* 67, 1185–1189, 1991.
163. Kannel, W.B. and Larson, M. Long-term epidemiologic prediction of coronary disease: the Framingham experience, *Cardiology* 82, 137–152, 1993.
164. Assmann, G. and Schulte, H. Identification of individuals at high risk for myocardial infarction, *Atherosclerosis* 110 (Suppl.), S11–S21, 1994.
165. Khovidhunkit, W. et al. Infection and inflammation-induced proatherogenic changes of lipoproteins, *J Infect Dis* 181 (Suppl.), S462–S472, 2000.
166. Ridker, P.M., Glynn, R.J., and Henekens, C.H. C-reactive protein adds to the predictive value of total and HDL cholesterol in determining risk of first myocardial infarction, *Circulation* 97, 2007–2011, 1998.
167. Shah, P. K. et al. Exploiting the vascular protective effects of high-density lipoprotein and its apolipoproteins: an idea whose time for testing is coming, part I, *Circulation* 104, 2376–2383, 2001.
168. Newton, R.S. and Krause, B.R. HDL therapy for the acute treatment of atherosclerosis, *Atheroscler Suppl* 3, 31–38, 2002.
169. Badimon, J.J., Badimon, L., and Fuster, V. Regression of atherosclerotic lesions by high density lipoprotein plasma fraction in the cholesterol-fed rabbit, *J. Clin. Invest.* 85, 1234–1241, 1990.

170. Rubin, E.M. et al. Inhibition of early atherogenesis in transgenic mice by human apolipoprotein A-I, *Nature* 353, 265–267, 1991.

171. Tangirala, R. et al. Regression of atherosclerosis induced by liver-directed gene transfer of apolipoprotein A-I in mice, *Circulation* 100, 1816–1822, 1999.

172. Shah, P.K. et al. High-dose recombinant apolipoprotein A-I(milano) mobilizes tissue cholesterol and rapidly reduces plaque lipid and macrophage content in apolipoprotein e-deficient mice: potential implications for acute plaque stabilization, *Circulation* 103, 3047–3050, 2001.

173. Eriksson, M. et al. Stimulation of fecal steroid excretion after infusion of recombinant proapolipoprotein A-I: potential reverse cholesterol transport in humans, *Circulation* 100, 594–598, 1999.

174. Angelin, B., Parini, P., and Eriksson, M. Reverse cholesterol transport in man: promotion of fecal steroid excretion by infusion of reconstituted HDL, *Atheroscler Suppl* 3, 23–30, 2002.

175. Schmitz, G., Kaminski, W.E., and Orso, E. ABC transporters in cellular lipid trafficking, *Curr. Opin. Lipidol.* 11, 493–501, 2000.

176. Oram, J.F. et al. ABCA1 is the cAMP-inducible apolipoprotein receptor that mediates cholesterol secretion from macrophages, *J. Biol. Chem.* 275, 34508–34511, 2000.

177. Clee, S.M. et al. Common genetic variation in ABCA1 is associated with altered lipoprotein levels and a modified risk for coronary artery disease, *Circulation* 103, 1198–1205, 2001.

178. Tall, A.R., Costet, P., and Wang, N. Regulation and mechanisms of macrophage cholesterol efflux, *J Clin Invest* 110, 899–904, 2002.

179. Barter, P.J. Hugh Sinclair Lecture: regulation and remodelling of HDL by plasma factors, *Atheroscler Suppl* 3, 39–47, 2002.

180. Trigatti, B. et al. Influence of the high density lipoprotein receptor SR-BI on reproductive and cardiovascular pathophysiology, *Proc Natl Acad Sci USA* 96, 9322–9327, 1999.

181. Graft, G.A. et al. ABCG5 and ABCG8 are obligate heterodimers for protein trafficking and biliary cholesterol excretion, *J. Biol. Chem.* 278, 48275–48282, 2003.

182. Yancey, P.G. et al. Importance of different pathways of cellular cholesterol efflux, *Arterioscler Thromb Vasc Biol* 23, 712–719, 2003.

183. Braun, A. et al. Loss of SR-BI expression leads to the early onset of occlusive atherosclerotic coronary artery disease, spontaneous myocardial infarctions, severe cardiac dysfunction, and premature death in apolipoprotein E-deficient mice, *Circ Res* 90, 270–276, 2002.

184. Cockerill, G.W. et al. High-density lipoproteins inhibit cytokine-induced expression of endothelial cell adhesion molecules, *Arterioscler Thromb Vasc Biol* 15, 1987–1994, 1995.

185. Mertens, A. et al. Increased low-density lipoprotein oxidation and impaired high-density lipoprotein antioxidant defense are associated with increased macrophage homing and atherosclerosis in dyslipidemic obese mice: LCAT gene transfer decreases atherosclerosis, *Circulation* 107, 1640–1646, 2003.

186. Panzenbock, U. et al. Oxidation of methionine residues to methionine sulfoxides does not decrease potential antiatherogenic properties of apolipoprotein A-I, *J Biol Chem* 275, 19536–19544, 2000.

187. Hyka, N. et al. Apolipoprotein A-I inhibits the production of interleukin-1-beta and tumor necrosis factor-alpha by blocking contact-mediated activation of monocytes by T lymphocytes, *Blood* 97, 2381–2389, 2001.

188. Holvoet, P. et al. Arg123–Tyr166 domain of human ApoA-I is critical for HDL-mediated inhibition of macrophage homing and early atherosclerosis in mice, *Arterioscler Thromb Vasc Biol* 21, 1977–1983, 2001.
189. Sirtori, C.R., Calabresi, L., and Franceschini, G. Recombinant apolipoproteins for the treatment of vascular diseases, *Atherosclerosis* 142, 29–40, 1999.
190. Chiesa, G. et al. Recombinant apolipoprotein A-I (Milano) infusion into rabbit carotid artery rapidly removes lipid from fatty streaks, *Circ Res* 90, 974–980, 2002.
191. Nissen, S. E. et al. Effect of recombinant ApoA-I Milano on coronary atherosclerosis in patients with acute coronary syndromes, *JAMA* 290, 2292–2330, 2003.
192. Yancey, P.G. et al. Efflux of cellular cholesterol and phospholipid to lipid-free apolipoproteins and class A amphipathic peptides, *Biochemistry* 34, 7955–7965, 1995.
193. Mishra, V.K. et al. Studies of synthetic peptides of human apolipoprotein A-I containing tandem amphipathic alpha-helixes, *Biochemistry* 37, 10313–10324, 1998.
194. Navab, M. et al. Oral administration of an Apo A-I mimetic peptide synthesized from D- amino acids dramatically reduces atherosclerosis in mice independent of plasma cholesterol, *Circulation* 105, 290–292, 2002.
195. Marcil, M. et al. Cellular phospholipid and cholesterol efflux in high-density lipoprotein deficiency, *Circulation* 107, 1366–1371, 2003.
196. Barter, P.J. et al. Cholesteryl ester transfer protein: a novel target for raising HDL and inhibiting atherosclerosis, *Arterioscler Thromb Vasc Biol* 23, 160–167, 2003.
197. Kerr, J.F., Wyllie, A.H., and Currie, A.R. Apoptosis: a basic biological phenomenon with wide-ranging implications in tissue kinetics, *Br J Cancer* 26, 239–257, 1972.
198. Bennett, M.R., Apoptosis in the cardiovascular system, *Heart* 87, 480–487, 2002.
199. Geng, Y.J. and Libby, P. Progression of atheroma: a struggle between death and procreation, *Arterioscler Thromb Vasc Biol* 22, 1370–1380, 2002.
200. Burke, A.P. et al. Coronary risk factors and plaque morphology in men with coronary disease who died suddenly, *New Engl J Med* 336, 1276–1282, 1997.
201. Geng, Y.J. et al. Fas is expressed in human atherosclerotic intima and promotes apoptosis of cytokine-primed human vascular smooth muscle cells, *Arterioscler Thromb Vasc Biol* 17, 2200–2208, 1997.
202. Bennett, M.R., Breaking the plaque: evidence for plaque rupture in animal models of atherosclerosis, *Arterioscler Thromb Vasc Biol* 22, 713–714, 2002.
203. Pollman, M.J. et al. Inhibition of neointimal cell bcl-x expression induces apoptosis and regression of vascular disease, *Nat Med* 4, 222–227, 1998.
204. Li, Q. et al. Overexpression of insulin-like growth factor-1 in mice protects from myocyte death after infarction, attenuating ventricular dilation, wall stress, and cardiac hypertrophy, *J Clin Invest* 100, 1991–1999, 1997.
205. Kockx, M., Princen, H.M., and Kooistra, T. Fibrate-modulated expression of fibrinogen, plasminogen activator inhibitor-1 and apolipoprotein A-I in cultured cynomolgus monkey hepatocytes: role of the peroxisome proliferator-activated receptor-alpha, *Thromb Haemost* 80, 942–948, 1998.
206. Kolodgie, F.D. et al. Localization of apoptotic macrophages at the site of plaque rupture in sudden coronary death, *Am J Pathol* 157, 1259–1268, 2000.
207. Chen, Z. et al. Photodynamic therapy with motexafin lutetium induces redox-sensitive apoptosis of vascular cells, *Arterioscler Thromb Vasc Biol* 21, 759–764, 2001.
208. Kereiakes, D.J. et al. Phase I drug and light dose-escalation trial of motexafin lutetium and far red light activation (phototherapy) in subjects with coronary artery disease undergoing percutaneous coronary intervention and stent deployment: procedural and long-term results, *Circulation* 108, 1310–1315, 2003.

209. Hayase, M. et al. Photoangioplasty with local motexafin lutetium delivery reduces macrophages in a rabbit post-balloon injury model, *Cardiovasc Res* 49, 449–455, 2001.

210. Rockson, S.G. et al. Photoangioplasty for human peripheral atherosclerosis: results of a phase I trial of photodynamic therapy with motexafin lutetium (Antrin), *Circulation* 102, 2322–2324, 2000.

211. Rabbani, R. and Topol, E.J. Strategies to achieve coronary arterial plaque stabilization, *Cardiovasc Res* 41, 402–417, 1999.

212. Brown, D.L. et al. Identification of 92-kD gelatinase in human coronary atherosclerotic lesions: association of active enzyme synthesis with unstable angina, *Circulation* 91, 2125–2131, 1995.

213. Carmeliet, P. et al. Urokinase-generated plasmin activates matrix metalloproteinases during aneurysm formation, *Nat Genet* 17, 439–444, 1997.

214. Lijnen, H.R. Extracellular proteolysis in the development and progression of atherosclerosis, *Biochem Soc Trans* 30, 163–167, 2002.

215. Fernandez, C.A. et al. Structural and functional uncoupling of the enzymatic and angiogenic inhibitory activities of tissue inhibitor of metalloproteinase-2 (TIMP-2): loop 6 is a novel angiogenesis inhibitor, *J Biol Chem* 278, 40989–40995, 2003.

216. Saren, P. et al. TNF-alpha and IL beta selectively induce expression of 92-kDa gelatinase by human macrophages, *J Immunol* 157, 4159–4165, 1996.

217. Galis, Z.S. et al. Increased expression of matrix metalloproteinases and matrix degrading activity in vulnerable regions of human atherosclerotic plaques, *J Clin Invest* 94, 2493–2503, 1994.

218. Nagaoka, I. and Hirota, S. Increased expression of matrix metalloproteinase-9 in neutrophils in glycogen-induced peritoneal inflammation of guinea pigs, *Inflamm Res* 49, 55–62, 2000.

219. Mach, F. et al. Activation of monocyte/macrophage functions related to acute atheroma complication by ligation of CD40: induction of collagenase, stromelysin, and tissue factor, *Circulation* 96, 396–399, 1997.

220. Wize, J. et al. Ligation of selectin L and integrin CD11b/CD18 (Mac-1) induces release of gelatinase B (MMP-9) from human neutrophils, *Inflamm Res* 47, 325–327, 1998.

221. Silence, J. et al. Persistence of atherosclerotic plaque but reduced aneurysm formation in mice with stromelysin-1 (MMP-3) gene inactivation, *Arterioscler Thromb Vasc Biol* 21, 1440–1445, 2001.

222. Williams, H. et al. Characteristics of intact and ruptured atherosclerotic plaques in brachiocephalic arteries of apolipoprotein E knockout mice, *Arterioscler Thromb Vasc Biol* 22, 788–792, 2002.

223. Curci, J. A. et al. Preoperative treatment with doxycycline reduces aortic wall expression and activation of matrix metalloproteinases in patients with abdominal aortic aneurysms, *J Vasc Surg* 31, 325–342, 2000.

224. Tyagi, S.C. and Hoit, B.D. Metalloproteinase in myocardial adaptation and maladaptation, *J Cardiovasc Pharmacol Ther* 7, 241–246, 2002.

225. Jackson, C. Matrix metalloproteinases and angiogenesis, *Curr Opin Nephrol Hypertens* 11, 295–299, 2002.

226. Moons, A.H., Levi, M., and Peters, R.J. Tissue factor and coronary artery disease, *Cardiovasc Res* 53, 313–325, 2002.

227. Wilcox, J.N. et al. Localization of tissue factor in the normal vessel wall and in the atherosclerotic plaque, *Proc Natl Acad Sci USA* 86, 2839–2843, 1989.

228. Kaiser, B., Hoppensteadt, D.A., and Fareed, J. Tissue factor pathway inhibitor: an update of potential implications in the treatment of cardiovascular disorders, *Expert Opin Investig Drugs* 10, 1925–1935, 2001.

229. Kockx, M.M. et al. Decreased apoptosis and tissue factor expression after lipid lowering, *Circulation* 102, E99, 2000.

230. Kockx, M.M. et al. Cell composition, replication, and apoptosis in atherosclerotic plaques after 6 months of cholesterol withdrawal, *Circ Res* 83, 378–387, 1998.

231. Moons, A.H. et al. Recombinant nematode anticoagulant protein c2, an inhibitor of the tissue factor/factor VIIa complex, in patients undergoing elective coronary angioplasty, *J Am Coll Cardiol* 41, 2147–2153, 2003.

232. Neumann, F.J. *Chlamydia pneumoniae*–atherosclerosis link: a sound concept in search for clinical relevance, *Circulation* 106, 2414–2416, 2002.

233. Kuo, C.C. et al. Demonstration of *Chlamydia pneumoniae* in atherosclerotic lesions of coronary arteries, *J Infect Dis* 167, 841–849, 1993.

234. Saikku, P. et al. Serological evidence of an association of a novel Chlamydia, TWAR, with chronic coronary heart disease and acute myocardial infarction, *Lancet* 2, 983–986, 1988.

235. Muhlestein, J.B. et al. Increased incidence of Chlamydia species within the coronary arteries of patients with symptomatic atherosclerotic versus other forms of cardiovascular disease, *J Am Coll Cardiol* 27, 1555–1561, 1996.

236. Muhlestein, J.B. Antibiotic treatment of atherosclerosis, *Curr Opin Lipidol* 14, 605–614, 2003.

237. Muhlestein, J.B. Chronic infection and coronary artery disease, *Med Clin North Am* 84, 123–148, 2000.

238. Sander, D. et al. Reduced progression of early carotid atherosclerosis after antibiotic treatment and *Chlamydia pneumoniae* seropositivity, *Circulation* 106, 2428–2433, 2002.

239. Neumann, F. et al. Treatment of *Chlamydia pneumoniae* infection with roxithromycin and effect on neointima proliferation after coronary stent placement (ISAR-3): a randomised, double-blind, placebo-controlled trial, *Lancet* 357, 2085–2089, 2001.

240. Cercek, B. et al. Effect of short-term treatment with azithromycin on recurrent ischaemic events in patients with acute coronary syndrome in the Azithromycin in Acute Coronary Syndrome (AZACS) trial: a randomised controlled trial, *Lancet* 361, 809–813, 2003.

241. Feldman, L.J. and Isner, J. M. Gene therapy for the vulnerable plaque, *J Am Coll Cardiol* 26, 826–835, 1995.

242. Baek, S. and March, K.L. Gene therapy for restenosis: getting nearer the heart of the matter, *Circ Res* 82, 295–305, 1998.

243. DeYoung, M.B. and Dichek, D.A. Gene therapy for restenosis: are we ready? *Circ Res* 82, 306–313, 1998.

244. Libby, P. Gene therapy of restenosis: promise and perils, *Circ Res* 82, 404–406, 1998.

245. Brieger, D. and Topol, E. Local drug delivery systems and prevention of restenosis, *Cardiovasc Res* 35, 405–413, 1997.

246. Klugherz, B.D. et al. Gene delivery from a DNA controlled-release stent in porcine coronary arteries, *Nat Biotechnol* 18, 1181–1184, 2000.

247. Klugherz, B.D. et al. Gene delivery to pig coronary arteries from stents carrying antibody-tethered adenovirus, *Hum Gene Ther* 13, 443–454, 2002.

248. Perlstein, I. et al. DNA delivery from an intravascular stent with a denatured collagen–polylactic–polyglycolic acid-controlled release coating: mechanisms of enhanced transfection, *Gene Ther* 10, 1420–1428, 2003.

249. Rutanen, J., Markkanen, J., and Yla-Herttuala, S. Gene therapy for restenosis: current status, *Drugs* 62, 1575–1585, 2002.
250. Janssens, S.P. Applied gene therapy in preclinical models of vascular injury, *Curr Atheroscler Rep* 5, 186–190, 2003.
251. Luo, Z. et al. Adenovirus-mediated delivery of fas ligand inhibits intimal hyperplasia after balloon injury in immunologically primed animals, *Circulation* 99, 1776–1779, 1999.
252. Mann, M. J. et al. *Ex vivo* gene therapy of human vascular bypass grafts with E2F decoy: the PREVENT single-centre, randomised, controlled trial, *Lancet* 354, 1493–1498, 1999.
253. Santiago, F.S. and Khachigian, L.M. Nucleic acid-based strategies as potential therapeutic tools: mechanistic considerations and implications to restenosis, *J Mol Med* 79, 695–706, 2001.
254. Pang, J.H. and Chau, L.Y. Copper-induced apoptosis and immediate early gene expression in macrophages, *Atherosclerosis* 146, 45–52, 1999.
255. McCaffrey, T.A. et al. High-level expression of Egr-1 and Egr-1-inducible genes in mouse and human atherosclerosis, *J Clin Invest* 105, 653–662, 2000.
256. Fahmy, R.G. et al. Transcription factor Egr-1 supports FGF-dependent angiogenesis during neovascularization and tumor growth, *Nat Med* 9, 1026–1032, 2003.
257. Lowe, H.C. et al. Catalytic oligodeoxynucleotides define a key regulatory role for early growth response factor-1 in the porcine model of coronary in-stent restenosis, *Circ Res* 89, 670–677, 2001.

Index